Hearing Aids for
Speech-Language Pathologists
A Guide to Modern Rehabilitative Audiology

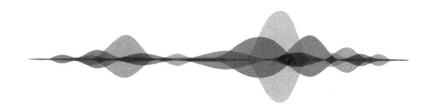

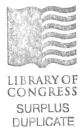

Editor-in-Chief for Audiology
Brad A. Stach, PhD

Hearing Aids for
Speech-Language Pathologists
A Guide to Modern
Rehabilitative Audiology

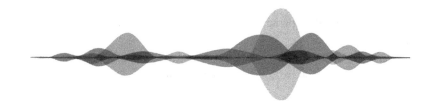

H. Gustav Mueller, PhD
Lindsey E. Jorgensen, AuD, PhD

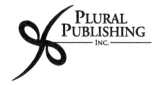

PLURAL
PUBLISHING
INC.

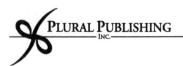

5521 Ruffin Road
San Diego, CA 92123

e-mail: information@pluralpublishing.com
Web site: https://www.pluralpublishing.com

Typeset in 10.5/13 Minion Pro by Achorn International
Printed in the United States of America by Integrated Books International

Library of Congress Cataloging-in-Publication Data
Names: Mueller, H. Gustav, author. | Jorgensen, Lindsey E., author.
Title: Hearing aids for speech-language pathologists : a guide to modern
   rehabilitative audiology / H. Gustav Mueller, Lindsey E. Jorgensen.
Description: San Diego : Plural Publishing, Inc., [2020] | Includes
   bibliographical references and index.
Identifiers: LCCN 2019035361 | ISBN 9781635502145 (paperback) |
   ISBN 1635502144 (paperback) | ISBN 9781635502152 (ebook)
Subjects: MESH: Hearing Aids | Correction of Hearing
   Impairment—instrumentation | Wireless Technology
Classification: LCC RF300 | NLM WV 274 | DDC 617.8/9—dc23
LC record available at https://lccn.loc.gov/2019035361

Contents

Preface

So . . . what do speech-language pathologists need to know about hearing aids and amplification devices? What do they *want* to know? While we had been told by many that a book such as this would be welcome in the speech-language community, carving out a plan of action required some careful thought. We of course consulted with our speech-language pathology colleagues who work with individuals wearing hearing aids; we reviewed publications and papers written on the topic; and we solicited the opinion of new grads in the profession, asking what information they wish they would have been provided during their training. We considered our own training from years ago in communication disorders, and one of us (HGM) even resorted to thinking back, albeit way back, to his days of working as a speech-language pathologist in the school system. And we even went the family route, with Gus seeking insights from his daughter Caitlin—a speech-language pathologist—while Lindsey went to her mother—a retired director of special education. So, did all this background research result in the production of the perfect book? Probably not, but we hope that we at least got close.

Whether you're a graduate student or a practicing speech-language pathologist, you will find this text provides you with the latest in concise and practical information in the areas of hearing aids, hearing assistive devices, and rehabilitative audiology. Hearing aid technology changes at a rapid pace. For speech-language pathologists who work with individuals with hearing loss, many of who use hearing instruments, keeping up with this new technology can be challenging, and sometimes even intimidating.

On any given day you might encounter a new hearing aid rechargeable system, a teenager asking for help setting up direct iPhone streaming, or an elderly patient trying to understand how to use his smartphone app to adjust directivity and noise reduction. This book is designed to remove the mystery and the confusing high-tech terms of the many new hearing aid algorithms and features by simply laying out the need-to-know aspects in an organized, easy-to-read, and easy-to-understand manner.

The core of this text focuses on how modern hearing aids work, both in function and in practicality, as well as the tests associated with the fitting of these instruments. Attention is given to both the school-age and adult hearing aid user. We recognize, however, that amplification is not just hearing aids, and therefore chapters have also been dedicated to implantable amplification strategies as well as FM and Bluetooth solutions.

Hearing aid fitting cannot be studied in isolation, but rather, how it fits into the complete treatment of the patient with hearing loss, including the audiologic rehabilitative process. For this reason, the beginning chapters of the text are devoted to a review of the basics of the modern audiologic evaluation and the associated auditory pathologies. In the final chapters of the book, we address hearing screening in the schools and the audiologic rehabilitative process from identification to treatment to (re)habilitation. Our goal with this text is for it to be a resource for the speech-language pathologist who works with people with hearing loss.

We want to thank our fellow Plural book authors Todd Ricketts, Ruth Bentler, Brad Stach, Brian Taylor, and Jerry Northern for allowing us to borrow material from their excellent texts. We also would like to thank Elaine Keogh and Jessica Messersmith for their valuable and constructive suggestions and for providing insight into the practicality and usefulness of the text in daily practice. Assisting in many of the fine pieces of putting this book together were University of South Dakota Department of Audiology graduate students Emily Benson and Michelle Novak. And, of course, a thanks to our families for their support and encouragement.

Gus Mueller
Bismarck, ND

Lindsey Jorgensen
Vermillion, SD

1 Provision of Hearing Aids: Who, What, and Where

The selection and fitting of hearing aids has been associated with audiology since . . . before audiology was called audiology. In fact, it is probable that the extensive work with hearing aids and aural rehabilitation by several individuals during World War II is what led to the coining of the words *audiology* and *audiologist*. But, when we talk of the provision of hearing aids, it quickly becomes clear that audiologists are only a part of the big picture. In this chapter, we talk about the variety of entities involved in hearing aid provision, how these may work together, or—in some cases—how they may be in direct opposition. Additionally, we'll discuss many of the overriding principles, guidelines, regulations that impact this relationship, and where and how the speech-language pathologist fits in.

A Little History (Big Thanks to a Speech Pathologist!)

Regardless of who actually coined the word audiology, there is little question that the advancement of the use of the term was linked directly to the establishment of rehabilitation centers during World War II. These sites were established to handle the large number of returning veterans suffering from hearing loss. Four major military regional sites were established: Hoff General Hospital (Santa Barbara, CA), Borden General Hospital (Chickasha, OK), Philadelphia Naval Hospital (PA), and Deshon General Hospital (Butler, PA). Captain Raymond Carhart—a 1936 doctoral graduate of Northwestern University (**majoring in speech pathology**, experimental phonetics, and psychology)—was assigned to Deshon Hospital from 1944 to 1946, and his work there has had a lasting effect on the field of audiology and, specifically, the selection and fitting of hearing aids.

Following World War II, there were several additional military audiology facilities established at major hospitals—Walter Reed Army Medical Center in Washington, DC being the most notable. We also saw the emergence of several U.S. Department of Veterans Affairs (VA) audiology clinics. All of these facilities employed audiologists, both military and civilian, who conducted hearing aid evaluations and also dispensed hearing aids to veterans, active duty, and retired military personnel. Because of the ethical constraints placed on audiologists fitting hearing aids outside of the government—which we will discuss shortly—these military and VA hospital clinics became known as an excellent training site for audiology students wanting to obtain hands-on experience with the selection and fitting of hearing aids. It was also during this time that audiology training programs began to emerge. These early programs were in the Midwest at locations such as Northwestern University, the University of Iowa, and Purdue University. The first doctorate granted in audiology was from Northwestern in 1946.

Although audiologists at military facilities enjoyed the benefits of directly dispensing hearing aids to their patients, until the 1980s, in the civilian sector, nearly all hearing aids were dispensed by hearing aid dealers, not audiologists. Like today, there were many storefront hearing aid sales facilities, many of them franchises. Audiologists' clinical activities regarding hearing aid dispensing were influenced greatly by the American Speech-Language-Hearing Association (ASHA), the primary professional organization for audiologists during this time frame. For arguably good reasons, the ASHA had the belief that it could be challenging to professional ethics if an audiologist were to evaluate a patient for a hearing aid, recommend a hearing aid, and then turn around and sell the patient the hearing aid they had just recommended. Selling hearing aids, therefore, was a violation of the ASHA ethical standards.

So it was that during this time frame that audiologists had a somewhat unusual role in the selection and fitting of hearing aids. During this era, although the majority of hearing aids were dispensed by a *dispenser* without the patient first going to an audiologist, there were situations when an audiologist was involved. When this happened, the general fitting process would go something like the following:

- The patient would go to a university or hospital clinic to have his or her hearing tested and be evaluated for hearing aids.
- After some limited testing, the audiologist would recommend a specific brand of hearing aid and specific settings.
- The patient was then referred directly to a given hearing aid dealer (nonaudiologist) who sold that brand (most dealers only sold one or two brands).
- The protocol for most facilities was that after the patient purchased the new

hearing aids, the patient would return to the audiology clinic for the audiologist to give the fitting his or her blessing.

This was a situation rife with conflict; as in many cases, the patient had purchased a hearing aid different from what the audiologist had recommended. The audiologist and dispenser would disagree regarding what was best, and the patient was caught in the middle.

ASHA Caves: *Selling* Is Not a Bad Word (Anymore)

Regarding the ASHA code of ethics mentioned earlier, it is important to point out that in the 1960s and 1970s state licensure for audiology did not exist for most states. Clinical audiologists, therefore, valued their ASHA certification and did not want to jeopardize their standing as an ASHA member. And, for the most part, audiologists not belonging to the ASHA were considered outsiders. Moreover, most audiologists, especially those in academia, tended to believe that selling hearing aids had a certain sleaze factor associated with it. There of course were audiologists who tested the system, and their expulsion from the ASHA was publicized. As time went on, however, more and more audiologists saw the benefits of providing complete services for their patients, and in the early 1970s, we started to see audiologists going into a dispensing private practice—with or without approval from the ASHA.

The movement to remove the violation for selling hearing aids from the ASHA code of ethics gathered steam in 1977 when a group of ASHA members formed the Academy of Dispensing Audiology (ADA). The name of the organization obviously was selected to make the point that selling hearing aids should be part of the audiologists' scope of practice (the name has since been changed to the Academy of Doctors of Audiology). Although you might think that this new organization was simply a handful of young maverick audiologists, it actually included several prominent members of the profession—most notably Leo Doerfler, PhD, who was not only the ADA's founding president, but also a former president of the ASHA.

While the internal pressure for change was resulting in many heated discussions at professional meetings, the event that probably triggered the change in ASHA policy was a 1978 U.S. Supreme Court ruling against the National Society of Professional Engineers, saying that their code of ethics could not be used to prohibit price interference for engineers' services. And so it was that selling hearing aids for profit became ethical. By the end of 1979, nearly 1,000 audiologists were selling hearing aids, and that number grew to 5,000 by the end of the 1980s (Harford, 2000).

Audiologists Selling Hearing Aids in the Workplace

Things have changed considerably since the days that audiologists only dispensed hearing aids in government facilities. Today, there are approximately 16,000 licensed audiologists in the United States, and 60% to 70% of these dispense hearing aids. (Note: by comparison, there are approximately 8,000 licensed hearing instrument specialists.) Audiologists dispense from a variety of settings ranging from their own private practice, to an otolaryngologist's practice, to a university or hospital clinic, to an office owned by a manufacturer, or—in more recent years—from chain department stores. Hearing aids are sold in university clinics as part of most AuD training programs. Shown in Figure 1–1 are the most recent data from the American Academy of Audiology (AAA) summarizing typical work

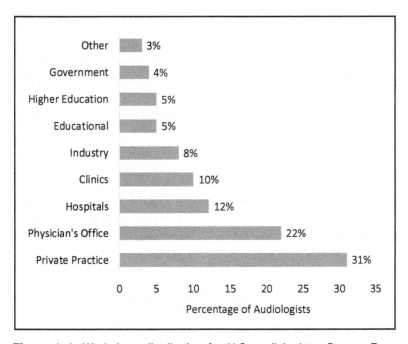

Figure 1–1. Workplace distribution for U.S. audiologists. *Source*: From *Essentials of Modern Hearing Aids: Selection, Fitting, and Verification* (p. 31), by T. A. Ricketts, R. Bentler, and H. G. Mueller, 2019, San Diego, CA: Plural Publishing. Reprinted with permission.

settings. Observe that the highest percent of audiologists are in privately owned audiology practices. Although this is the most common workplace, data from the ADA suggests that only 15% to 20% of audiology offices are owned and controlled by audiologists, much lower than other similar professions (e.g., optometry 75% and dentistry 93%). Private practice ownership among audiologists has been decreasing significantly in recent years, as offices are being purchased by manufacturers and other buying groups. Many of those not directly purchased by a hearing aid manufacturer, are financed by the manufacturer, and as a result, the practice more or less becomes a "company store," as hearing aid purchases from the company help repay the loan.

THINGS TO REMEMBER: Who Is Selling Hearing Aids?

While audiologists would like to think that they are the "gatekeepers" in the hearing aid delivery system, this is far from true. When you encounter a patient who owns hearing aids, there are several possibilities regarding the source. It is important to point out that regarding patient benefit, two factors are in play: the technology of the instrument itself and the programming of the instrument for the patient's individual needs (assuming the instrument is programmable). The best hearing aid in the world is of little or no benefit when programmed incorrectly, and on the other hand, a relatively inexpensive product might function quite well when programmed by a knowledgeable professional. With this is mind, logic would suggest that patient benefit is the highest when hearing aids are purchased from an audiologist—they sell top-end technology and have the most education and training regarding the fitting of hearing aids. Here is a review of the three most common purchase sources:

■ **Audiologist.** In most states, audiologists must a have a dispensing license separate from their audiology license. This means that they have passed a written and practical exam. While for most states the audiology license requires a doctoral degree, this of course isn't true for the dispensing license. Dispensing audiologists may belong to the ASHA and hold the CCC-A, or belong to the AAA and hold board certification, but neither of these is required for the practice of audiology or the sale of hearing aids.

■ **Hearing Instrument Specialist (HIS).** Most states have similar requirements for becoming a licensed hearing aid dispenser. A typical example reads: "Be 18 years of age or older. Have a high school diploma or its equivalent. Have not committed acts or crimes constituting grounds for denial of licensure (convicted felon). Have passed a written and practical test." There are many licensed dispensers who of course far exceed the education requirements. For example, in some states there are otolaryngologists who have a dispensing license. It's not uncommon for other professionals to adopt selling hearing aids as a part-time second career following retirement. HISs can become certified with the National Board for Certification in Hearing Instrument Sciences (NBC-HIS), an organization affiliated with the International Hearing Society (IHS).

■ **Internet/Mail Order.** A third source of hearing aid purchase is through the Internet or newspaper and direct mail advertising. A recent search of "hearing aids" on eBay provided 24,899 matches! These sales ads ranged from $9.99 products to a $9,000 Phonak product from India (free remote programming!). Now, we need to mention that these are not all "hearing aids" according to the strict definition, but the lines of this definition become more blurred each year (see our later definition of a personal sound amplifier product [PSAP]). And what about the licensure issue? Well, if it is truly a hearing aid, then whoever is selling it should be a licensed dispenser in the state in which the prospective owner lives. Until we have hearing aid sniffing dogs at UPS, FedEx, and the post office, enforcement of this simply isn't going to happen.

In most cases, the hearing aid purchased through the Internet will need programming by an audiologist, not to mention that the patient will also need long-term follow-up rehabilitation care. How this is accomplished often becomes a sticky issue for dispensing audiologists. How are these patients handled when they show up for an appointment carrying their newly purchased hearing aids with them? Some Internet hearing aid sales sites have attempted to partner with dispensing audiologists—that is, the patient brings in the Internet-purchased hearing aids and the audiologist conducts the programming. In general, audiologists have not been receptive to this arrangement. However, Internet sales are not going to go away, so we expect that some type of arrangement will evolve so that this group of patients can receive effective benefit from their instruments.

■ **Over-The-Counter (OTC).** This delivery system will be with us starting in 2020. At this writing, we do not know the details, but we expect that this category of hearing aids will be available for purchase at major retail outlets. Audiologists and HISs may elect to also offer OTCs in their clinics and offices. A developing situation.

Hearing Aid Distribution Channels

Indirectly and sometimes directly related to the workplace where we find audiologists dispensing hearing aids is the overall hearing aid distribution system. Where does the audiologist buy their hearing aids to sell?

Where do they buy products that are "sort of" hearing aids?

Hearing Aid Manufacturers

Regarding major hearing aid manufacturers, we have what is referred to as the *Big Five*, composed of Demant (primary brand

Oticon), WS Audiology (primary brands Widex and Signia), Starkey, GN Store Nord (primary brand ReSound), and Sonova (primary brands Phonak and Unitron). Between them, these companies own or manage 15 to 20 other brands of hearing aids. In addition, there are probably another 25 to 30 lesser-known hearing aid manufacturing companies. Today, most audiologists have one or two favorite companies and buy directly from these manufacturers, with more than 90% of total hearing aid sales from the Big Five.

Buying Groups

Some audiologists find it advantageous to work with a buying group. That is, because of the increased volume, the groups can demand discounts from the manufacturers and pass these savings on to members of the group. There are several different groups and different types of groups to choose from. Examples are Audigy, AUDNET Hearing Group, Elite, EarQ, and Consult YHN. Many of the groups offer a range of practice assistance other than just hearing aid purchases. Some of the buying groups, however, more or less work exclusively with the brands of one or two manufacturers.

Retail Outlets

All of the Big Five have retail outlets, which may consist of established stores such as Beltone (owned by GN), companies with multicenter clinical sites such as Newport Audiology (Sonova) or HearUSA (WS Audiology), or the manufacturer may be more subtly involved through corporate-owned, independent practices. Many practices that

appear to be owned and operated by audiologists have been financed by a major hearing aid company, and the audiologist is more or less obligated to dispense the hearing aids of that company. In addition to the Big Five, retail offices also are operated by Amplifon (Miracle Ear), Costco, and Sam's Club (and probably several more since the writing of this book). All the retail outlets employ audiologists, although the audiologist or hearing instrument specialist mix varies considerably among sites.

Internet Sales

We talked about this briefly in the previous "Things to Remember" box. An Internet purchase is possible by simply going to eBay or to Internet sites specializing in Internet sales. Although, most—if not all—manufacturers have issued a statement saying that they will not sell hearing aids to retailers who do not conduct an in-person fitting, this is difficult to control. For example, if a regular customer of a hearing aid manufacturer purchases 10 BTE hearing aids, how does the company know how and when they were sold? Internet sales also may be illegal in some states, but again, enforcement is difficult.

OTCs, PSAPs, and Hearables

We recognize that these are products and not distribution channels, but we explain the connection soon. When is a product a personal sound amplifier product (PSAP) and when is it a hearing aid? The distinction becomes more blurred each year. In March 2009, the Food and Drug Administration (FDA) issued guidance describing how hearing aids and PSAPs differ. This guidance

---

KEY CONCEPT: To Bundle or Not?

Surveys indicate that 80% to 85% of audiologists who sell hearing aids use a *bundled* approach. That is, a single, inclusive price that includes the audiologist's cost for the product, fitting fees, counseling, and follow-up visits (either throughout the life of the hearing aid, or, in some cases, only during the warranty period). The patient is not informed what percent of the total cost is for the product or what costs are for services, although our experiences suggest that the average patient believes the bulk of the cost is the product (which usually isn't true).

Audiologists who use an *unbundled* approach, sometimes called "fee-for-service," break out the cost of the product, accessories, fitting fees, consulting, and follow-up services. This has the advantage of clearly showing the value of the fitting and counseling that goes along with dispensing hearing aids.

Additionally, it eliminates the patient's concern that the audiologist is upselling when he or she recommends more features, as the fitting fee would likely stay the same (e.g., it does not require more time or counseling to fit a 20-channel product than a 4-channel product). Some audiologists, however, shy away from the unbundled approach because they believe that when the patient sees the true cost of the hearing aid, they will consider the audiologist's fees to be unreasonable. Also, audiologists fear that the patient may not return for the necessary follow-up visits because of the cost involved, and the end result will be dissatisfaction with amplification. Because of this, some audiologists use a partly unbundled approach. All of this will become a much greater business concern when over-the-counter (OTC) hearing aids and more sophisticated PSAPs occupy a larger market share.

---

defines a hearing aid as a sound-amplifying device intended to compensate for impaired hearing. PSAPs, the guidance states, are not intended to make up for impaired hearing. Instead, they are intended for non-hearing-impaired consumers to amplify sounds in the environment for a number of reasons, such as for recreational activities. You maybe have seen advertisements for such devices as "Game Ear" or "Hunter's Ear." Some PSAPs are more or less novelty items, but today, we also have advanced PSAPs advertised as having 14 bands and channels, digital noise reduction, feedback reduction, and a volume control wheel. Sounds a lot like a hearing aid to us, but such products are being sold over-the-counter at retail outlets.

A category of PSAPs, or what some might consider a category of hearing aids, are what are called "hearables." The exact definition is somewhat fluid, but in general, a hearable is an earpiece that uses wireless communication to enhance a listening experience. Hearing aid companies are using hearing aids to do more than simply amplify sound (monitor movement, detect falls, translate a foreign language, etc.).

Commercial electronic companies also see the advantage of using earbuds to measure biometrics, and are designing products of this type that also have the ability to amplify sound. Starting to sound like a hearing aid? Or, a converging of products?

And then we have OTC products. In the past, we have referred to many PSAPs as OTC hearing aids, as in function they were. In 2017, we had the FDA Reauthorization Act, which stated that there will be a new official class of hearing aids, authorized by the FDA, which will be sold over-the-counter. The FDA is expected to publish proposed regulations for the new category of hearing aids by August 18, 2020—so depending on when you are reading this, these products may be on the market. The general guidelines say that these OTC products will have the same fundamental scientific technology as current hearing aids, but will be available over-the-counter, without the supervision, prescription, or other order, involvement, or intervention of a licensed person—to consumers through in-person transactions, by mail, or online. They will be for adults (18 and older), and will be designed to provide adequate amplification for mild-to-moderate hearing losses. They may include self-assessment tests, and the user will be able to control their OTC hearing aids and customize them as they see fit (probably via a smartphone app).

The impact that the new OTC category will have on hearing aid distribution is unknown. Will this attract a new group of hearing aid users who would have never gone through traditional distribution channels? Will new users try these, like the results, and then purchase traditional hearing aids? Or, will the current hearing aid patients of audiologists abandon them for this low-cost option? And who will be the major manufacturers? Our current Big Five? Or companies like Bose, Samsung and Apple? Stay tuned.

Laws, Regulations, Rules, and Guidelines Related to the Fitting of Hearing Aids

There are many rules and regulations that go along with the practice of dispensing hearing aids. While it's unlikely that you will be selling hearing aids, it's very possible that you could have a patient who uses hearing aids, and knowledge of some of these regulations may come in handy.

Scope of Practice

A good starting point for this section is the scope of practice for audiology. Although we do not usually think of these as regulations or rules, they do serve as a foundation for the development of other documents. All major audiology organizations have a published scope of practice. For example, the AAA's scope of practice (last updated January 2004) states as part of its purpose:

> This document outlines those activities that are within the expertise of members of the profession. This Scope of Practice statement is intended for use by audiologists, allied professionals, consumers of audiologic services, and the general public. It serves as a reference for issues of service delivery, third-party reimbursement, legislation, consumer education, regulatory action, state and professional licensure, and inter-professional relations.

Regarding the fitting of hearing aids, the document states:

> The audiologist is the professional who provides the full range of audiologic treatment services for persons with impairment of hearing and vestibular function. The audiologist is responsible for the evaluation, fitting, and verification of amplification devices, including assistive listening devices. The audiologist determines the appropriateness of amplification systems for persons with hearing impairment, evaluates benefit, and provides counseling and training regarding their use. Audiologists conduct otoscopic examinations, clean ear canals and remove cerumen, take ear canal impressions, select, fit, evaluate, and dispense hearing aids and other amplification systems.

Copies of the scope of practice for audiology from the AAA and the ASHA can be found in Appendix A and B, respectively.

Licensure

As mentioned earlier, certainly, one of the most important concerns regarding the sale of hearing aids is obtaining appropriate licensure, which is controlled on a state-by-state basis. For audiologists, this could simply mean obtaining your *audiology license* for a given state; however, at the time of writing this text, in 13 states, it also is necessary to obtain a second hearing aid dispensing license. These state laws do change fairly frequently, so if you are concerned regarding the credentials of someone selling hearing aids, we suggest that you check with the AAA or the ASHA to obtain the current status for specific states. In some states, even when the hearing aid dispensing license is not necessary, additional requirements to the standard audiology license do apply.

Board Certification

Some type of certification in audiology is available from both the AAA and the ASHA, although it is not necessary to belong to the organization to obtain and hold the certification. The AAA certification is granted by the American Board of Audiology, and hence it often is referred to by the abbreviation ABA. The ASHA certification is the Clinical Certificate of Competence in Audiology, or CCC-A. Some audiologists have both, so paging through the yellow pages you might see an audiologist listed as AuD, ABA, CCC-A. Of note, ABA certification does require additional continuing education and exams while CCC-A does not require any additional testing or continuing education beyond those required for ASHA membership. Board certification is not required for dispensing hearing aids, and holding such certification, for the most part, is only indirectly related to the services provided.

Hearing Aid Fitting Guidelines

As with other areas of clinical audiology, over the years, various guidelines have been established regarding the selection and fitting of hearing aids. Typically, these guidelines are developed by a group of key experts and reflect what is considered good practice at the time of the writing. Whether these guidelines have had an impact on clinical practice

KEY CONCEPT: Practice Patterns

- Scope of practice statement: A list of professional activities that define the range of services offered within the profession of audiology.
- Preferred practice patterns: Statements that define generally applicable characteristics of activities directed toward individual patients.
- Position statements: Statements that specify an organization's policy and stance on a matter.
- Practice guidelines: A recommended set of procedures for a specific area of practice, based on research findings and current practice.
- Promising practice: At least preliminary evidence of effectiveness in small-scale interventions or evidence for which there is potential for generating data that will be useful for making decisions about taking the intervention to scale and generalizing the results to diverse populations and settings.
- Gold standard: The highest level of practice founded in research practices.

DID YOU KNOW: Watch Out for False Idols!

Directly related to "Best Practice" is "Evidence-Based Practice," which dates back to the mid-1800s in clinical medicine, but only recently has been emphasized in the fitting of hearing aids. Noted expert in this area, David L. Sackett, MD, describes it as the conscientious, explicit, and judicious use of current best evidence in making decisions about the care of individual patients. Frank C. Wilson, MD, also an authority in *evidence-based practice* once wrote: "Neither unaudited experience nor logical thought can replace controlled clinical trials, so until documentation of a procedure's effectiveness can be demonstrated, it should be considered a false idol and worship withheld."

is debatable. Portions of guidelines, however, have found their way into the body of state license documents.

The AAA Fitting Guidelines

We mentioned earlier that *fitting guidelines* are only best practice guidelines if they are constructed using the rules of evidence-based practice. The 2006 hearing aid fitting guidelines for adults published by the AAA used this approach, as did their June 2013 document on pediatric amplification. If you happen to question the fitting process of an adult or a child, these documents provide a review of "preferred practice" supported by research evidence.

For adults
https://audiology-web.s3.amazonaws.com
/migrated/haguidelines.pdf_53994876e92e42
.70908344.pdf

For children
https://www.audiology.org/sites/default
/files/publications/PediatricAmplification
Guidelines.pdf

FDA Regulations

As you might expect, there are government regulations relating to the manufacture, sale, and fitting of hearing aids. These issues are addressed by the medical devices regulations (subchapter H, revised April 1, 2010) of the U.S. Food and Drug Administration (FDA), Department of Health and Human Services. This regulation has definitions of both audiologist and dispenser. In general, the term dispenser is used in the regulation, and this term would apply to audiologists involved in selling hearing aids.

FDA Red Flags

One of the things outlined in the FDA regulation are the eight *red flags* for referral (not to be confused with the *Red Flag Rules* issued by the Federal Trade Commission

[FTC] in 2010). The regulation states that a dispenser should advise a prospective hearing aid user to consult a licensed physician (preferably an otolaryngologist) promptly if any of the following are observed through record review, case history, or testing:

1. Visible congenital or traumatic deformity of the ear.
2. History of active drainage from the ear within the previous 90 days.
3. History of sudden or rapidly progressive hearing loss within the previous 90 days.
4. Acute or chronic dizziness.
5. Unilateral hearing loss of sudden or recent onset within the previous 90 days.
6. Audiometric air-bone gap equal to or greater than 15 dB at 500 hertz (Hz), 1000 Hz, and 2000 Hz.
7. Visible evidence of significant cerumen accumulation or a foreign body in the ear canal.
8. Pain or discomfort in the ear.

In general, even if these eight conditions were not present in the regulation, the prudent audiologist would probably refer to a

---

KEY CONCEPT: Medical Clearance for Hearing Aid Purchase?

For many years, the FDA required a medical clearance (from an MD) for anyone buying a hearing aid. Patients did have the option to bypass this requirement by signing a waiver, which commonly happened. In December 2016, the FDA issued a statement saying that they no longer intend to enforce this requirement. This was no doubt related to the new OTC hearing aid category that was brewing at the time (which we discussed earlier). Children (under 18) will continue to have the medical evaluation requirement without the option of a waiver. The FDA statement did say, however, that dispensers are still required at this point to make available, and provide consumers the opportunity to review, the User Instruction Brochure that contains information about possible red flags prior to the sale of a hearing aid.

physician if any of these conditions existed anyway. A referral would not be needed if there was documentation of physician referral for a continuation of the same condition (e.g. congenital malformation). Depending on your definition of significant, one exception might be cerumen accumulation, which often does not require a medical referral and easily can be handled by most audiologists (assuming it is allowed by the state's licensure law).

HIPAA

The Health Insurance Portability and Accountability Act (HIPAA) became law in 1996. The part of HIPAA that has the most impact on audiology practice is the Accountability or Administrative Simplification section. Contained in this section are rules regarding transactions and code sets, privacy, and security. There also are rules mandating that that the Employer Identification Number provided to the IRS be utilized when submitting claims to insurers, and a rule that mandates the use of the National Provider Identifier (NPI) by audiologists when submitting claims to all insurers including Medicare and Medicaid. Each clinic or facility must also obtain an NPI.

FTC

The FTC has issued a set of regulations, effective in June 2010, known as the Red Flag Rules. These rules apply to any audiology practice that accepts and processes third-party payments or insurance, or acts as a creditor for its patients. This rule requires practices to create and implement written identity theft prevention, detection, and management policies and procedures in an attempt to protect their patients from iden-

tity theft. The Red Flag Rules can be considered an expansion of the HIPAA privacy rules. As with the HIPAA Privacy Policy, the audiology practice needs to create office policies and procedures that outline how the practice intends to identify, detect, and respond to identity theft red flags.

Laws and Statutes

There are several laws and statutes that have the possibility to directly relate to the sale of hearing aids. In particular, they apply when the audiologist is involved with reimbursement through Medicare or Medicaid.

- Antikickback Statute: We are referring to the Medicare and Medicaid Patient Protection Act of 1987, as amended, 42 U.S.C. §1320a-7b. The section of this statute that relates directly to the sale of hearing aids prohibits the offer or receipt of certain remuneration in return for referrals or recommending purchase of supplies and services reimbursable under government healthcare programs.
- Stark Law: The federal statute dealing with physician self-referral is generally referred to as the *Stark Law*, although there have been modifications. Congress included a provision in the Omnibus Budget Reconciliation Act of 1989, which barred self-referrals for clinical laboratory services under the Medicare program, effective January 1, 1992. This provision is known as *Stark I*. Under this law, if a physician or a member of a physician's immediate family has a financial relationship with a healthcare entity, the physician may not make referrals to that entity for the furnishing of designated health services under the Medicare program.

- False Claims Act: The False Claims Act (31 U.S.C. §§ 3729–3733, also called the *Lincoln Law*) is a federal law that imposes liability on persons and companies who defraud governmental programs. As it relates to audiology and hearing aids, the False Claims Act deals with audiologists who submit claims for services that were not done or were not necessary.

- Gifts or Inducements to Beneficiaries. Ever see a newspaper ad advertising "free hearing tests?" Of course you have—the ad in Figure 1–2 is very typical. Are those "free tests" offered to get people in the door to sell them hearing aids? Of course. Gifts and inducements to beneficiaries is included under section 1128A(a)(5) of the Social Security Act, enacted as part of HIPAA. Specifically the law states: "It is unlawful to knowingly offer or give remuneration to Medicare or Medicaid beneficiaries to influence their choice of provider for any item or service covered by Medicare or a state health care program."

Ethics

As with all areas of clinical audiology, ethical guidelines relate to several different aspects of dispensing hearing aids. Are the patients treated properly? Do the fitting and verification procedures assure that the patients obtained what is best for them? Are there outside incentives that influence clinical decisions? Ethical guidelines related to hearing aid fitting can also originate from several sources: professional organizations, state licensure documents, hearing aid manufacturers, and health-care organizations.

Code of Ethics of Professional Organizations

When we think of a code of ethics, we usually first associate them with professional organizations. You might even know of someone who was removed from an organization because of a violation of a given organization's standards. We have included the

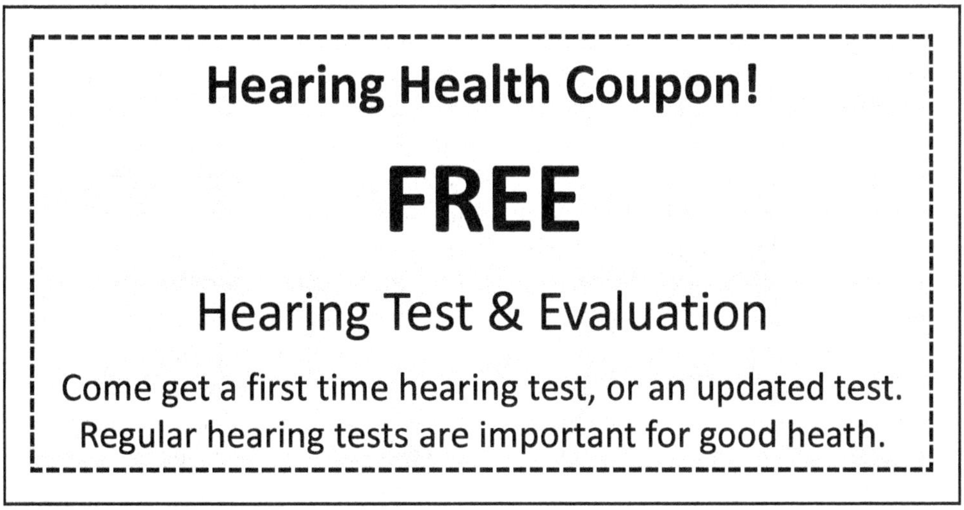

Hearing Health Coupon!

FREE

Hearing Test & Evaluation

Come get a first time hearing test, or an updated test.
Regular hearing tests are important for good heath.

Figure 1–2. Dispensers placing this ad might want to remember that the law states: "It is unlawful to knowingly offer or give remuneration to Medicare or Medicaid beneficiaries to influence their choice of provider for any item or service covered by Medicare or a state health care program."

ethical guidelines for the AAA (Appendix C). The code of ethics covers a wide range of activities that can be related to the sale and fitting of hearing aids: maintaining high standards of professional competence, maintaining patient confidentiality, providing appropriate services and products, making accurate public statements, avoiding commercial interests that could impact patient care, and abstaining from dishonesty or illegal conduct that could adversely affect the profession. The code of ethics for the ASHA is very similar to the AAA and can be found at: https://www.asha.org/Code-of-Ethics/

In recent years, there has been an increased effort by training programs to set a high ethical-standards bar when it relates to students and their relationship (real or perceived) with manufacturers of hearing aids and audiometric test equipment. And it's not just about the free pizza provided during a luncheon seminar by a company rep. Manufacturers offer many incentives, which might include small gifts (pens, backpacks, etc.), but often involve relatively expensive items such as free trips to the manufacturer-sponsored "summer camp." Would attendance at a mountain retreat, all expenses paid, influence a stu-

---

POINTS TO PONDER: Okay to Have a Favorite Manufacturer?

You maybe know an audiologist who fits nearly all their patients with the same brand of hearing aids. Is this okay? Many audiologists purchase 80% or more of their hearing aids from a single manufacturer. Although some might frown on this, we certainly do not consider this unethical, as long as the amplification needs of each patient are being met. There are many advantages of using a primary manufacturer. The most significant is the greater familiarity with the products and the fitting software. Fine-tuning hearing aids quickly on a busy day can be quite challenging for even the seasoned audiologist if several different manufacturers are used. Not only does manufacturer software differ greatly in how changes are made to different hearing aid features, but those features probably will be given different names. In addition, controls with the same name (e.g., gain for soft) may have different effects on compression parameters depending on the specific manufacturer. Another advantage of only using one or two manufacturers is the increased familiarity with the manufacturer's support staff, which can help solve fitting, ordering, repair, and administrative problems. Additionally, hearing aid technology is rapidly changing, often every six months. Keeping up to date on manufacturer hearing aid platforms and function is essential to appropriate selection and fitting. Therefore, audiologists often choose to use only one or two manufacturers in order to keep up with the changing technology. Finally, if enough hearing aids are purchased each month, there also will likely be a reduction in the cost of the products, which can be passed along to the patient.

dent when they are deciding what hearing aids to sell in later years? For these reasons, several universities prohibit their students from accepting gifts and attending such events, and some training institutions do not even allow students to have any item, such as a pen, with the logo of an audiology-related manufacturer. (Note: medical center research has shown that a free pen will influence what medicine a medical student will prescribe). There has been considerable research regarding how gifts can influence professional behavior. Here is a summary:

- Companies work harder to influence you than you work to resist their efforts.
- You probably believe that your professional colleagues will be influenced, but that you will not.
- You are probably more influenced than you think.
- Small gifts pack about the same punch as larger ones.

Regarding the sale and dispensing of hearing aids

- Dispensing more of a given brand without complete consideration of options
- Dispensing a higher tier product (more channels, features, etc.) than is needed for certain patients
- Inability to recognize false claims from a favorite brand
- Developing a close relationship with the manufacturer's rep

In Closing

As we have discussed, there is a long history between audiology and the fitting of hearing aids. There is a long and storied history regarding audiology and hearing aid dispensing too. Consider that as recent as the late 1970s, it was considered unethical for audiologists to sell hearing aids, compared with today, when a large portion of hearing aids sold in the United States are by audiologists who own and operate their own private practice, and the profit from these sales contributes significantly to the audiologists income.

Regarding the distribution and manufacturing of hearing aids, we now have the Big Five companies, which includes more than 90% of the hearing aids sold. But, as you might expect, the landscape is constantly changing. It's anyone's guess how the new OTC category will influence dispensing practices. And, what about the increasing number of private practices owned by manufacturers? Are we going back to the days of mostly *franchise offices*?

We have reviewed many of the related background issues that need to be considered: licensure, certification, guidelines, regulations, laws, reimbursement, and ethics. These topics are maybe not as intriguing as what we'll cover in later chapters, but important nonetheless. As a speech pathologist, although you might be on the periphery of these issues, it may be necessary to refer to some of these when working with your patients using hearing instruments.

2 The Routine Audiologic Evaluation: A Review

From our friend Bobby Boyle: *"If you want to improve something, you first have to measure it."* Robert Boyle was the scientist who discovered the inverse relationship between the pressure and volume of a gas, which explains, among many other things, the relationship between ear canal volume and sound pressure level—an important concept when fitting hearing aids to children. His work has become known as "Boyle's Law." During Sir Robert's laboratory experiments (ca. 1660), he also discovered that to better understand something you first have to measure it. This concept certainly holds true for hearing care professionals because when we take the time to accurately measure hearing, we better understand how a hearing loss affects communication. And of course, even the most basic audiologic measures impact the fitting of hearing aids, not only in determining candidacy, but in programming the appropriate gain and output.

The aim of this chapter is to briefly review the basic procedures of the hearing test battery, helping you understand why each test needs to be completed, and how the results of each test might impact the hearing aid fitting. This basic test battery is designed to identify the type and degree of hearing loss. There are other, more advanced audiologic tests; however, these tests typically do not play a significant role in the fitting of hearing aids.

Otoscopy

Any audiologic exam starts off with a good otoscopic examination of the ear. When working with patients wearing hearing aids, it's always important to have an otoscope handy—what might be perceived as a "broken" hearing aid, might just be an ear canal full of cerumen. Otoscopes come in a large variety of styles and sizes. They, of course, also vary significantly in cost, ranging from a disposable otoscope for under $10 that you can purchase on Amazon to the common Welch-Allyn clinical models in the $100 to $200 range. Some are wall mounted (which makes them easier to find in a busy office), whereas others are portable. Wall-mounted otoscopes are attached by a flexible power cord to a base, which serves to hold the otoscope when it's not in use and also serves as a source of electric power, being plugged into an electric outlet. Portable models, the type most likely used by speech-language pathologists, are powered by batteries in the handle; these batteries may be changed or are rechargeable and can be recharged from a base unit.

In addition to or instead of traditional otoscopy, it's possible to use video otoscopy, an otoscope attached to a video monitor so that the observations can be easily observed and stored. These are becoming more and more popular in audiologists offices, and recent surveys have shown that about 50% of dispensing offices use this equipment. There are several advantages to using this equipment. First, it is much easier to visualize minor abnormalities on the large video screen than when using the traditional handheld otoscope. Secondly, the patient is able to see what you see. If there is something abnormal (e.g., an ear canal plugged with cerumen), this assists greatly in counseling. Sometimes, after using hearing aids, new users develop pressure sores in the ear canal; these also may be visible. A third advantage is that the "view" of the patient's ear canal and eardrum can be printed for part of their permanent record. This is useful for follow-up visits, or, if you refer the patient for medical care, they can take a photo of their ear canal along to their primary physician or otolaryngologist. Using a special attachment, which you can purchase from Oaktree Products, you can turn your iPhone into an otoscope. Simply purchase the optical otoscope attachment and specula, download the app, and you can perform otoscopy with your smartphone.

The Audiometer and the Pure-Tone Audiogram

The typical audiometer will have an output for air conduction, bone conduction, and speech; the ability to have either pulsed or warble pure tones; and a variety of different masking noises (e.g., narrowband, white noise, and speech noise). There is a frequency selection dial and a hearing level dial (often referred to as an attenuator) for selecting the intensity level. Some audiometers are PC-based and actually may not have a "dial" for some of these functions— you would simply use your mouse. There

also is a talk-forward/talk-back feature that allows you to talk to the patient through the earphones (or loudspeakers if you have them), and also hear what the patient is saying using a monitor microphone. It is best to have a "two channel" audiometer, which means that different input signals and intensities can be delivered independently (e.g., speech from one channel, noise from the other, both delivered to the same ear).

Like everything else, audiometers have become a lot more automated and portable over the past few years. Using any type of computer-based audiometric system is very helpful in maintaining patient records in an easily accessible, organized manner. Today, you can purchase and download an audiometer and essentially turn your iPad into a basic audiometer. However, beware of calibration when using a tablet or phone-based audiometer as any bumps to the volume control will change the output of the sounds thus changing the calibration.

About Earphones

The selection of earphones is critical as these earphones are part of the calibration of the audiometer. And, yes, earphones are color coded: red for right and blue for left. Historically, the most commonly used earphones have been the Telephonics supra-aural TDH-series (e.g., Model 39, Model 49P, etc.). These earphones are attached to a rubber cushion and are held in place using headband designed with a specific tension. While still used by some audiologists, these are not the preferred earphones for routine use. The preferred earphones for audiometric testing are called "insert earphones," most commonly used are those from Etymotic Research. With this type of earphone, the signal is taken from the receiver box (clipped on to the patient clothes) via a tube, which then terminates in a foam plug (similar to what we use for hearing protection). This foam plug is "rolled down," and then inserted into the ear canal. These earphones are calibrated in a 2-cc coupler, just like hearing aids, which helps when conversion between the two is needed.

There are several advantages of insert earphones compared to the older TDH styles:

- Improved interaural attenuation (less sound leaking to other ear around the head)
- Improved patient comfort (the tight fitting headband of the TDH earphones is very uncomfortable for some patients)
- Improved infection control (the foam tips are designed for one-time use and are discarded following testing)
- Better attenuation of ambient room noise; the foam tips, when expanded in the ear canal, serve as an earplug
- Elimination of collapsed canal
- Increased reliability due to better placement; when supra-aural earphones are used, thresholds can vary by 10 dB or more in the high frequencies simply because the earphone was not aligned properly

Air Conduction Testing

We perceive sounds in two different ways. Sound can be either transmitted via sound waves in the air through the outer ear (ear canal to the eardrum), through the middle ear, and to the inner ear (cochlea); or sound can be directly transmitted to the cochlea via bone conduction. When testing a patient's hearing using the air conductive pathway of sound from the outer to the inner ear, we use earphones and perform what is termed "air conduction audiometry." The pure tone

or speech stimulus that we introduce via the earphones travels through the outer ear and middle ears, to the inner ear, then along the eighth nerve, the brain stem, and finally to the auditory cortex of the brain where it is perceived.

Bone Conduction Testing

When we deliver pure tones or speech signals by placing a bone conduction oscillator directly on the mastoid bone behind the ear (or on the forehead), we are bypassing the outer and middle ear structures. A properly placed oscillator literally vibrates the bones of the skull, stimulating neural activity in the cochlea, then sending the neural signal on to the auditory cortex via the eighth nerve (or auditory nerve) and the brain stem auditory centers. These vibrations directly move the structures of the inner ear and allow us to eventually perceive sound in the exact same way we perceived the air conducted signal.

During a routine hearing test, we usually conduct different procedures in which either air conducted or bone conducted sounds are presented to the ears. Comparing air and bone conduction thresholds helps us to determine the site of lesion of the hearing loss. Site of lesion testing tells us very important information about where the problem contributing to the hearing loss lies: the outer, middle, or inner ear. For example, if person has a significant loss by air conduction but excellent hearing by bone conduction, we know that the problem must lie in either the outer or middle ear (you should be able to confirm or eliminate the outer ear through otoscopy). On the other hand, if the results indicate that air conduction and bone conduction thresholds are exactly the same, we can assume that the problem is at the cochlea, nerve, or even in the brain. In Chapter 9 we will discuss some of the conditions that may lead to disorders of the outer, middle, and inner ear.

The Audiogram

The audiogram tells us the threshold of hearing for a series of frequencies we present to the patient during a routine hearing test. Threshold is a measure of sensitivity and corresponds to the softest sound a person hears half the time it is presented. The audiogram and its symbols have been around for decades. Instead of spending time on their origins, let's just say that most symbols on the audiogram are internation-

ally recognized to stand for *something*. An audiogram should have a key on it describing what each symbol represents. Over the years, several different types of forms and symbols have been used. For example, we happen to prefer to put the right and left ear results on different audiograms displayed side by side, as we find this easier to interpret and less messy. Some put the right and left ear plots on the same chart. Others simply write the thresholds in rows—no graphing, symbols, or audiograms at all.

But, like most things, it's usually best to go along with some type of consensus. We have that for audiometric symbols, and they are shown in Figure 2–1. This chart of standard symbols is from the American Speech-Language-Hearing Association (ASHA).

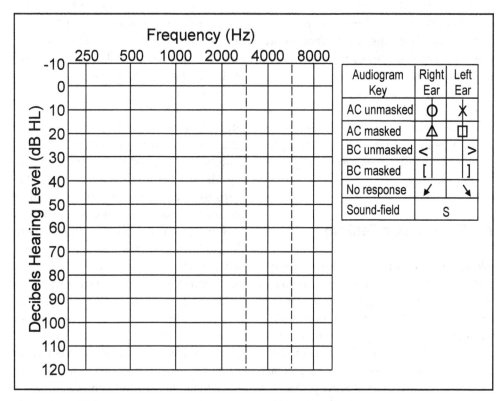

Figure 2–1. The standard audiogram and symbols for air and bone conduction testing. *Source*: From *Audiology: Science to Practice* (3rd ed., p. 130), by S. Kramer and D. K. Brown, 2019, San Diego, CA: Plural Publishing. Reprinted with permission.

> ### *TAKE FIVE: Anecdote About the Audiogram and Symbols*
>
> The audiogram is as old and established as dirt, so there are, of course, a lot of tales about it. Normally, the discussion centers on why it's upside down. Audiologists might be the only people in the world who believe that on a chart, big numbers should go on the bottom and small numbers should go on the top. Here's a little tale that you might like: We know of an audiologist who was given an official "letter of reprimand" (from her boss, "the ENT Doctor") because she refused to graph the audiogram with a red pen for the right ear and a blue pen for the left ear; she did them both in black. Hopefully she has found a new job! Okay—here is one more: Have you ever seen an audiogram where the air conduction and bone conduction thresholds were exactly the same for both ears? We have. Many times. In theory, this should happen when the loss is cochlear. But what is the probability of this *really happening* for 500 Hz, 1000 Hz, 2000 Hz, and 4000 Hz for both ears? We got the answer to this question from audiologist Bob Margolis, who apparently had time one day to do some calculations. His findings were that it would happen in once in every 250,000 patients. In practical terms, if a clinical audiologist saw 10 patients a day, it would happen every 104 years.

The "Normal" Audiogram

Let's get started with a normal audiogram, shown in Figure 2–2. You will notice on this audiogram that the *O* denotes the right ear and the *X* represents the left ear. We have handwritten the symbols on the audiogram to add an element of realism, even though we know many clinicians now record perfect *X*s and *O*s with the aid of their computerized audiometer. As mentioned earlier, historically, the right ear is displayed in red and the left ear is displayed in blue, although if a person cannot tell the difference between a black *O* and *X*, we might question if they really are qualified to interpret an audiogram in the first place (see our "Take Five" on this topic). These two symbols, regardless of color, are what we use for plotting air conducted sounds. The other thing you should notice is that in this case, all the symbols are at the top of the audiogram, between 0 dB HL and 20 dB HL. If the symbols representing the left and right ear are between 0 dB and 20 dB, the hearing thresholds are considered normal, although whether the cut-off for "normal" should be 15 dB or 20 dB is debatable. We do know that if someone who has had thresholds of 0 dB wakes up one morning with thresholds of 20 dB, they will *not* consider their hearing "normal." Figure 2–3 provides the commonly accepted classification of degree of hearing loss, although since most hearing loss is downward sloping, for a given patient, the loss might be mild in the low frequencies, moderate in the mid-frequencies, and severe in the high frequencies.

Notice on Figure 2–2 that there are six *X*s and *O*s plotted on the audiogram. For simplicity in this example, we have used only six key frequencies. In most cases,

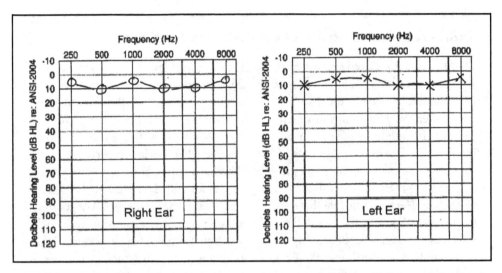

Figure 2–2. An example of normal hearing recorded on the audiogram. Note how all the thresholds for both ears are between 0 and 20 dB HL in this example. *Source*: From *Fitting and Dispensing Hearing Aids* (2nd ed., p. 99), by B. Taylor and H. G. Mueller, 2017, San Diego, CA: Plural Publishing. Reprinted with permission.

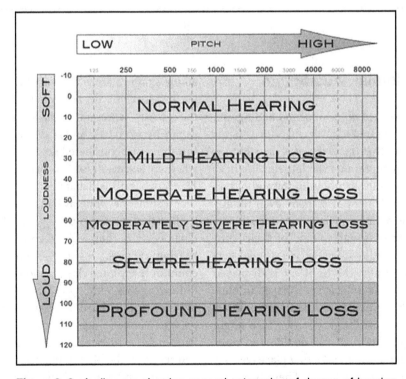

Figure 2–3. Audiogram showing general categories of degree of hearing loss. There is no "standard" for these categories, and they may vary by 5 dB to 10 dB based on different data sets. For example, some have suggested that 15 dB should be used as the cutoff for normal hearing.

however, the audiologist will also want to do testing at other frequencies. For example, thresholds at 1500 Hz, 3000 Hz, and 6000 Hz often are helpful in the programming of hearing aids and patient counseling.

The next set of essential symbols represents the threshold for bone conducted sounds. These should be normal for people with hearing loss confined to the middle or outer ear who have normal inner ear thresholds. In the example in Figure 2–4, the patient has a conductive hearing loss in both ears. This patient was a 5-year-old with bilateral middle ear effusion. Notice now how the air conduction symbols are around 30 to 40 dB, but the bone conduction symbols are around 5 to 10 dB, causing a "gap" between the two symbols. This is referred to as the air-bone gap: a telltale sign of a conductive hearing loss, typically involving the middle ear.

There are two broad classifications of audiogram shapes: flat and sloping. A sloping audiogram means the degree of hear-ing loss is much greater in one frequency region than another, highs versus lows. Typically, the hearing loss is greater in the high frequencies compared to the lows. Figure 2–5 is an example of downward slop-ing (high frequency) hearing loss. Notice that as the frequency becomes higher, more sound pressure (intensity) is needed to reach threshold—this is a common audio-gram type observed in most clinics, as it is the signature of presbyacusis. On the other hand, a "flat" hearing loss means that all the thresholds fall around the same inten-sity level. From a diagnostic standpoint, we rarely see a flat hearing loss that is either noise-induced or presbyacusis, so we are more apt to suspect some other pathology.

Now that we are on the subject of shapes, it's a good time to mention some other impor-tant shapes and terms that are commonly used:

▪ Symmetric hearing loss: Hearing loss is similar in both ears (usually 10 to 15 dB at all frequencies).

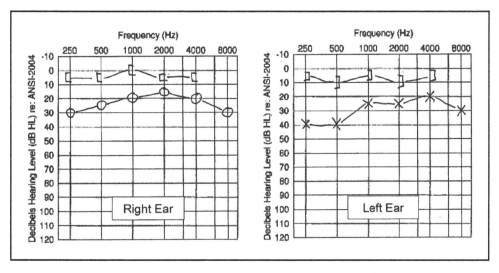

Figure 2–4. Mild conductive hearing loss in both ears. Note the difference between the air conduction and the bone conduction thresholds. This is a typical audiogram observed for a child with middle ear effusion. *Source*: From *Fitting and Dispensing Hearing Aids* (2nd ed., p. 100), by B. Taylor and H. G. Mueller, 2017, San Diego, CA: Plural Publishing. Reprinted with permission.

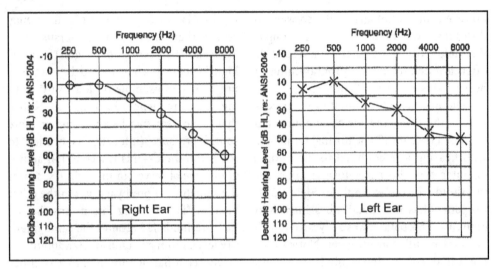

Figure 2–5. Mild sloping high-frequency hearing loss in both ears. This is a very typical pattern observed with presbycusis, and a common hearing loss of an individual fitted with bilateral hearing aids. *Source*: From *Fitting and Dispensing Hearing Aids* (2nd ed., p. 101), by B. Taylor and H. G. Mueller, 2017, San Diego, CA: Plural Publishing. Reprinted with permission.

- Asymmetric hearing loss: One ear is significantly different than another (usually 20 dB or more) for a range of frequencies. Pay attention to these, as most "routine" patients will have a symmetrical loss.

- Flat: Relatively equal hearing loss (within 20 dB or so) across frequencies 500 Hz to 4000 Hz.

- Gradually sloping: Hearing loss becomes progressively, but gradually, worse as the frequencies become higher.

- Presbycusic: General pattern of a gradually downward-sloping hearing loss, observed in older individuals.

- Precipitously sloping (ski slope): Hearing loss becomes rapidly worse as frequencies become higher (e.g., change of 20 dB per octave).

- Reverse slope: Significant hearing loss in lower frequencies with hearing loss becoming better (or normal) in higher frequencies.

- Noise notch: Normal or relatively normal hearing in the low and midrange, with a hearing loss in the 3000 Hz to 6000 Hz range, and then improved thresholds for 8000 Hz.

- Cookie-bite: Normal or near-normal hearing in the low frequencies, a significant loss in the 1000 Hz to 4000 Hz range, then returning to normal or near-normal in the high frequencies (when plotted, gives the appearance that a "bite" has been taken out of normal hearing).

- Reverse cookie-bite: Significant loss in low frequencies and high frequencies, but normal or near-normal hearing in the mid-frequencies.

- Corner audiogram: Hearing loss in the very low frequencies, with no measurable hearing in the higher frequencies (the entire audiogram is plotted in the "lower-left corner" of the audiogram).

The air conduction pure-tone thresholds tell you how *much* hearing loss a person has. In simple terms, the amount of hearing loss is the difference (in dB) between 0 dB HL (average hearing level for people with excellent hearing) and the patient's threshold at each frequency. As we mentioned earlier, in order to communicate the amount of hearing loss to other professionals and to the patient, there are general categories that are used (see Figure 2–3). The average air conduction hearing loss for the speech frequencies is usually calculated using the three-frequency pure-tone average (PTA). You can calculate the PTA by adding the thresholds obtained at 500 Hz, 1000 Hz, and 2000 Hz then divide the sum by 3. This is the PTA for each ear. In some cases, we use the PTA and the degree of hearing loss chart to summarize the amount of hearing loss for each ear. In downward sloping hearing losses, which are what we commonly see when fitting hearing aids, it has been suggested that a better indication of the patient's amplification needs is represented with a high-frequency PTA (HF-PTA). For the HF-PTA we use the average of the frequencies of 1000 Hz, 2000 Hz, and 4000 Hz. Consider a patient who has thresholds of 5 dB at 500 Hz, 15 dB at 1000 Hz, 40 dB at 2000 Hz, and 70 dB at 4000 Hz. This is a very common hearing loss that is routinely fitted with hearing aids. If we simply take the PTA, which is 20 dB, it gives the impression that we are fitting hearing aids to someone with near-normal hearing, when in fact, this patient's HF-PTA is 42 dB.

While the audiologic battery keeps expanding and dozens of tests have been developed since the time that pure-tone thresholds were first used, these basic threshold measures are still the cornerstone of the hearing aid fitting. As we'll discuss in Chapter 4, pure-tone thresholds are used to program today's digital products, as algorithms exist that predict the necessary gain for soft, average, and loud speech based on these values. Once the thresholds have been entered, with a simple mouse click the hearing aids are programmed. For verification purposes, these same thresholds are converted to ear

---

KEY CONCEPT: Mild Losses and Hearing Aids

A common question, even among audiologists, is how bad does a hearing loss have to be before hearing aids are needed? There is no simple answer—a quick calculation of the patient's unaided speech intelligibility index (SII) helps a little, but does not provide a definite answer; we'll talk more about that in Chapter 4 when we introduce the count-the-dots audiogram. In general, we want to look at the audibility of speech, including soft speech, for the important speech frequencies (Reminder: soft speech is around 20 to 25 dB HL). Because most hearing losses are downward sloping, we often are looking at the degree of hearing loss in the 2000 Hz to 4000 Hz range for marginal candidates. Do we fit hearing aids to someone with normal hearing through 2000 Hz? Probably. With normal hearing through 3000 Hz? Maybe, but usually not. For these marginal cases, the patient's perceived handicap, measured speech recognition in background noise, and his or her listening needs play a big role in the decision-making process. This may have an even larger impact for children who are developing speech and language, where audibility of soft speech can be critical.

THINGS TO REMEMBER: Masking Is Not Just for Halloween Anymore!

When viewing an audiogram or when reading an audiologic report, it's possible that you will see reference to "masking." In the world of audiometry, masking is defined as the condition in which one sound (some type of noise) is introduced into one ear while measuring the threshold (or speech recognition) of the other ear. When conducting a hearing test, it is important to test each ear independently—when a threshold is noted for the right ear, it is critical to ensure that indeed it was the right ear, not the left ear that was responding. When sound reaches a certain intensity level, it will "cross over" to the opposite ear. For air conduction testing (either pure tones or speech), this usually happens when the difference between ears is 50 dB to 60 dB (assuming that insert earphones are used—the values are smaller for supra-aural earphones). Given that most hearing losses are relatively symmetrical, masking does not come into play too often for air conduction testing. For bone conduction measures, however, the "crossover" point is at or near 0 dB (because the entire skull is in vibration regardless if the bone oscillator is placed behind the right or left ear). Masking, therefore, is nearly always needed.

If you are viewing an audiogram from an audiologist, you can assume that they knew what they were doing and used effective masking. The concept of masking, however, is often not well understood by audiometric technicians and others conducting hearing testing (e.g., hearing instrument specialists), so you might view these audiograms a little more suspiciously if there is asymmetry and the thresholds don't seem quite right.

---

canal SPL, and through real-ear measures, hearing aid output is measured to ensure the ear canal values agree with prescribed values.

Hearing Screening: School-Age Children

As early as 1924, a recently invented instrument called an "audiometer" was suggested for use in testing school-age children. The procedure has been in place ever since. We will discuss in depth how you can set up a screening in Chapter 9 as it's unusual for this testing to be conducted by an audiologist and usually the testing is by technicians and volunteers overseen by an audiologist or speech-pathologist. In some facilities, however, speech-language pathologists also become involved, simply because of their proximity and their knowledge of audiometry. ASHA Guidelines for audiometric screening call for this testing to be conducted on initial entry into school and annually in kindergarten, first, second, and third grade; then screened again in 7th and 11th grades.

Pure-tone screening is the method of choice. Manual testing under earphones should be conducted for each ear at test frequencies of 1000 Hz, 2000 Hz, and 4000 Hz at a level of 20 dB. While a lower level (e.g., 15 dB) may be even a better for identifying mild hearing loss, ambient noise in most locations prevents testing at that level. Also, it is because of the ever-present ambient noise that 500 Hz is not included as a test frequency. Allowable ambient noise should not exceed the following: 49.5 dB SPL at 1000 Hz, 54.5 dB SPL at 2000 Hz, and 62 dB SPL at 4000 Hz.

A lack of response from the child for any frequency in either ear constitutes failure of the screening, and follow-up screening should be conducted. If the child also fails on retest, they should be referred to an audiologist for a complete diagnostic evaluation. The basic test protocol is as follows:

- Instruct the child regarding the task. They may be asked to raise their hand, or push a button whenever they hear the "beep," even if it is very soft. This is a task that even kindergarten children should be able to perform successfully.
- Place the earphones on the ears—ensure that they are centered.
- To ensure the child understands the task, present a tone of 40 dB at 1000 Hz in both the right and left ear.
- Decrease the dial setting to 20 dB, and present tones at each screening frequency in each ear. If reliability is in question (some children are anxious and give false-positive responses), two credible responses at the same frequency would indicate good reliability.

- Any child who does not hear each tone in each ear should be identified for repeat testing.
- The entire screening process should not take more than 1 to 2 min.

With any type of testing, there are potential pitfalls. The following is a list of some of the pitfalls for hearing screening.

- Observing you pushing the buttons or changing the dials. The child may respond to the visual cues. To correct this, you would want to seat the child at an angle so the tester and audiometer are out of their visual field.
- You giving visual cues through your facial expressions, looking up and down with presentations, or other eye or head movement.
- Headband or earphone is not placed correctly. Make sure that the earphone is placed so that the output of the sound is directly over the ear canal.
- Not clear instructions.
- Distractions or noise in the testing area.

Speech Audiometry

Speech audiometry has a long history related to fitting hearing aids. Several decades ago, speech audiometry was developed as a diagnostic tool (e.g., middle ear vs. cochlea vs. 8th nerve). Today, to a limited extent, that is still the primary purpose for conducting speech audiometry; however, it also can be part of the prefitting hearing aid assessment and counseling for appropriate expectations. Although there are dozens of speech tests to choose from that can be conducted in quiet or in noisy conditions, our focus here simply will be a quick review of the two most basic speech audiometry procedures:

speech recognition threshold and word recognition testing.

Speech Recognition Threshold (SRT)

The main purpose of the speech recognition threshold (SRT), sometimes called the speech reception threshold, procedure is to check the reliability of the pure-tone thresholds. The SRT should be within +/−10 dB of the average of the pure-tone thresholds at 500 Hz, 1000 Hz, and 2000 Hz for each ear, or for a precipitous downward sloping hearing loss, within +/−10 dB of the 500 Hz and 1000 Hz average. The stimuli used for SRT testing are spondees, which are two-syllable words that have equal stress on both syllables (e.g., baseball, cowboy, hotdog, sidewalk, etc.).

The SRT is often the first test of the audiologic battery. When it is completed first, there is no bias in the testing, which can occur if pure-tone thresholds are already known, and it can be used as a reliability check, as described earlier. Speech can be delivered using recorded material or by monitored live voice (MLV). MLV is the process of reading the words using a microphone with careful visual attention paid to the volume units (VU) meter of the audiometer. Recorded speech is the preferred method for more reliable results. However, particularly for children, those with cognitive problems, or poor understanding, MLV may be used.

Related to the fitting of hearing aids, the SRT has little use. As mentioned earlier, most hearing losses are downward sloping and, therefore, the SRT (which depends heavily on hearing in the low frequencies) provides little information regarding the amount of gain or output needed by the patient. As you view audiograms, however,

it's probable that you will see that most audiologists do complete the SRT. We're not sure exactly why, but one reason probably is simply out of habit, and it's part of most billing codes. As we stated earlier, the SRT should agree with the PTA, so if there is a case where it is suspected that a patient is exaggerating his or her hearing loss, the SRT serves as a good cross-check.

Word Recognition Tests

Word recognition (WR) testing is the first suprathreshold test in the audiometric evaluation. Suprathreshold means the test is conducted at an intensity level above threshold. It is typically performed at a presentation level that is somewhat louder than "comfortable" (or slightly "loud, but okay") to the patient—it's important to maximize audibility, which usually doesn't happen at the patient's MCL. The purpose of the WR testing is to evaluate an individual's ability to recognize single-syllable words from a phonetically balanced (PB) word list. The testing is sometimes casually referred to as a "PB" score, or incorrectly as "discrimination." (See associated Things to Remember box on this topic.)

Importance of Presentation Level

The purpose of the word recognition test is to assess cochlear function—that is, how good does it get when the signal is loud enough—this is commonly referred to as PB-Max. In no way is this intended to represent how a person understands in their daily environment. That is not the purpose of the test. We know that in most cases, they will do worse in everyday listening, as people do not talk as loud as the level that the test is conducted

---

THINGS TO REMEMBER: It's Not a Discrimination Task

In the "old days" (1950s to 1980s), it was common for audiologists to call word recognition testing speech discrimination testing, and simply refer to the outcome as a "discrim score." Fortunately, to keep us from continuing to embarrass ourselves, some wise opinion leaders, led by Fred Bess we believe, pointed out that what we were doing was certainly not a discrimination task. A discrimination task would require some sort of word differentiation, something to discrimi-nate (e.g., beer vs. deer). What we were doing clearly was word recognition. Today, hearing an audiologist call word recognition "discrim" is like fingernails on a chalkboard for some of us—akin to someone calling flip-flops, thongs. If some of you younger readers have not heard the sound of fingernails on a chalkboard, check it out: https://tinyurl.com/chalkboardnails. By the way, most all extremely annoying sounds are in the frequency range of 2000 Hz to 5000 Hz.

(e.g., common presentation levels for WR testing are 75 to 80 dB HL). Moreover, listening to monosyllables, under earphones, in quiet, in a test booth does not correlate well with any real-world listening experience that we are aware of. To state the obvious, it is therefore critical that WR testing be conducted at a level in which the words are loud enough to be audible. If possible, audible in the higher frequencies (e.g., 2000 to 3000 Hz), as many of the words contain high-frequency consonants. We state this because when you are viewing an audiogram and see a score that is unusually low, it is important to see if the testing was conducted at a loud enough level (usually the presentation level is indicated on the audiogram). An incorrect procedure that shows up now and then is adding 40 dB to the SRT to determine the presentation level. If you see an audiogram and the audiologist actually notes that WR testing was conducted +40 above the SRT, interpret the percentages recorded with considerable skepticism.

Importance of Recorded Lists

There are several different monosyllabic words lists, often named after the laboratory where they were developed. The lists are similar, but slightly different WR scores will result. Most audiologists use the Northwestern University List #6 (NU-6), which by far is the most researched. While we once used records, then cassettes, then CDs, today these word lists are available as electronic files that can be added to a computer-based audiometer. It is important to point out that it is not only the list that is important, but who recorded the list. The list which has the most research support is the Auditec of St. Louis recording. Different recordings of the same list can result in differences in scores of 20% or greater. Remember this adage: *"The words are not the test—the test is the test."*

This is why all best practice documents state that WR testing must be conducted using standardized recorded material, although it is possible to conduct the test with the audiologist using live voice. Would any audiologist violate best practice and conduct the testing live voice? Unfortunately, yes! If you see an audiogram and the audiologist actually notes that WR testing was conducted live voice, interpret the percentages recorded with considerable skepticism (typically, live voice scores are better than the patient's true scores, sometimes by 30% to 40%).

Importance of Using Full List

Also related to the validity of the WR scores, standard word lists are 50 words in length, and all best practice guidelines state that 50 words are presented to each ear for each patient (with a value of 2% per correct word). Unfortunately, sometimes examiners "feel the need for speed" and only use 25 words. The latter is referred to as using a "half-list." Although using a half-list does save a little time, accuracy is sacrificed. The words differ in difficulty, and because the lists were not intended to be halved, the most difficult words may not be equally distributed between the first and second half. On one list, for example, of the ten most difficult words, eight of them are on the second half of the list. The full 50-word lists always should be used. If you see an audiogram and the audiologist actually notes that they took a shortcut and only used half of the list, interpret the percentages recorded with considerable skepticism.

10-Word List for Screening Purposes. This is going to sound like we are contradicting what we just said in the previous paragraph, but stick with us. There are times when a 10-word list is just fine. There are special recordings of the 50-word NU-6 words lists that have the 10 most difficult words presented first. Research has shown that if a patient gets 10 out of 10 or 9 out of 10

of these words correct, there is a 95% probability that if we gave them all 50 words, they would score 96% or better; and therefore, there is no reason to deliver all 50 words. Now, of course most patients do not score 10/10 or 9/10, but when they do (usually someone with normal hearing), this saves a little test time for the audiologist. More and more, audiologists are using the "ordered-by-difficulty" list, so you might start seeing some 10-word list results on audiograms. The exact score isn't known, but really, who cares if it's 96%, 98%, or 100%?

Interpreting WR Test Scores

We typically report the WR score on the audiogram as a percent correct as well as giving a brief description of the degree of impairment. When talking to the patient or other professionals, it sometimes is helpful to use general terms to describe a percentage range. Table 2–1 gives some common categories used to describe the degree of impairment for a given percent score. These are only general guidelines—you may see somewhat different ranges published elsewhere, as there is no standard for these classifications. For example, we would consider the "good" category to extend too low (recall that this testing is conducted at a loud level). When we see patients with word recognition of 80%, neither the patient nor us typically thinks of this as "good." But, the chart does provide some general guidance.

One of the common questions associated with WR testing is, "When is a difference really a difference?" In other words, when you are viewing an audiogram that shows a patient has a score of 72% in the right ear and 56% in the left ear, is speech understanding really better in the right ear, or does it simply reflect normal variability between scores. We have the answer—something called the binomial distribution

Table 2–1. Commonly Used Categories to Summarize Word Recognition Scores, and the Degree of Impairment That Often Is Associated with This Word Recognition Performance

WRS (% Correct)	Degree of Impairment	Word Recognition Ability
100–90	None	Excellent/Normal
89–75	Slight	Good
74–60	Moderate	Fair
59–50	Poor	Poor
<50	Very Poor	Very Poor

Source: From *Audiology: Science to Practice* (3rd ed., p. 168), by S. Kramer and D. K. Brown, 2019, San Diego, CA: Plural Publishing. Reprinted with permission.

is a statistically derived table of probabilities that is used to determine a real difference from normal variability.

The variability in WR testing that is significant decreases as the number of words increases. Therefore, a 50-word list has less variability than a 25-word list, yet another reason why a 50-word list always should

be used. Using Table 2–2, you can take the scores that you are viewing from the right and left ears, or compare different scores for the same ear from tests in the past, to see if there is a critical (real) difference.

Using Table 2–2 to see if a difference really is a difference is fairly simple. Just take the lower of the two scores you are comparing

---

CASE STUDY: Real Difference or Not?

Here is a little case study related to the binomial model data—see Table 2–2. You are working with a teenager with a bilateral hearing loss, who wears hearing aids. He tells you that he doesn't think he is doing as well in his left ear as he was doing in the past. This could be a function of the left hearing aid, or maybe he actually has had a change in his speech recognition ability. Fortunately, he goes in for annual audiologic testing. You see that when he was tested a year ago, his PB-Max was 84% in his left ear. He was tested again a few weeks ago, and now his score is 62%. Is this significantly worse than 84%? Let's find out. Go to Table 2–2

and locate 62% (it was the lower of the two scores). Now, move over three columns to the right to the "50" column (that's the number of words used for the testing). Notice that the number is 80%. Was the score from a year ago larger than 80%? Yes, it was! This means that the two scores are indeed significantly different, and you know it's probably not an issue with the left hearing aid. Pretty simple, huh? Observe, however, that if the audiologist doing the testing had been looking for a shortcut and only conducted 25 words, now these two values are no longer different (see the "25 word" column, where the value is 87%)

Table 2–2. Critical Difference Values for Monosyllabic Words Based On the Binomial Distribution (95% Confidence)

95% Confidence		**Number of Items (phoneme scoring = 2.5 number of words)**									
		10	25	50	63			10	25	50	63
The lower	0	33	15	8	6	The lower	50	91	77	70	68
of the two	1	36	17	10	9	of the two	51	91	78	71	68
scores being	2	38	20	12	11	scores being	52	92	79	71	69
compared	3	40	22	14	13	compared	53	93	80	72	70
(in %)	4	41	23	16	14	(in %)	54	93	81	73	71
	5	43	25	18	16		55	94	81	74	72
	6	45	27	19	17		56	95	82	75	73
	7	47	29	21	19		57	95	83	76	74
	8	48	30	22	20		58	96	84	77	75
	9	50	32	24	22		59	96	84	78	76
	10	51	33	25	23		60	97	85	78	77
	11	53	35	27	25		61	97	86	79	77
	12	54	36	28	26		62	98	87	80	78
	13	55	38	29	27		63	98	87	81	79
	14	57	39	31	29		64	99	88	82	80
	15	58	40	32	30		65	99	89	83	81
	16	59	42	33	31		66	100	90	83	82
	17	61	43	34	32		67	100	90	84	82
	18	62	44	36	34		68	100	91	85	83
	19	63	45	37	35		69	100	92	86	84
	20	64	47	38	36		70	100	92	87	85
	21	65	48	39	37		71	100	93	87	86
	22	66	49	41	38		72	100	93	88	86
	23	68	50	42	40		73	100	94	89	87
	24	69	51	43	41		74	100	95	89	88
	25	70	53	44	42		75	100	95	90	89
	26	71	54	45	43		76	100	96	91	89
	27	72	55	46	44		77	100	96	92	90
	28	73	56	47	45		78	100	97	92	91
	29	74	57	48	46		79	100	97	93	92
	30	75	58	50	47		80	100	98	94	92
	31	76	59	51	48		81	100	98	94	93
	32	77	60	52	50		82	100	99	95	94
	33	77	61	53	51		83	100	99	95	94
	34	78	62	54	52		84	100	100	96	95
	35	79	63	55	53		85	100	100	97	96
	36	80	64	56	54		86	100	100	97	96
	37	81	65	57	55		87	100	100	98	97
	38	82	66	58	56		88	100	100	98	97
	39	83	67	59	57		89	100	100	99	98
	40	83	68	60	58		90	100	100	99	98
	41	84	69	61	59		91	100	100	100	99
	42	85	70	62	60		92	100	100	100	99
	43	86	71	63	61		93	100	100	100	100
	44	87	72	64	62		94	100	100	100	100
	45	87	73	65	63		95	100	100	100	100
	46	88	74	66	64		96	100	100	100	100
	47	89	75	67	65		97	100	100	100	100
	48	89	75	68	66		98	100	100	100	100
	49	90	76	69	67		99	100	100	100	100

Note. To obtain the upper critical value, determine where the lower of the two word recognition scores (row) intersects with the number of words used in the testing (column).

Source: Courtesy of Arthur Boothroyd and Carol Mackersie. From *Audiology: Science to practice* (3rd ed., p. 170), by S. Kramer and D. K. Brown, 2019, San Diego, CA: Plural Publishing. Reprinted with permission

and find it on the chart. (Hint: it's a number between 0 and 100.) Next, look under one of the four columns (10, 25, 50, or 63) that designates the number of words used in the testing (note: 63 is for phoneme scoring, which is rarely conducted). For example, if a 50-word list was used and the lower of the two scores is 52%, the other score has to be greater than 71% for the difference to be significant. When scores exceed the critical difference and it's not explained by the audiogram (e.g., the thresholds of one ear are significantly worse than the other), it's a "red flag" for a possible medical problem causing the low score, and a medical referral is probably warranted.

Immittance Battery

The immittance battery is considered a part of the routine audiologic examination by most audiologists. While this is not directly related to the fitting of hearing aids, the results could impact some of the fitting decisions. It's common that you will see immittance results in a report or charted on an audiogram, so we'll briefly review some of the components. Immittance testing usually involves three separate measures: tympanometry, equivalent volume, and the acoustic reflex.

Tympanometry

Tympanometry is the best know component of immittance audiometry. There are many different tympanometry screeners on the market, which are easy use, and even conduct an interpretation for the examiner. Because of this, you will find pediatricians, nurses, and, yes, even speech-language pathologists conducting screening tympanograms. The tympanogram measures how the admittance (impedance) of the middle ear system changes as a function of different amounts of applied air pressure. To obtain this measure, a probe is placed in the ear with an airtight seal. Within the probe are three small tubes which have the function to a) change pressure, b) present a continuous low-frequency probe tone, and c) assess the changes of the probe tone as it is reflected by the TM as the pressure within the ear canal is altered via a microphone.

KEY CONCEPT: Immittance, Impedance, or Admittance?

The first immittance units introduced in the early 1970s recorded tympanograms using impedance values. The test itself soon became known as "impedance audiometry." It was only a year or two later, however, when other equipment was introduced that didn't measure impedance; rather, it measured the opposite—admittance. When you were using this equipment, you were not doing impedance audiometry, but admittance audiometry. As you might guess, this led to considerable confusion, especially in clinics that had both types of equipment. In the later 1970s a group of wise audiologists suggested that we pull out the electrical engineering term "immittance," coined in 1945. Immittance is the preferred term when something can be expressed in either impedance or admittance. Immittance does not have units, as it applies to both of the other measures, which have different units. And so, immittance it is!

Commonly, the pressure is changed from +200 daPa to –300 daPa.

For a normal TM and middle ear, we would expect the admittance of the system to be the highest at or around 0 daPa, and then become worse when pressure is applied on the TM (+200 daPa) or when a negative pressure is applied (–300 daPa). Today's equipment adjusts the absolute values obtained to an adjusted scale, which makes it much easier for all of us to interpret the findings. A commonly used adjusted scale goes from 0.0 to 2.5. This scale then also allows us to observe the amplitude change from +200 (calibrated to 0.0) to the maximum peak of the tympanogram, which we'd like to see around 0 daPa at an amplitude of .5 to 1.5 (this may vary for different equip-ment, and usually is indicated on the tympanogram form).

For the normal TM and middle ear, we would expect a peak around 1.0 to 1.5 occurring around 0 daPa. An example of this is shown in Figure 2–6. This is often referred to as a Type A tympanogram (A = good, and it looks sort of like an A; easy to remember). If the patient has negative middle ear pressure (but little or no middle ear effusion), there will still be a peak, but it will occur when negative pressure is placed in the ear canal (pulling the TM back to its normal position). The peak could be at –50 to –100, or as negative as –300 daPa with more severe retraction. This is a Type C tympanogram. If significant middle ear effusion is present, or some other form of otitus

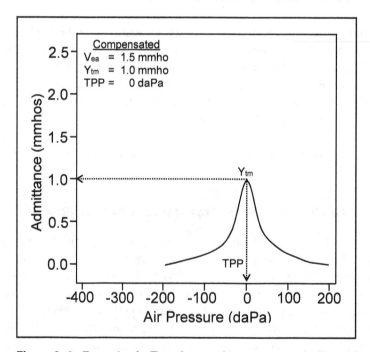

Figure 2–6. Example of a Type A normal tympanogram (calibrated to 0.0 mmhos for the +200 daPa for display purposes). The air pressure where the tympanogram peak occurs is referred to as the "tympanometric peak pressure." *Source*: From *Audiology: Science to Practice* (3rd ed., p. 218), by S. Kramer and D. K. Brown, 2019, San Diego, CA: Plural Publishing. Reprinted with permission.

media, there is little change from +200 to −300, and the tympanogram will be more or less "flat." This is referred to as a Type B tympanogram. There also are a couple other types of tympanograms, observed less often, and they are displayed in Figure 2–7.

The following is a summary of the different tympanogram types (see Figures 2–6 and 2–7 to observe associated shape).

▦ Type A: Expected finding for normal TM and middle ear.
▦ Type B: Commonly seenw with middle ear effusion or other types of otitis media, which has restricted the mobility of the middle ear system. Note: this also is the pattern observed when the probe is not placed correctly and is against the canal wall.

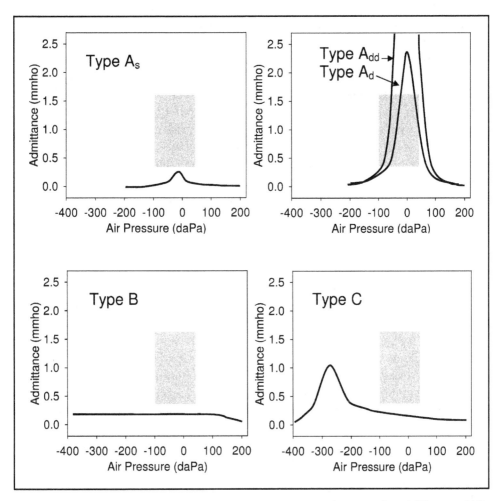

Figure 2–7. Example of four different tympanogram types, each suggestive of different middle ear pathologies. See text for description of the types. *Source*: From *Audiology: Science to Practice* (3rd ed., p. 222), by S. Kramer and D. K. Brown, 2019, San Diego, CA: Plural Publishing. Reprinted with permission.

CLINICAL TIP: Flat Can Be Good Too!

Pediatricians, parents, and patients are not experts on interpreting tympanograms, nor should they be, but the one thing most of them do know is that "flat is bad." But flat isn't always bad. Consider a young kid with pressure equalizing (PE) tubes and an audiologist conducting immittance to obtain the equivalent volume—a good test to determine if the tube is open. The expected finding is that you would have a flat tympanogram, as the open tube prevents there being a positive or negative pressure on the TM and therefore the admittance doesn't change as function of air pressure. So "flat" would be the expected finding for an open tube, which should be confirmed with a larger-than-average equivalent volume. In this case, flat is good!

Now, one might ask, why was the audiologist even doing a tympanogram if there was a tube in place? The test outcome would be obvious (flat if the tube was open, also flat if the tube was closed). There are a couple reasons why. First, with today's automated systems, the tympanogram simply might be automatically measured as part of the equivalent volume assessment. But there is a better reason. Sometimes, to the unsophisticated eye looking through the otoscope, a PE tube that is lying in the ear canal looks very much like a PE tube that is inserted in the TM. If it really is lying in the canal, you just might obtain a Type A tympanogram—a rather important (pleasant) finding!

- Type C: Observed when there is a retracted TM (usually because of poor Eustachian tube function). In untreated cases, the Type C often gradually becomes a Type B, as fluid is collected in the middle ear cavity.
- Type A_S: Reduced amplitude usually caused by a middle ear condition—often associated with early otosclerosis. S = "shallow" or "stiffness."
- Type A_D: Increased amplitude due to a hyper-mobile system. Most often associated with a disarticulation of the ossicular chain, but also can be seen with TM conditions (e.g., monomeric membrane). D = "deep" or "disarticulation."

Equivalent Volume Measures

Most immittance systems automatically provide an equivalent volume measure when the airtight seal is obtained. It is estimated from the +200 daPa, and for adults (10 years and older), normal values are from around 0.80 cc to 2.20 cc. As you would expect, the normative values are considerably smaller for young children—for example, 0.60 cc to 1.20 cc for children 18 months to 10 years. The equivalent volume can be handy to check for different conditions, especially if it is larger than normal.

If equivalent volume is larger than normal, it is most likely due to

- TM perforation
- PE tube in place, and it is open

If the equivalent volume is smaller than normal, it is most likely due to

- Impacted cerumen (or other foreign object in canal)
- Probe assembly pushed against canal wall

The most common use of the equivalent volume measure is to monitor the "openness" of PE tubes. You probably have worked with children who have PE tubes in place—for the middle ear condition to resolve, it is important for the tubes to stay open. While a skilled otolaryngologist can probably discern this using an operating microscope, it also is very obvious using the equivalent volume measure. If the equivalent volume for a 5-year-old is 2.0 cc, we can be quite certain that we are including the volume of the middle ear cavity, and not just the ear canal. As discussed earlier with hearing screening, tympanometry screening also has some pitfalls. We have listed a few common pitfalls for tympanometry screening:

- Clogged probe and probe tip. Routinely visually inspect the area to ensure that there is not any earwax.
- Using too large or too small of a probe tip. All people have a different shape and size of ear canal. You may need to try several different sizes or shapes to get the right seal and get an accurate reading.
- Child is moving too much; this includes head movement, swallowing, talking, and so forth.
- Probe tip is pressed against the ear canal wall. Try to go directly into the ear canal; when it is pressed against

the wall, you will not get an accurate reading.
- Debris in the ear canal. Look in the ear and make sure that there is nothing that could get stuck in the probe. Minimal wax is fine, a Barbie shoe is not.

Acoustic Reflex

The third component of the immittance battery is the measurement of the acoustic reflex (some simply call it the stapedial reflex, but the tensor tympani does play a small role). This test primarily is used to differentiate cochlea from retrocochlear pathology, but it also can be useful in determining the presence or extent of conductive pathology, and provides information regarding facial nerve function. The probe assembly is placed as it would be for tympanometry, and a loud signal is presented, usually 80 dB HL or louder. If the reflex contracts and the middle ear is normal, we then see a change in admittance (a stiffening). For individuals with normal hearing and normal middle ears, we expect this to happen around 75 dB HL to 95 dB HL. Acoustic reflex testing is normally conducted for the pure tones of 500 Hz, 1000 Hz, and 2000 Hz.

When observing or reading about acoustic reflex results in a report, note that there is a standardized method for reporting the findings—hopefully, this was used by your favorite audiologist:

- Right Contralateral: Stimulus in right ear, probe in left ear.
- Right Ipsilateral: Stimulus in right ear, probe in right ear.
- Left Contralateral: Stimulus in left ear, probe in right ear.
- Left Ipsilateral: Stimulus in left ear, probe in left ear.

If you see in a report that acoustic reflexes are absent, it could be for a variety of reasons. Here are a few examples:

- Conductive loss of 30 dB to 40 dB (stimulus ear)
- Cochlear hearing loss greater than 50 dB to 60 dB (stimulus ear)
- Nerve VIII pathology—hearing may be normal or near normal (stimulus ear)
- Low brain stem disorder (e.g., MS)—hearing may be normal or near normal (stimulus ear)
- Conductive loss causing an abnormal tympanogram (probe ear)
- Facial nerve pathology (e.g., Bell's palsy)—hearing may be normal (probe ear)

There are clinical cases, where for practical reasons, the audiologist may forego acoustic reflex testing. For example, if a child has a history of bilateral middle ear effusion and audiometry shows a bilateral conductive hearing loss, we know that the reflexes will be absent. It may not be worth the effort, for either the child or the audiologist, to conduct the measure. While acoustic reflexes do have a reasonably good sensitivity for detecting nerve VIII pathology, the test has become less relied on in recent years because of the common use of MRI whenever there is a hint of a retrocochlear pathology. There is, however, an increase is the use of acoustic reflex testing related to cochlear implants (see Chapter 7).

Otoacoustic Emissions

Otoacoustic emissions (OAEs) are considered to be related to the amplification function of the cochlea. In the absence of external stimulation, the activity of the cochlear

---

KEY CONCEPT: When Absent Isn't Really Absent!

As we discussed, in the immittance battery, a common procedure is the assessment of the acoustic reflex. When audiologists report these findings, terms such as present, elevated, and absent are commonly used. Let's take the example of a large nerve VIII tumor on the right side. It is very possible that because of the reduction of neural synchrony at the level of the cochlear nucleus, the acoustic reflex will be absent when the stimulus is presented to that ear (right contralateral and right ipsilateral test conditions). Makes sense. Now, let's take the example of severe serous otitis in the right ear. It is very likely (like 99%) that the reflex will be absent when the probe is in the right ear (left contralateral and right ipsilateral test conditions). The middle ear condition prevents movement of the TM, and hence, no reflex is recorded. But is the reflex really absent? Certainly not—there is nothing neurologically wrong with the acoustic reflex arch. This sort of thing often requires some explanation to a puzzled neurologist (and maybe speech-language pathologists too)—why do we record it as absent when it isn't absent? Because it helps with the diagnosis of middle ear pathology on the right side, and since we can't measure it, we don't really know if it's absent or not. But yes, it can be confusing.

DID YOU KNOW: The Predictions of Thomas Gold

In 1951, astrophysicist Thomas Gold proposed at a national meeting that recently detected radio signals originated from outside of the Milky Way Galaxy. A little far-fetched perhaps? How about this one—in May of 1960, Gold published a paper suggesting that the origins of life on earth were from a pile of waste products accidently dumped by extraterrestrials long ago. And here is another—in the late 1940s, he published papers suggesting that there is a mechanical resonator within the cochlea, which could actually cause the ear to produce sounds. Wait. There might be something to that one. While all of Gold's predictions may well be true, the last one we are quite certain about. The ear does indeed create its own sounds, and we call them otoacoustic emissions or OAEs. They were first described by David Kemp in 1978, clinically friendly equipment for their measurement became available in the late 1980s, and an OAE CPT code was established in 1995.

---

amplifier increases, leading to the production of sound. Research suggests that outer hair cells are the elements that enhance cochlear sensitivity and frequency selectivity, and act as the energy sources for amplification. These low-intensity acoustic signals can be measured in the ear canal. The emissions travel outward along the basilar membrane, through the middle ear, and vibrate the TM. The measurement of OAEs is efficient and fast, which has made it a popular clinical test; in fact, it is what is often used as a part of a newborn hearing screening.

These measures only indirectly relate to the selection and fitting of hearing aids. The primary connection is that this test is used for most newborn screening programs. Because of the relatively good sensitivity and specificity, the results of the testing can be used to determine who should be referred for further evaluation. There are many factors that can cause the OAE to be absent, so it's important to remember that this is just a screening test, and does not reveal the magnitude or etiology of the hearing problem.

OAEs also are used in many clinics, and you may see the results in reports for both children and adults. Dhar (2014b) wrote an excellent article summarizing what these findings might mean, and these are summarized in the following text:

If OAEs are present, you can be fairly certain that one or more of the following is true:

- The patient has no major middle ear pathology. There are reports of recordable OAEs with small perforations or mild pressure deviations from atmospheric pressure. However, it is improbable that OAEs will be recordable in full-blown cases of otitis media.
- The patient has a functional complement of outer hair cells.
- Because outer hair cell pathology is highly correlated with most common forms of hearing loss (e.g., noise induced or age related), it is safe to assume that the patient's hearing is most likely within the normal range.
- Using that same logic, it is also probably safe to assume that the patient will demonstrate normal frequency

discrimination or even speech perception ability in noise.

- However, present OAEs do not guarantee normal function of the entire auditory system. For example, auditory brain stem responses would be necessary to garner confidence that inner hair cell and auditory nerve function is normal in a patient.

If OAEs are absent, you can be fairly certain that one or more of the following is true:

- The patient has degradation of outer hair cell function.
- The patient may have a middle ear condition preventing the forward transmission of stimuli and the reverse transmission of the OAEs.
- The patient most likely has hearing thresholds worse than 20 dB HL.

Dhar (2014b) does go on to add:

> While it is fun to give you bullet points to create a decision tree, I would be remiss if I did not point out that conditions such as auditory neuropathy could yield perfectly normal OAEs and the disorder would not be diagnosed without the use of other tools that specifically target other parts of the auditory system. So the bottom line is that OAEs are an important part of an audiologist's test battery but cannot be used as the one test for all purposes.

This of course is true for all audiologic tests.

Auditory Brain Stem Response

Audiologists conduct a variety of electrophysiologic tests, but the most common is the auditory brain stem response (ABR)—sometimes referred to as BSER (brain stem evoked response) or BAER (brain stem auditory evoked response) by other specialties. The response is an indication of neural activity and synchrony of nerve VIII and the low brain stem. It occurs with a very short latency (within 10 ms) following the stimulation signal, which also must be of very short duration. The presentations typically are 11 to 41/s, with 1,500 to 2,000 presentations for a single measure. The signals typically are clicks or tone pips presented at a relatively loud level, unless a threshold search is being conducted.

The ABR is characterized by a series of six to seven peaks, which in general represent different neural centers of nerve VIIII and the brain stem. For clinical purposes, we only focus on the first five peaks, and for some testing, only Wave V, as it is the most robust. Some researchers have attempted to specifically relate the different peaks to neural structures—with the general conclusion of Wave I: nerve VIII (distal); Wave II: nerve VIII (proximal); Wave III: cochlear nucleus; Wave IV: superior olivary complex; and Wave V: lateral lemniscus and input to the inferior colliculus. The classic ABR for someone with normal hearing, obtained by presenting clicks at a relatively high input level, is shown in Figure 2–8.

At one time (1980s), the ABR was **THE** test used to detect retrocochlear disorders. Because of the frequent use of MRI, those days are gone, but the ABR still plays a very prominent role, and it is related to hearing aid fitting. When a hearing loss is expected and the patient is not able to provide reliable behavioral responses (usually because he or she is an infant or toddler), the ABR is an effective tool to estimate hearing thresholds. For these patients, tone-burst stimuli are used, and commonly the frequencies of 500 Hz, 1000 Hz, 2000 Hz, and 4000 Hz are

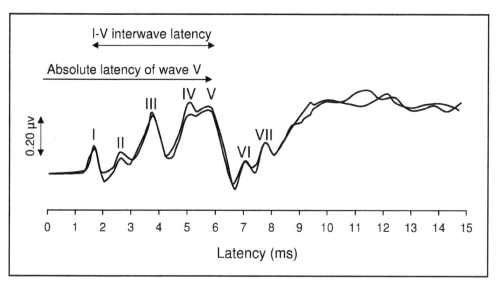

Figure 2–8. A normal ABR response (both amplitude and latency) to click stimuli delivered at a relatively high input level. The waves I to VII are labeled. Clinically, interest typically only is with waves I to V. Diagnostically, important measures are the latency of Wave V, and the I–V interwave difference. *Source*: From *Audiology: Science to Practice* (3rd ed., p. 253), by S. Kramer and D. K. Brown, 2019, San Diego, CA: Plural Publishing. Reprinted with permission.

DID YOU KNOW: For the Bumpologists

The individual usually credited with first describing the ABR is Don Jewett, who at the time was at the University of San Francisco. Interestingly, Jewett was not an audiologist, hearing scientist, or physiologist, but rather an orthopedic surgeon. Because of the five ABR peaks that he described in his classic article, audiologists soon began to call these notable responses "Jewett Bumps." The audiology pioneers conducting ABRs in these early years (ca. 1975) were a close knit group, and proudly referred to themselves as "Bumpologists." Most of the original clan of Bumpologists have now retired, but you still may see one or two at an ASHA convention.

---

tested. The most resilient Wave of the five is Wave V, and the input signal is lowered to the softest point that Wave V still can be observed. There are correction factors that are used to convert the ABR values to estimated thresholds in HL (termed eHL) for the patient, and these values then can be used to program the hearing aids. Figure 2–9 shows an example of a threshold search using the ABR. This happens to be someone with normal (or near normal) hearing, as you can see that Wave V was tracked with inputs as low as 10 dB to 20 dB. Note, however, that as the input becomes

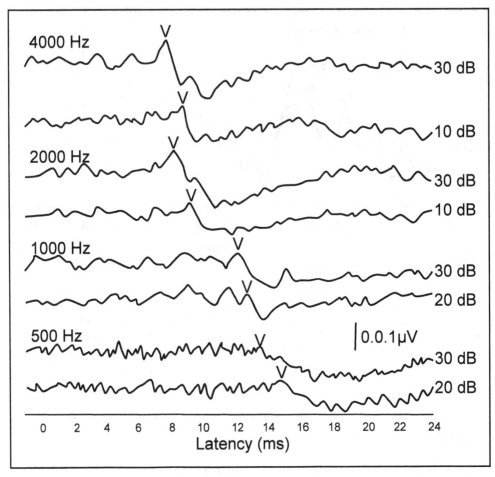

Figure 2–9. Tone-burst ABR waveforms recorded in "threshold search" ABR testing for four different key frequencies. These findings suggest normal or near-normal hearing. This is the type of ABR testing conducted for infants and toddlers to obtain an estimate of hearing thresholds, which then can be used to program hearing aids. *Source*: From *Audiology: Science to Practice* (3rd ed., p. 257), by S. Kramer and D. K. Brown, 2019, San Diego, CA: Plural Publishing. Reprinted with permission.

softer, the amplitude of Wave V decreases and the latency increases—this is the expected finding. This technique has been extremely helpful as we do the initial programming of hearing aids for very young children. Follow-up studies have shown that these ABR-based threshold estimates agree quite well with measured behavioral thresholds obtained when the child is older.

In Closing

In many areas of speech-language pathology, it is common to encounter audiograms and audiology reports on a regular basis. The purpose of this chapter was to provide some general background regarding the different tests, and offer a few tips regarding

---

CLINICAL TIP: ABR Threshold Measures—A Caveat

In this chapter, we have discussed how the ABR can be used to substitute for behavior auditory thresholds when it is not possible to conduct traditional testing—such as the case with an infant or toddler. We need to point out that the ABR simply is a representation of neural function reflecting cochlear output and low brain stem synchrony. It is *not* a measure of conscious hear-ing. There are a number of central auditory conditions which can impact the perception of sound. Conversely, it is possible to have normal behavioral hearing and an abnormal ABR, which is observed in some cases of auditory neuropathy. Clearly, the ABR is just one test in a battery that can be used to differentiate normal hearing from different hearing disorders.

---

interpretation. We even provided a little guidance regarding the assessment of credibility (e.g., don't believe a word recognition score conducted live voice!).

Interestingly, the most basic of all the tests, the pure-tone air conduction audiogram, is the most important in the selection and fitting of hearing aids, as it is what we use to select different products and it guides us in the programming. The ABR, of course, is also a critical tool when behavioral testing is not possible. On the other hand, some of the tests we discussed, such as acoustic reflexes and OAEs are not all that related to the fitting of hearing aids, but do enter into the decision process on occasion. We hope that this information will assist you the next time you encounter an audiogram or audiologic report.

3 Common Causes of Hearing Loss

Before we specifically get started talking about hearing aids in Chapter 4, we would like to review some of the common causes of hearing loss, and how these different types of losses might impact amplification decisions. The primary purpose of this chapter is to simply provide you with a quick reference regarding hearing disorders, characteristics of the hearing loss, and the audiometric configuration that is most closely associated to the disorder. As you are working with patients with various speech disorders, you may find in their case history mention of a given audiologic pathology—this chapter will help you relate the pathology to. the potential hearing handicap.

Symptoms Versus Etiology

Before reviewing the various types of hearing disorders, let's discuss the difference between a symptom and an etiology. Understanding the difference between a symptom and an etiology is important. When one of your patients complains to you about a possible hearing loss, they may be experiencing several symptoms related to any number of possible hearing disorders.

- A symptom is a description by the patient of what they are feeling, or an observation you make (e.g., dizziness, pain, etc.).

- An etiology is the underlying cause for the disorder. It is only through an accurate hearing test, which may lead to a diagnosis by a physician, that you may know the cause or etiology.

In some cases, the etiology is never known. It is common to conduct medical tests to "rule out" pathologies that require further medical attention. A person with an unexplained unilateral loss, for example, may have an MRI to rule out a space occupying lesion. Once the MRI shows there is no obvious pathology, the patient is cleared for the fitting of a hearing aid, although the true cause for the hearing loss still remains unknown. In most cases, regardless of the etiology, once a treatable medical problem involving the ear has been ruled out, the patient will be fitted with hearing aids. When we think of hearing aid patients, typically the hearing disorders will involve the inner ear. Not only are these disorders much more common (e.g., presbycusic, noise induced, etc.), but disorders of the cochlea usually require the use of hearing aids as part of the treatment process, and for the most part, hearing aids are the only treatment. The following symptoms are ones you will frequently encounter, and are used by physicians and audiologists on a regular basis.

Tinnitus

This is the perceived sensation of ear noise, often described as a ringing or buzzing in the ear. It is not a disorder, just the sensation to hear sounds generated by the auditory system—in fact, recent research suggests that this sound is generated by areas of the brain, not the ear. For example, people with a severed acoustic nerve may still experience tinnitus. Tinnitus, however, is often associated with hearing loss and hearing disorders. For example, most people with noise-induced hearing loss have tinnitus. In this case, there is no medical treatment. On the other hand, someone with an acoustic nerve neuroma also may have tinnitus and, in this case, a medical workup is critical. Tinnitus can be an occasional occurrence, or it can be constant. Tinnitus is actually more common than hearing loss, as it believed that more than 50 million Americans experience tinnitus to some degree. In case you're wondering, tinnitus can be pronounced either as ti-NIGHT-us or TIN-i-tus; the latter is preferred by most professionals.

Vertigo and Dizziness

True vertigo is a severe spinning (person spinning or room spinning) sensation usually of a short duration. It can be spontaneous or associated with head movement. The patient can have the sensation of spinning themselves or that the room is spinning around them. There are almost as many causes of dizziness as there are ways in which patients describe it. It is fairly common to encounter patients with hearing loss (especially if it is of relatively sudden onset) who are also experiencing vertigo.

Otalgia

Simply put, this is ear pain, sometimes called an "earache." Otalgia is not always associated with hearing disorders, as it can

be caused by conditions such as impacted teeth, sinus disease, and inflamed tonsils. If directly related to the ear, it may be due to middle or outer ear pathology. It's common for there to be a generalization of pain. That is, the external ear could be painful, resulting from an ear canal problem.

Aural Fullness

The perceived sensation of a plugged ear often accompanies vertigo and sudden hearing loss. Aural fullness can also be a symptom of a problem involving the middle ear, often related to poor Eustachian tube function. However, some patients with an acoustic nerve neuroma also report fullness in the ear.

Hyperacusis and Mysphonia

Hyperacusis is an abnormal sensitivity to sound. It is an internal overamplification of environmental sounds by the auditory system. Environmental sounds of ordinary intensity that do not bother most people really bother those suffering from hyperacusis—for example, a sound of 65 dB SPL might be perceived like a 100 dB SPL input. This is different than people who simply are "bothered" by loud noise. In extreme cases, the patient is so bothered by the sounds that they avoid all situations where sound is above average levels.

Mysphonia is a strong reaction to a specific sound. More than a mild irritation or annoyance to sounds, like fingernails on a chalkboard, mysphonia is a condition in which an individual becomes enraged or panicked from a specific sound. Repetitive sounds such as water dripping, gum chewing, or a refrigerator hum are known triggers of this rare condition. Both hyperacu-

DID YOU KNOW: More on Tinnitus

Tinnitus is a condition that still is not completely understood. In fact, experts are still not in complete agreement regarding the underlying causes of tinnitus. No two patients and no two tinnitus cases are alike. As such, the "best" treatment option is often contingent on an array of factors unique to each patient. Moreover, successful management of tinnitus may require overlapping layers of treatment. Some common treatments for tinnitus are summarized by the American Tinnitus Association:

■ General wellness. The perceived intensity of tinnitus can fluctuate depending on many factors, including the patient's overall well-being. There are simple things patients can do that may alleviate some of the burden such as diet, exercise, and stress reduction.

■ Hearing aids. Tinnitus often is associated with hearing loss. Using hearing aids to augment the reception and perception of external noise can often provide relief from the internal sound of tinnitus.

■ Sound therapies. Tinnitus is a non-auditory internal sound. But patients can use real external noise to counteract their perception and reaction to tinnitus. There are four different types of sound therapy:

□ Masking: exposing the patient to an external noise at a loud enough volume that it partially or completely covers the sound of their tinnitus

□ Distraction: using external sound to divert a patient's attention from the sound of tinnitus

□ Habituation: helping the patient's brain reclassify tinnitus as an unimportant sound that should can be consciously ignored; this is often referred to as tinnitus retraining therapy or TRT

□ Neuromodulation: the use of specialized sound to minimize the neural hyperactivity thought to be the underlying cause of tinnitus

■ Behavioral therapies. Tinnitus can generate strong, negative emotions like anxiety, depression, and anger. Patients can learn to control their emotional reactions and thereby disassociate tinnitus from painful negative behavioral responses.

■ Drug therapies. There are currently no FDA-approved drugs specifically for tinnitus. However, there are pharmacological options to address the stress, anxiety, and depression that are caused by (and can sometimes exacerbate) tinnitus.

sis and mysphonia are conditions that are managed by audiologists who specialize in its treatment. This treatment might involve sound therapy or lifestyle recommendations, such as using sound protection or creating "noise-free" zones within living spaces.

Interest in hyperacusis has increased significantly in recent years. As reported by Hall (2019), a search of the literature with PubMed using the key word "hyperacusis" showed that barely 100 articles were published back in the 1990s, whereas more than 200 articles were published between 2000 and 2009. He states that we're on track to reach least 450 peer-reviewed journal articles in the decade from 2000 through 2019. This growing literature includes prevalence studies, investigations on the mechanisms or pathophysiology of hyperacusis, and a number of papers on management options.

Excellent, easy-to-read summary articles on this topic have been written by audiologist James Hall (Hall, 2013, 2019). Table 3–1 is summary of the different disorders from Hall (2013). In his 2019 article, Hall outlines a possible treatment plan for someone who has loudness concerns. His systematic process is outlined in Figure 3–1.

General Classification of Hearing Disorders

In general, we use different terms to classify hearing disorders. These terms relate to the assumed location of the pathology. We say "assumed," as in some cases, the exact anatomical cause of the hearing loss is not known.

- Conductive/middle ear: This suggests that the cause of the hearing loss is related to the "conduction" of the signal to the inner ear (cochlea). This means that the problem exists lateral to the cochlea: in the outer or middle ear. Most of these disorders can be resolved through medical or surgical treatment. All middle ear pathologies that we will discuss later fit into this category.

Table 3–1. Definitions of Common Terms Associated with Decreased Sound Tolerance

Decreased Sound Tolerance (DST): Any reduction in the ability to tolerate sound. Sound produces negative reactions. There are different groups of patients with DST.

Hyperacusis: Lowered tolerance or a sense of discomfort to external sounds that do not trouble most people. Negative reactions depend on the physical characteristics of the sounds.

Misophonia: Negative reactions to specific categories or types of sounds but not all sounds. Misophonia is often context specific—such as a negative reaction to sounds like a family member eating, but not to similar sounds during dinner at a friend's house. Patients with misophonia can tolerate high levels of other sounds such as music or environmental noise.

Phonophobia: Negative reaction to certain sounds, including anxiety and fear that is intensified with anticipation of the sound. Phonophobia is a psychological phenomenon. Neurologists sometimes use the term to describe sound tolerance problems in patients with migraine.

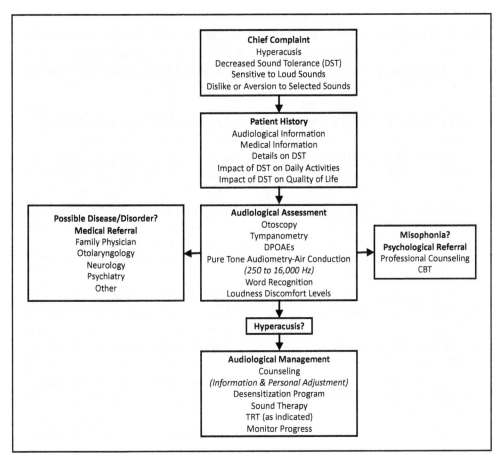

Figure 3–1. Protocol for assessment of a patient with concerns regarding loud sounds. *Source*: Adapted from Hall, 2019.

▓ Cochlear/inner ear: Many pathologies are very specific to the cochlea. These typically cannot be resolved through medicine or surgery, and the fitting of hearing aids (or cochlear implants) is the preferred treatment. You will sometimes hear patients say they have a "nerve" loss, and maybe they have been told this by their physician, but in most cases, the 8th nerve is functioning properly—the problem lies with the sensory hair cells of the cochlea. A noise-induced hearing loss typically would be classified as a "cochlear" pathology.

▓ Sensorineural: In some cases, it is difficult to determine if the pathology is limited to the cochlea, or if fibers of the 8th nerve also are involved. A more cautious description in this case would be the term "sensorineural" (sensori = cochlea), meaning it could be one or the other, or both.

▓ Mixed: As the term suggests, this is hearing loss that has both a conductive and a sensorineural component. A person with a noise-induced hearing loss (cochlear) who developed middle ear infusion (conductive) would fit into this category.

■ Neural (8th nerve): While neural could be anywhere between the cochlea and the auditory cortex, when this term is used, it commonly is referring to the 8th nerve. There are audiologic tests which certainly strongly indicate 8th nerve pathology (vs. cochlear), but today, with the common use of MRI scans, this classification would not be used until confirmation with these studies.

■ Central: A hearing pathology usually is classified as "central" when it is believed that the origin lies above the level of the cochlear nucleus. It could be low brain stem, high brain stem, or cortical. In some cases, these pathologies are not lesion or disease specific, but rather involve a generalized processing deficit, such as in the common auditory processing disorder classification (APD), which decades ago was referred to as CAPD—the "C" for central. Because some people still refer to APD as CAPD, you may see it as (c)APD.

Hearing loss is also classified by the time in which the hearing loss is acquired. Of course, one important reason for knowing when a hearing disorder is acquired is related to language development.

■ Congenital hearing loss: A hearing loss acquired at birth. Common causes include bacterial or viral infection, or ingestion of ototoxic medications.

■ Prenatal: A hearing loss that has developed before birth in which the mother has passed the hearing disorder on to the child. In other words, the hearing loss was acquired while the baby developed in utero. The most common prenatal hearing disorders are viral or bacterial infections. Many hereditary hearing disorders are acquired prenatally.

■ Perinatal: The hearing loss develops during or shortly after birth. Many of the same conditions causing a prenatal loss can occur perinatally.

■ Acquired or postnatal: A hearing loss that develops later in life. Prelingual

---

POINTS TO PONDER: Does Terminology Matter?

As you will notice, we used the term "sensorineural" to describe hearing loss that could possibly be of both the cochlea and the 8th nerve, or for cases where the exact etiology is unknown. In a 2014 editorial, Clark and Martin suggest we abandon the use of this term. Their editorial was endorsed by 19 key opinion leaders in audiology, including the guru of audiology terminology, James Jerger. The authors point out that the clear shortcoming of this one-word term is that it does not separate the two possible sites of lesion. They contend that today's diagnostic capabilities have greatly increased the audiologist's ability to accurately separate sensory from neural lesions. They suggested the use of a slash, as in sensory/neural hearing loss, meets the criteria for accurate terminology in audiology. They believe that this spelling better reflects an "and/or" situation when a clear differentiation between sensory and neural cannot be made. While perhaps a reasonable thought, as far as we can tell, since the 2014 publication, little traction has been made in changing the sensorineural terminology.

hearing loss is a hearing loss acquired during the critical language development years of between birth and about 12 years of age. Postlingual hearing loss is acquired after the most critical language years.

Unilateral Hearing Loss

In this chapter we will be discussing many types of hearing loss, some confined to the middle ear and others to the cochlea. While the majority of older people with hearing loss have a loss in both ears (this is related to the common etiologies of noise-induced and presbycusis), it is common to encounter unilateral hearing loss in school-age children. For that reason, we want to make some specific points regarding children with unilateral hearing loss. Unfortunately, many professionals underestimate the handicap that it presents.

For many years, the professional community, more or less, thought that "one good ear was good enough." Things began to change, however, in the early 1980s, spearheaded by research at Vanderbilt University. Within a few years we started to see publications by lead researcher Fred Bess, and his colleague Anne Marie Tharpe. Their pioneering work centered on 60 children (aged 6 to 18) who had been diagnosed with a unilateral loss of 45 dB or greater in the poorer ear, and thresholds no worse than 15 dB in the normally hearing ear. One of the many noteworthy findings from this research was the revelation that only half of these children were performing satisfactorily in school. Moreover, 35% of the children had repeated at least one grade, and an additional 13% required resource assistance. This was especially concerning given that the failure rate in that metropolitan area for the general elementary school population was only 3.5%. We will discuss further in Chapter 9 about

---

TAKE FIVE: Two Interesting Cases

Case #1
Audiologist: I see in your history that you're having some problems hearing?
Patient: Yes, I've noticed it the past few years.
Audiologist: Your right ear or your left ear?
Patient: Well, I guess it's neither.
Audiologist: Neither?
Patient: I just saw the doctor, and he said it was my "middle ear!"
Case #2
Audiologist (talking to grandmother on phone): I heard that cousin Keven

recently had some kind of ear surgery? Do you know what it was for?
Grandmother: I knew you were going to ask, so I wrote down some notes when I talked to him . . . he read part of the report to me . . . it had to do with some bone.
Audiologist: Probably one of the middle ear bones. Do you have the name of the bone?
Grandmother: I think so . . . just a minute. Yes, it was the "air bone."
Audiologist: What? The air bone?
Grandmother: Yes, something must not have been connected, as he said there was an "air-bone gap!"

the diagnosis and treatment of children with hearing loss, including those with unilateral hearing loss.

Anne Marie Tharpe (2018) recently provided an update on the progress that has been made since the Vanderbilt research of the 1980s. She states that today, unilateral hearing loss is typically being identified much earlier. Parents, teachers, and other professionals are aware of the problem earlier in children's lives. There are more opportunities for early intervention. She adds, however, that challenges remain, as despite the earlier identification and improved hearing technology, some children with unilateral losses are still struggling academically and behaviorally. This is partly because there are still a lot of professionals who do not think that unilateral hearing loss is problematic for children—that might include pediatricians or otolaryngologists or educators, and perhaps a segment of the audiologists and speech-language pathologists. Tharpe (2018) highlighted the need for parents to be involved in the management decisions for their children. This might involve the trial use of hearing technologies by their children or other strategies. It also means that audiologists and speech-language pathologists need to listen to and talk with parents about their concerns before deciding together on a management strategy.

Hearing Disorders of the Outer Ear

The following section is a summary of some of the most common hearing disorders you will encounter in your daily practice. To help make things fairly straightforward, we have organized the disorders as they relate to parts of the ear, starting with the outer ear. Most disorders of the outer ear are easy to observe, respond to treatment, and usually do not cause significant hearing loss. We review five of the most common in this section.

Impacted Cerumen

Cerumen (or earwax) is a normal by-product of a healthy ear. It lubricates the ear canal and protects the canal and tympanic membrane. As cerumen is produced by the subcutaneous glands of the ear canal, it migrates out of the ear canal by way of the tiny hairs lining the outer layer of the external ear canal. Some people produce more cerumen than others, especially the elderly. Additionally, other people may disturb the natural cerumen excretion process by inserting Q-tips and other foreign objects into their ear canal, attempting to remove the cerumen. These objects often irritate the canal, which then results in increased cerumen production, which then results in more probing by the individual—not a good thing.

For individuals who produce excessive cerumen, impaction sometimes also occurs because of hearing aid use. That is, the hearing aid (in the case of a custom instrument) or the earmold, at the time of each insertion, continues to push the cerumen to a given point (usually about 10 mm to 15 mm from the ear canal opening) and, eventually, a total (or near total) blockage will occur.

Impacted cerumen results in a temporary conductive hearing loss of varying degree (in severe cases, an air-bone gap as large as 30 dB to 40 dB will be present). Once the cerumen is removed by a qualified professional (some audiologists conduct cerumen removal), hearing returns to preimpact levels. A good otoscopic examination will reveal if impacted cerumen exists. If the ear canal is only partially blocked, this probably will have little or no impact on the patient's hearing.

External Otitis

Otitis externa is an inflammation of the outer ear and ear canal. Along with otitis media, which we address shortly, external otitis is one of two conditions commonly referred to as an "earache." External otitis can be an extremely painful condition requiring treatment from a physician. Hearing tests sometimes cannot be conducted on patients with severe external otitis because the ear is too painful to allow for the placement of earphones.

Acute external otitis often occurs suddenly, rapidly worsens, and becomes extremely painful. Because the tissues lining the external ear canal are extremely thin, they are easily torn or abraded by minimal force. Inflammation of the ear canal can begin when someone tries to self-clean their ear canal with a cotton swab or other small implement (we hear that car keys are popular!). Another cause of external otitis is prolonged exposure to water or extreme humidity. Regardless of the cause, external otitis occurs when active bacteria or fungus begins to infect the skin of the ear canal.

Pain that worsens on touching of the outer ear is the predominant complaint associated with external otitis. Patients may also experience discharge from the ear canal and itchiness. Swelling of the ear canal is another symptom, and when the swelling is severe enough, a conductive hearing loss may occur. In more advanced cases of external otitis, pain may radiate to the jaw and neck.

Topical solutions or suspensions in the form of ear drops typically are used to treat mild and moderate cases of otitis externa. In more advanced cases, a physician may have to use a binocular microscope to clean the ear canal and insert what is called an ear wick to deliver medication to the infected area. In general, we would not expect external otitis to cause a hearing loss. If the swelling was such that there was complete closure of the ear canal, then a mild conductive loss would be expected (probably greatest in the higher frequencies). In general, however, expect normal hearing with this pathology.

Tumors of the External Ear Canal

Both malignant and benign tumors have been found in the external ear canal. Bony tumors, called osteomas, are sometimes seen in the ears of people who have done a lot of swimming in cold water—also referred to as exostosis. You may not observe a tumor, in itself, but rather just a narrowing of the canal. Irritation from cold wind and water exposure causes the bone surrounding the ear canal to develop lumps of new bony growth which constrict the ear canal, sometimes referred to as "Surfer's Ear. Unless the bony growth or tumor closes off the entire external ear canal, they do not cause hearing loss. A detailed otoscopic exam should reveal this, and, unless this is a long-standing condition reported by the patient, a physician referral is appropriate.

Perforated Tympanic Membrane

There are several ways the tympanic membrane (TM) can become perforated. A perforated eardrum is a rupture or perforation (hole) of the eardrum that can occur as a result of infection, trauma (e.g., by trying to clean the ear with sharp instruments, or even a Q-tip), explosion, barotrauma, or surgery (accidental creation of a rupture).

Because traumatic perforations often alter otherwise normal tissue, they often heal spontaneously. One common cause of TM perforations is related to the buildup of excessive pressure in the middle ear as a result of a middle ear disorder (e.g., Eustachian tube dysfunction, infection, effusion, etc.). In these cases, the excess pressure causes the TM to rupture. Because of the underlying middle ear disorder, TM perforations caused from this excessive pressure need to be managed medically.

Surgical repair of a perforated TM is called myringoplasty or tympanoplasty. In some cases, the "surgical patching" procedures are not successful, and the patient will, more or less, have a "permanent" perforation. Those with more severe and long-standing ruptures may need to wear an earplug to avoid water (or other liquids) making contact with the eardrum and entering the middle ear cavity.

Perforation of the eardrum usually leads to conductive hearing loss. The amount of hearing loss caused by a perforated TM varies by both the size of the perforation and the location of the opening. Some perforations can be so small that they cannot be detected during routine otoscopy. With large perforations, it's common to see a conductive hearing loss of 30 dB to 40 dB. Once the perforation heals, hearing is usually recovered fully (maybe with a slight 5–10 dB drop due to scarring), but chronic infection over a long period may lead to permanent hearing loss, as the structure of the TM is altered.

Disorders of the Middle Ear

Recall that the purpose of the middle ear is to transmit the airborne sound from the ear-drum to the cochlea. This is accomplished quite effectively through the aerial ratio of the TM compared to the oval window, and through the lever action of the ossicular chain. As you would expect, anything that disrupts this flow will cause a middle ear (conductive) hearing loss. We'll describe some of the most common.

Otosclerosis

Otosclerosis is caused by two main sites of involvement of the sclerotic (or scar-like) lesions. The best understood mechanism is fixation of the stapes footplate to the oval window of the cochlea. This greatly impairs movement of the stapes and therefore transmission of sound into the inner ear ("ossicular coupling").

Additionally, the cochlea's round window can also become sclerotic, and in a similar way, impair movement of sound pressure waves through the inner ear ("acoustic coupling"). There is some documentation of sclerotic lesions that also are within the cochlea, sometimes referred to as "cochlear otosclerosis."

Treatment of otosclerosis often involves a surgical procedure called a stapedectomy. A stapedectomy consists of removing a portion of the sclerotic stapes footplate and replacing it with an implant that is secured to the incus. This procedure restores continuity of ossicular movement and allows transmission of sound waves from the eardrum to the inner ear. A modern variant of this surgery called a stapedotomy is performed by drilling a small hole in the stapes footplate with a micro drill or a laser, and inserting a pistonlike prosthesis.

Otosclerosis can be hereditary, and at least in the early stages, results in a conductive hearing loss of mild to moderate-severe

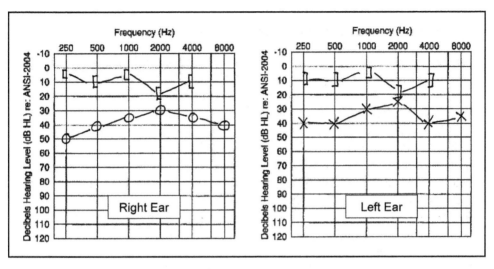

Figure 3–2. A bilateral conductive hearing loss consistent with bilateral otosclerosis. Notice the 2000 Hz notch in the bone conduction scores in both ears, a historic "signature" of otosclerosis, sometimes referred to as "Carhart's Notch" in reference to Raymond Carhart, father of audiology, who was one of the first to write about this finding. *Source*: From *Fitting and Dispensing Hearing Aids* (2nd ed., p. 139), by B. Taylor and H. G. Mueller, 2017, San Diego, CA: Plural Publishing. Reprinted with permission.

degree, usually with the greatest loss in the lower frequencies. It more often presents in women during child-bearing years or during/after a recent pregnancy. In the later stages, a mixed hearing loss may be present. Figure 3–2 gives an example of otosclerosis that you might see on an audiogram. While this patient certainly is a hearing aid candidate and probably would be a successful user of hearing aids, some patients opt for surgical treatment. The more cautious surgeon may simply recommend hearing aids for some of the patients as there are risks involved with the surgery; the outcome of the surgery (closure of the air-bone gap) varies significantly among surgeons—like most things, surgical experience is very important. Typically, following successful surgery there is a significant improvement in air conduction thresholds, although the patient may not have completely "normal" hearing.

Negative Middle Ear Pressure and Middle Ear Effusion

The Eustachian tube equalizes the pressure between the air filled middle ear and outside air pressure. This tube is normally closed, but when healthy, opens frequently when we talk, chew, yawn, and so forth. When the Eustachian tube becomes blocked or swollen from an allergy or common cold, the air pressure outside the middle ear is greater than the air pressure within the middle ear space. Children are more prone to negative middle ear pressure and effusion because the Eustachian tube has not had the opportunity to grow to the proper angle (~45°) and is much more horizontal.

Eustachian tube dysfunction causes the air trapped inside the middle ear to become absorbed by the tissues lining the middle ear space, resulting in a drop in pressure within

---

CLINICAL TIP: Our Friend Antonio Valsalva

Patients with Eustachian tube dysfunction may be asked by their physician to auto-inflate their Eustachian tube by attempting to force air into the middle ear space while holding their nostrils shut (they actually are instructed to try to blow air out of their nose, while holding their nose shut). This is called the Valsalva maneuver, named after Italian anatomist Antonio Valsalva who conducted extensive study of the ear and throat anatomy in the early 1700s. Divers use the Valsalva procedure to equalize pressure as they descend or surface. It also works very nicely for most all of us to equalize pressure at any time, such as when descending in an airplane. The procedure can do no harm, although it might generate some stares from onlookers on a crowded plane. Unfortunately, not everyone is able to open their Eustachian tube using this technique. There is even a Valsalva device used in spacesuits to allow astronauts to equalize the pressure in their ears by performing the maneuver inside the suit without using their hands to block their nose.

---

the middle ear space. The greater pressure from the outside air causes the tympanic membrane to become retracted, or pushed, into the middle ear space. This condition can be observed with otoscopy, although sometimes it is quite subtle. A specific audiologic test battery called immittance audiometry is used to measure the function of the entire middle ear system. Tympanometry, which is part of this battery, easily will reveal a retracted TM, or a middle ear system that is not moving effectively.

If negative middle ear pressure continues to develop and is present for an extended time, the fluids normally secreted by the mucous membranes are collected in the middle ear cavity, resulting in a condition called serous effusion or middle ear effusion. When fluid partially fills the middle ear space, a mild to moderate conductive hearing loss can occur. Often, when a young child has fluid in their middle ears, it is referred to by the layperson (e.g., parents) as an "ear infection."

Middle ear effusion, however, is not necessarily infectious, and in fact, usually it isn't.

The audiogram for this patient is directly related to the amount of retraction and/or the amount of fluid in the middle ear. If the patient only has a retracted TM, there probably will be little effect on hearing thresholds. If fluid begins to collect, expect thresholds, especially in the low frequencies, to drop accordingly.

There is a test that an audiologist can conduct to look at Eustachian dysfunction. They run a tympanogram to look at TM movement. Then they have a patient do a Valsalva procedure (plug nose and blow). This forces air up the Eustachian tube and the peak of the tympanogram should shift to the positive. The patient is then asked to do a Toynbee (plug nose and swallow). Another tympanogram is run, and the results should show a shift to the negative as the Toynbee pulls air out of the middle ear space. If the maneuvers both move the tympanogram, the Eustachian tube is functioning appropriately.

Otitis Media

If middle ear effusion is allowed to continue unabated, otitis media can develop. Otitis media is any infection of the mucous-membrane lining of the middle ear space. Recent evidence suggests that chronic otitis media during childhood may impact speech and language development, and if left untreated, can have a long-term impact on central auditory processing. Although otitis media is thought of as a disease of childhood, it can occur at any age and can be quite painful. When these tissues become infected, they become swollen, interfering with its pressure equalization function. During this process, the tympanic membrane becomes very vascular, resulting in the TM's red appearance.

There are two types of otitis media: chronic and acute. As you might imagine, acute otitis media has a very rapid onset time; whereas chronic conditions of otitis media are long-standing. In some cases, the fluid in the middle ear becomes thick and sticky, and, hence, the nonmedical term "glue ear" sometimes has been used to describe the condition. Like many pathologies of the middle ear, the audiogram will vary with the severity of the problem. It's reasonable to expect a conductive hearing loss of 20 dB to 30 dB, or worse. The configuration might be similar to that shown in Figure 3–2. In severe cases, air-borne gaps of 30 dB or greater are common.

Current recommendations from the American Academy of Pediatrics suggests no treatment for the first seven days of the infection. Research out of Mayo Clinic showed no significant rates of improvement of the infection with or without antibiotics if the infection cleared within seven days. If the infection does not clear within the first week, antibiotics are used in the treatment of otitis media. If otitis media persists, however, pressure equalization (PE) tubes are inserted into the TM by an otolaryngologist. This procedure is called myringotomy with PE tubes. These tubes are also referred to as grommets or tympanostomy tubes. If the tubes are open during audiometric testing (they sometimes become plugged), you would expect to see relatively normal hearing. In the pediatric population, recommendations for PE tubes are more than 3 infections in a 6-month period. If immittance testing is conducted, volume measures will quickly indicate if the tube is open or closed. The tubes are brightly colored and are usually easy to see when you do a routine otoscopy. Additionally, if you continue to see what appears to be infection, don't delay on referring to a physician as the child may need to see an ENT for PE tube placement.

Cholesteatoma

In general, cholesteatomas are the result of a long-standing middle ear condition. Cholesteatomas form a sac with concentric rings consisting of a protein called keratin; there is some evidence to classify them as low-grade tumors. In patients with TM perforations, the tissue may enter the middle ear through the perforation, producing a cholesteatoma. Cholesteatomas may also be caused by chronic episodes of otitis media. Cholesteatomas are dangerous because they eventually can erode the bones of the middle ear. They potentially also could damage the facial nerve, and if left untreated over several years, will even invade the nose and brain cavity in rare instances. In most cases, cholesteatoma are removed with surgery. As with other middle ear pathologies, the patient will have a conductive hearing loss, although the patient with a cholesteatoma will typically have a more severe loss than most other middle ear conditions, due to the extent of the disease. It's common to observe air-bone gaps of 30 dB to 40 dB.

Tympanosclerosis

Tympanosclerosis is characterized by white plaques on the surface of the tympanic membrane and deposits on the ossicles. It often is the result of chronic otitis media, which when untreated, leaves this white residue. Tympanosclerosis can have a stiffening effect on the TM, which may result in a mild conductive hearing loss in the low frequencies. As mentioned earlier, PE tubes are a common treatment for otitis media. It's common for these patients (~30%–40%) to have resulting tympanosclerosis after the PE tubes have fallen out or have been removed.

Ossicular Disarticulation

This is also referred to as ossicular "dislocation" or "discontinuity." As the name indicates, this condition results in one of the two joints between the three ossicles being pulled apart or disarticulated (the incudostapedial juncture is the most common). It can produce a wide variety of conductive hearing losses depending on the location and extent of the disarticulation. The most common causes of ossicular disarticulation are degenerative diseases and trauma to the head. In severe head trauma, a TM perforation also might be observed. Interestingly, the largest hearing loss (conduc-

tive) from disarticulation is present when the TM is intact, not perforated. In these cases, it is possible for an ossicular disarticulation to cause up to a 50 dB to 60 dB conductive hearing loss. This sometimes has been referred to as "maximum" conductive loss, as the cochlea is stimulated via bone conduction for higher presentation levels.

Disorders of the Cochlea

For adults, sensorineural hearing loss resulting from cochlear pathology is by far the most common type of hearing impairment. In this section, we spend some time reviewing the most common types of sensorineural hearing loss resulting from cochlear pathology. Because there is very limited medical or surgical treatment of cochlear hearing loss, these are the people that are most frequently fitted with hearing aids.

Presbycusis

If your patient is beyond the age of 60 years old, it's possible that the hearing sensitivity has progressively worsened over the years, and this will now be reflected in the audiogram, especially in the higher frequencies. This gradual deterioration of hearing is often a result of prebycusis (sometimes written "presbyacusis"). Simply stated, presbycusis is hearing loss caused by the cumulative effects of the aging process. This progression is somewhat more rapid for men than for women, although this partially could be due to the fact that men experience more noise exposure than women, which is difficult to separate from the aging effects on the inner ear structures.

KEY CONCEPT: Aging or Simply Low-Level Noise?

As you know, presbycusis is normally thought of as hearing loss due to the natural aging process. An intriguing question, however, that often comes up regarding presbycusis is whether this is indeed the result of aging by itself, or the result of aging in a noise- and stress-filled society. Is presbycusis just a different type of noise-induced hearing loss? An often-cited study related to this topic dates back to 1962, and was conducted with the Mabaan tribe in Sudan. Because of their isolation, there was very little noise in their lives. And guess what—there was little or no hearing loss for even the older members of the tribe (~75 years old). Interpretation of this is a little tricky, as there were also other differences (e.g., general health, diet, etc.), but it certainly is something to think about.

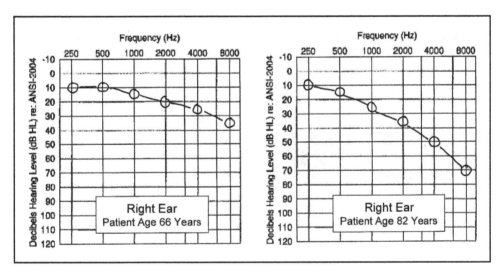

Figure 3–3. The progressive nature of presbycusis for an individual's right ear. The audiogram on the left is from a 66-year-old male. The audiogram on the right is for the same male patient at the age of 82. We only show the right ear thresholds, but typically a symmetrical pattern is observed. *Source*: From *Fitting and Dispensing Hearing Aids* (2nd ed., p. 144), by B. Taylor and H. G. Mueller, 2017, San Diego, CA: Plural Publishing. Reprinted with permission.

Presbycusis affects all parts of the ear, including neural transmissions to the brain, but the primary site of lesion is the cochlea. The outer hair cells within the cochlea are particularly sensitive to the wear and tear associated with the aging process. As a general rule, the higher the frequency, the greater effect of presbycusis (even people in their 20s and 30s experience loss of sensitivity in the >16,000 Hz range).

The classic presbycusis audiogram will show a gradually sloping downward pattern; nearly always, as the frequency becomes higher, the hearing loss becomes worse (Figure 3–3). Because this is a generalized aging process, we would also expect the loss to be

---

DID YOU KNOW: Commercial Exploitation of Presbycusis

Given the known effects of presbycusis on high-frequency hearing, a cell phone ring has been developed with a center frequency around 16,000 Hz. The notion is that school children can use it to call each other during class or in places where the phone is supposed to be turned off, and their teachers won't hear it! Another technology application related to presbycusis has been to use a very loud, high-pitched signal in stores where teenagers loiter— the device is named the "Mosquito." The sound is very annoying and drives away the younger folk, but the older adult customers can't hear it! Sometimes presbycusis can be a good thing.

---

quite symmetric. In fact, if the loss is downward sloping but *not* symmetric, other etiologies should be considered.

Noise-Induced Hearing Loss (NIHL)

Exposure to loud sounds can result in temporary or permanent hearing loss. This condition is called noise-induced hearing loss (NIHL). Around 30 million adults in the United States are exposed to hazardous sound levels in the workplace. Among these 30 million people, it's estimated that one in four will acquire a permanent hearing loss as a result of their occupation.

The degree of hearing loss caused by NIHL depends on the intensity of the sound, duration of the exposure, frequency spectrum of the sound, individual susceptibility, along with other variables. Usually, this type of hearing loss is due to continued exposure to work or recreational noise exposure that has occurred over several years. It is possible, however, for NIHL to occur for only a very short duration of exposure, or even a single blast (referred to as "acoustic trauma"). Because of the shape of the cochlea and the resonant effects of the outer ear, most cases of NIHL show a high-frequency hearing loss, with maximum loss in the 3000 to 6000 Hz range, and usually with some recovery at the highest frequencies. This pattern on the audiogram often is called a "noise notch" (Figure 3–4). NIHL can affect people of all ages.

There is a direct relationship between the intensity of noise, the duration of the exposure, and the degree of potential NIHL. When counseling patients about noise exposure, it's good to have a general idea of what is "safe," and when hearing protection is needed. The Occupational Health and Safety Agency (OSHA) is an arm of the federal government responsible for ensuring that workers are safely protected from dangerous amounts of noise. Table 3–2 indicates when the intensity and duration of exposure becomes dangerous for individuals. If a worker is exposed to levels of sound greater than 90 dB for 8 hr per day, they are

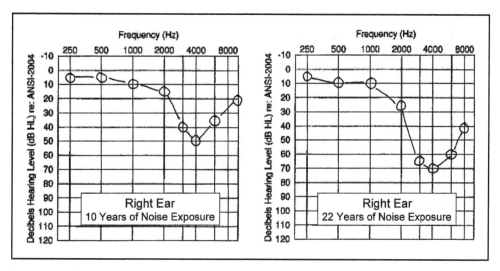

Figure 3–4. The effects of NIHL over time for one individual's right ear. Thresholds were measured 12 years apart for a male patient working in a condition of intense noise (daily carpentry with skill saw). The audiogram on the right shows the progressive nature of the hearing loss consistent with the patient's history of noise exposure. Notice how the dip at 4000 Hz deepens, and other frequencies become more involved. The left ear had the same pattern but was not as severe; perhaps there was some attenuation of the noise from head shadow for this ear. *Source*: From *Fitting and Dispensing Hearing Aids* (2nd ed., p. 145), by B. Taylor and H. G. Mueller, 2017, San Diego, CA: Plural Publishing. Reprinted with permission.

Table 3–2. Maximum Permissible Noise Levels	
90 dB	8.0 hours
92 dB	6.0 hours
95 dB	4.0 hours
97 dB	3.0 hours
100 dB	2.0 hours
102 dB	1.5 hours
105 dB	1.0 hour
110 dB	30 minutes
115 dB	15 minutes

Source: Downloaded from http://www.quietsolution.com /Noise_Levels.pdf. *Source:* From *Fitting and Dispensing Hearing Aids* (2nd ed., p. 146), by B. Taylor and H. G. Mueller, 2017, San Diego, CA: Plural Publishing. Reprinted with permission.

KEY CONCEPT: Personal Music Systems and Hearing Loss

In the past few years, there has been a lot of discussion regarding young people obtaining noise-induced hearing loss from listening to iPods and other personal stereo systems via earphones. It probably isn't as bad as suggested by some of the articles, but there is a real problem in that many of these devices can be turned up quite loud and many people use them for several hours continuously without giving their ears a "rest." This is particularly a problem for people who listen in background noise (e.g., factory workers), as they need to turn the music to a level to overcome the noise. A rest period each hour is critical (and less loud, of course, is good too). Some of these devices have default lower output levels, or provide a warning when it is set too high.

---

required to wear hearing protection. Notice that as the intensity increases, the exposure time needed to cause damage is reduced.

Ototoxicity

There are several drugs used for therapeutic treatment of diseases that have the potential side effect of causing damage to the inner ear. Because the cochlea is such a delicate organ, it is susceptible to damage from medications and chemical agents. Such drugs and agents are considered to be ototoxic or poisonous to the ears.

Ototoxic drugs have one thing in common: they cause a sensorineural hearing loss. The amount of ototoxic hearing loss depends on the exact dosage and duration of use. When you encounter a patient who has used or been exposed to an ototoxic medication or agent, you should consult a physician or pharmacist. An ototoxic hearing loss can present itself in different ways, but, typically, the high frequencies are the first affected, and the hearing loss is usually downward sloping. Some facilities conduct high-frequency audiometry (10,000 to 18,000 Hz) to monitor early changes in hearing.

There are hundreds of ototoxic medications and agents. The most common ones along with their therapeutic uses are listed in Table 3–3. Also listed is whether the drug causes a permanent or reversible hearing loss. The majority of drugs cause a permanent hearing loss, but some cause reversible hearing loss. This list is by no means exhaustive; rather, it is designed to represent a sample of the most common ototoxic agents you will encounter. Because new medications are always being introduced into the market, it is best to consult with your local physician or pharmacist for the most current information.

Sudden Hearing Loss

Sudden hearing loss is usually defined as greater than 30 dB hearing reduction, over at least three contiguous frequencies, occurring over a period of 72 hr or less. Some patients describe that the hearing loss was noticed instantaneously (usually when they wake up in the morning) and others report that it rap-

Table 3–3. A Summary of Common Drug Types and Their Effects on Hearing

Type of Drug	Type of Hearing Loss	Reversible? (Y/N)
1. Aminoglycoside Antibiotics ▪ streptomycin ▪ gentamycin ▪ kanamycin ▪ vancomycin	Sensorineural	No
2. Cancer Chemotherapeutics ▪ cisplatin ▪ carboplatin	Sensorineural	No
3. Loop Diuretics (Furosemide) ▪ lasix ▪ bumax	Sensorineural	Yes
4. Salicylates ▪ aspirin	Sensorineural	Yes
5. Quinine	Sensorineural	Yes

Source: From *Fitting and Dispensing Hearing Aids* (2nd ed., 148), by B. Taylor and H. G. Mueller, 2017, San Diego, CA: Plural Publishing. Reprinted with permission.

idly developed over a period of hours or days. Typically, only one ear is affected, and the severity of the hearing loss varies considerably. It's common for the patient to also experience tinnitus. The average age at onset is individuals in their 40s and 50s. Often, this strikes people who are otherwise healthy, and the experience usually is quite traumatic. Imagine going to sleep and all is well, and then waking up not being able to hear in one ear!

There are many causes for sudden hearing loss; the most common three being viral, circulatory, or metabolic. In many cases, the cause is recorded as idiopathic (unknown) in the health records, as test results are inconclusive and the true cause is never known.

About two-thirds of people who experience sudden hearing loss have their hearing spontaneously recover. In most cases, however, an otolaryngologist will consider some treatment, if for no other reason than doing something seems better than doing nothing. A common treatment is oral corticosteroid

therapy. Some research evidence is available supporting the benefit of this regimen, and it is most effective when started immediately after the hearing loss is noticed. It is important, therefore, that if you are the first professional to see one of these patients, that you aggressively encourage them to see a physician immediately, even if it means that you assist them in obtaining the appointment. It might be time to call in a chip from the neighborhood otolaryngologist. We've seen general practitioners shrug it off as something as minor as Eustachian tube dysfunction, and the patient isn't seen again for a month.

Viral and Bacterial Diseases

There are several viral and bacterial infections that can result in sensorineural hearing loss. Infections, such as cytomegalovirus, can be transmitted to the child from the mother in utero. This is a condition known as prenatal. The following diseases are considered prenatal conditions that can result in a congenital hearing loss:

- Syphilis
- Rubella
- Toxoplasmosis
- Cytomegalovirus (CMV)
- Herpes simplex virus

There also are several viral and bacterial infections that occur after a child has been born that can produce sensorineural hearing loss. In most cases, these postnatal infections enter the inner ear through the blood supply that is carrying the infection. The following are some of the most common diseases acquired after birth (postnatal) causing hearing loss:

- Mumps
- Measles
- Bacterial meningitis
- Herpes zoster oticus

Ménière's Disease

Ménière's disease is named after the French physician Prosper Ménière who first reported that vertigo was caused by inner ear disorders in an article published in 1861. Ménière's disease, in its "classic form," is used to describe a hearing disorder with one or more of the following characteristics:

1. A hearing loss (usually in one ear) of sudden or rapid onset.
2. A fullness or pressure sensation in the ear.
3. Brief and sudden episodes of severe dizziness (vertigo).
4. A roaring (tinnitus) in the affected ear.

THINGS TO REMEMBER: "Hidden Hearing Loss"

There has been a lot of discussion in recent years regarding "hidden hearing loss." Simply stated, this usually is in reference to a patient who enters the clinic complaining of having a hearing loss, but routine audiometric findings are normal. Recent findings from animal studies of noise-induced and age-related hearing loss suggest that cochlear synapse loss is a likely contributor to difficulties understanding speech in noise, and may be an instigating factor in the generation of tinnitus and hyperacusis—even when hearing thresholds are normal. This cochlear synaptopathy may be widespread in acquired sensorineural hearing loss; it has been referred to as "hidden hearing loss" in that test results using the traditional audiologic battery often will be normal. Unfortunately, most audiologists do not routinely conduct word recognition in background noise, which in many cases would identify the pathology. While the dysfunction may be hidden to the audiologist, it's very real for the patient. There has been some success fitting hearing aids to these patients, even though their audiometric thresholds are normal.

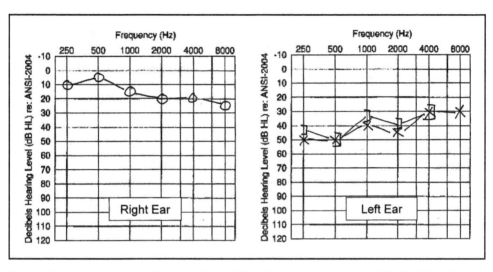

Figure 3–5. Asymmetric left sensorineural hearing loss consistent with Ménière disease. *Source*: From *Fitting and Dispensing Hearing Aids* (2nd ed., p. 151), by B. Taylor and H. G. Mueller, 2017, San Diego, CA: Plural Publishing. Reprinted with permission.

One or all of the symptoms require an immediate referral to a physician. There are many subcategories of Ménière's disease beyond the scope of this chapter. Some types of cochlear hearing losses of sudden onset, such as Ménière's, although they are sensorineural, may actually return to normal levels.

The exact cause of Ménière's disease is not known, but it is believed to be related to *endolymphatic hydrops* or excess fluid in the inner ear. It is thought that endolymphatic fluid bursts from its normal channels in the ear and flows into other areas, causing damage. This is called "hydrops." This may be related to swelling of the endolymphatic sac or other tissues in the vestibular system of the inner ear, which is responsible for the body's sense of balance.

There is no standard "signature" audiogram for Ménière's, but in general, there tends to be more low-frequency hearing loss than observed for most other sensorineural pathologies. That is, the audiogram often appears "flat" or upward sloping rather than the more common downward sloping pattern. Figure 3–5 shows an audiogram of a patient diagnosed with Ménière's disease. Note the asymmetric (unilateral) nature of the hearing loss. After this hearing loss has stabilized, this person might be fit with a hearing aid in the affected ear.

Retrocochlear Disorders

In general terms, retrocochlear disorders or pathology refers to damage to the nerve fibers along the ascending auditory pathways, running from the internal auditory canal to the auditory cortex. In other words, we might be quite certain that the problem does not lie within the middle ear or the cochlea and, therefore, the locus must be somewhere more medial. Commonly, in audiologic practice, retrocochlear is used to refer to the eighth nerve and the low brain

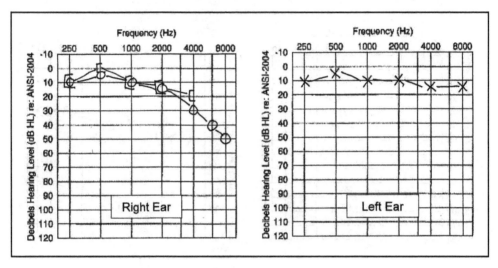

Figure 3–6. A mild, right asymmetric sensorineural hearing loss consistent with possible retrocochlear pathology. *Source*: From *Fitting and Dispensing Hearing Aids* (2nd ed., p. 152), by B. Taylor and H. G. Mueller, 2017, San Diego, CA: Plural Publishing. Reprinted with permission.

stem, and auditory dysfunction at higher auditory levels is referred to as "central."

In most cases, eighth nerve retrocochlear pathologies involve tumors. Retrocochlear tumors—referred to as acoustic schwannomas, acoustic neuromas, neurinomas, or neurilemomas—typically (but not always) produce unilateral high-frequency hearing loss in their more advanced stages. And, unlike presbycusis and many other types of *cochlear* pathology, it is unlikely that there would be uniform symmetric tumors, so there usually is asymmetry between ears in the audiogram (Figure 3–6).

The signs and symptoms of eighth nerve retrocochlear pathology are subtle and difficult to identify with conventional audiometry. In many cases, in the early stages, there is no significant hearing loss (although there may be a reduction of speech understanding for speech in noise, or other difficult speech tests). Many patients will complain of tinnitus on the affected side, vertigo or dizziness, fullness, or speech not sounding clear. In cases where retrocochlear pathology is suspected, a complete audiologic diagnostic battery and otologic referral is needed.

Hereditary Hearing Loss

Hearing disorders can be classified into two types of groups: exogenous (outside the genes) and endogenous (within the genes).

- Exogenous hearing disorders are those caused by toxicity, noise, accident, or injury that damage the inner ear. We have already summarized many exogenous factors of hearing loss in this chapter.
- Endogenous hearing disorders originate in the genes of the individual. An endogenous hearing disorder is transmitted from the parents to the child as an inherited trait. Hearing losses resulting from hereditary

factors comprise a significant number of all hearing disorders.

It is estimated that there are more than 400 different genetic syndromes in which hearing loss is either a regular or occasional feature. During a routine case history with adults, you may encounter various genetically transmitted syndromes that have hearing loss as one of their characteristics. Some patients may have a hearing loss that is genetic that the patient was unaware of because many progress at a very slow rate.

Nonorganic Hearing Loss

There are cases when a hearing loss may be measured on the audiogram, but there is no organic basis to explain the impairment. Some of the terms used to describe this include nonorganic hearing loss, pseudohypocusis, and functional hearing loss. If indeed the patient knowingly is exaggerating their hearing loss, the term malingering is used.

Aside from the cases of malingering (adults' exaggeration of the hearing loss often is related to financial compensation), the reasons for nonorganic hearing loss are not clearly understood. A common population to present with suspected nonorganic responses is teenagers, who often are experiencing other emotional problems, or are having difficulty in school. In some cases, there may be an underlying hearing loss, and the patient is simply adding to it. There are specific audiologic tests that nearly always identify the patient presenting with a nonorganic hearing loss. This frequently leads to very interesting counseling sessions, as some parents would rather believe that their child has a hearing loss, than that their child is pretending to have a hearing loss.

Central Auditory Disorders

There are two ways that we can look at central auditory disorders relative to this chapter. First, we could point out that audiologists rarely test for a central auditory disorders prior to fitting hearing aids, so there is not a lot of reason to discuss them. On the other hand, we could mention that most hearing aids are fitted to older individuals, and many of these have some form of cognitive decline. When we say "central" auditory disorder we are referring to levels above the cochlear nucleus. This could be some type of disease or space-occupying lesion, but most commonly it is a processing deficit of cortical origin. To remind you of the complexities of the central auditory system, we have included Figure 3–7.

You no doubt have heard that the most common complaint from hearing aid users, or prospective hearing aid users, is understanding speech in background noise. What we call "noise" can have two different kinds of masking effects. We first have "energetic masking." This is noise of most any type that "covers up" the desired speech signal. That is, the noise is louder than the speech, at least at some frequencies. Another type of masking is what is referred to as informational or perceptual masking. As the name suggests, in this case, the noise usually is other speech or portions of speech, something that has meaning (talking to someone at a party with background babble, or when the TV is playing in the background). In this case, the noise might not be louder than the desired speech signal, but the brain has trouble separating the wanted speech signal from the unwanted speech signal. As you might guess, this latter type of masking becomes worse as people age, and their central auditory separation abilities decrease.

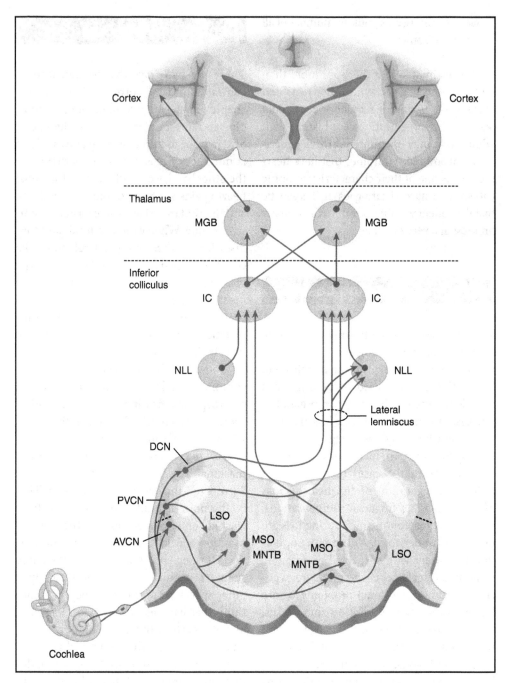

Figure 3–7. An anatomic illustration of the central auditory system. *Source*: From *Comprehensive Dictionary of Audiology: Illustrated* (3rd ed., p. 50), by B. A. Stach, 2019, San Diego, CA: Plural Publishing. Reprinted with permission.

And this becomes worse when cognitive disorders are present.

In Chapter 6, we will review a test that you might see mentioned in audiology reports. The test is called the QuickSIN. It is a test where sentences are delivered at different signal-to-noise levels, with the purpose to determine how much handicap the patient has for understanding speech in background noise. Normal-hearing individuals may score around +2 dB SNR (speech is just 2 dB above the noise), whereas someone with a hearing loss and poor speech-in-noise processing may score +12dB SNR to 16 dB SNR (they need the speech signal to be that much louder than the noise to score 50% correct). Why this test relates to our discussion here is that the background noise for the QuickSIN is not noise, rather four talkers. So indeed, informational masking is in play, and people with cognitive decline do not do well on this test. The results of this test are a relatively good predictor of how someone will do understanding speech in background noise in the real world, and to some extent, it is a central auditory test (although not used as a diagnostic tool to identify specific pathologies).

Hearing Loss, Hearing Aids, and Cognitive Decline

As mentioned, when we work with people with cognitive decline, we often are also are working with an older individual. Within the United States, approximately 5.7 million people are living with dementia. Alzheimer's disease accounts for approximately 60% to 70% of these cases, followed by vascular dementias. These numbers are expected to rise in the next few decades, as life expectancy increases. The older the individual, the more likely he or she will be affected by dementia. It is rare for someone under the age of 65 to have dementia, but approximately 1 in 70 people aged 65 to 69 have this disorder, and nearly 1 in 4 people aged 85 to 89 have dementia. Given the aging demographic of Americans, the number of patients with cognitive concerns will only grow. We also know that approximately one in three people between the ages of 65 and 74 has hearing loss, and nearly half of those older than 75 have difficulty hearing. When comparing these hearing loss data to the dementia prevalence findings, we see that for older individuals, there is a relatively high probability of having *both* dementia and hearing loss. There is also a growing body of literature suggesting some interaction between a person having hearing loss and the likelihood of them also presenting with dementia.

Several factors related to dementia work against successful hearing aid use

- Poor central separation of signals— informational masking has greater impact
- Poor short-term memory—unable to fill in the blanks of missing words fast enough to keep up with conversations
- Listening effort increases—the patient has to work harder to keep up, making communication situations stressful and tiring
- Listening fatigue—the increased effort to keep up leads to listening fatigue, which encourages the patient to "tune out," or simply give up

An expert in this area is Frank Lin, M.D., Ph.D. who is the director of the Cochlear Center for Hearing and Public Health and a Professor of Otolaryngology, Medicine, Mental Health, and Epidemiology at Johns Hopkins. In a recent article (Lin, 2019) he reviews three areas which link cognitive decline to hearing loss. The following is paraphrased from his article.

■ **Cognitive load.** When you can't hear well, the ear is constantly sending a garbled auditory signal to the brain. Does the brain constantly have to work harder to process that poor signal? Is the brain reallocating resources, per se, to constantly dealing with that garbled auditory signal and does it come at the expense of other systems? Cognitive resource capacity is the idea that we have a pool of cognitive resources for thinking, planning, memory. We now know that over time with aging, we can lose some of these resources from things such as synaptic loss of the brain. The brain is constantly having to re-allocate resources to help with deciphering and decoding that much more garbled auditory signal. The prefrontal cortex part of the brain is typically not needed for sound processing, and yet we are seeing an activation of this part of the brain in people with even a mild to moderate hearing loss (as compared to normal hearing individuals). In other words, different regions of the brain are being recruited for auditory and language stimuli in order to compensate for a reduced auditory signal, and the brain needs to expend more effort to decode the signal. This is one pathway through which hearing loss could directly impact cognitive decline and dementia.

■ **Brain structure/function.** A second, related pathway connecting hearing loss with cognitive decline is the idea that hearing loss in and of itself may lead to changes in terms of brain structure and, as a result, brain function. This finding is based on studies conducted on large groups of older adults with hearing loss over many years using brain MRI scans. In several different studies, they found that people with hearing loss have faster rates of brain atrophy. The structural integrity of the brain dictates its function. The two most important conditions that can damage the brain over time are microvascular disease (i.e., small vessel disease from high blood pressure, diabetes, etc.) as well as the more classic Alzheimer's neuropathology.

■ **Social isolation.** The third mechanism which has been hypothesized is the idea that for some people, hearing loss can lead to social isolation problems. In the field of gerontology, studies have repeatedly shown that social isolation is arguably one of the biggest predictors of morbidity and mortality in older adults. Health and behavioral pathways are affected by things such as adherence to medical treatments, as well as smoking, diet, and exercise. In addition, psychological pathways are impacted by a person's self-esteem, self-efficacy, sense of well-being and the ability to cope. Recently, however, one of the more compelling theories is the idea that social isolation or loneliness is directly linked to physiologic changes in the body, which precipitates adverse events. Research has suggested that socially isolated people have an increased upregulation of pro-inflammatory genes and increased inflammation, which causes a lot of adverse events and aging processes in the body.

Considerable research has been conducted searching for the relationship between hearing loss and dementia. What we really don't know is if it's an association, a link, or a causation. As reviewed by Lin (2019), what we do know is that there is some link—and

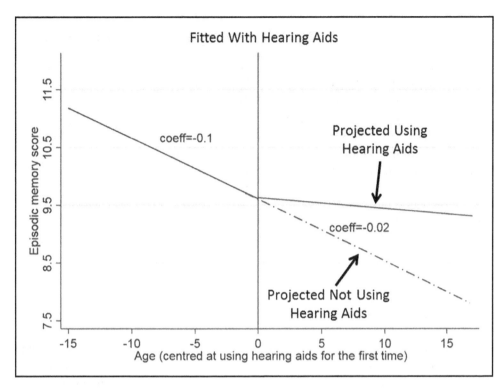

Figure 3–8. Illustration of the projected trajectory decline in memory relative to aging, and the change of trajectory when hearing aids are fitted.

that hearing loss impacts cognition, cognition impacts hearing, and common factors influence both hearing and cognition. One intriguing aspect of this research is the question of whether the fitting of hearing aids will change the predictable downward spiral of cognition for people with hearing loss. The answer might be "yes." We are referring to the recent findings of the large-scale Sense-Cog Project (Dawes, Maharani, Nazroo, Tampubolon, & Pendleton, 2019). Trajectories of cognitive function were plotted based on memory test scores before and after using hearing aids. Adjusting for potential confounders—including gender, education, smoking, alcohol consumption, marital status, employment, physical activities, symptoms of depression, and number of health comorbidities—they found that the rate of cognitive decline on a memory test was slower following the adoption of hearing aids (Figure 3–8). All good news, so stay tuned for further developments.

Syndromes and Disorders Associated with Pediatric Hearing Loss

What we have discussed to this point are pathologies that are relatively common in an audiology clinic, especially if it is affiliated with a medical center. Also, many of these

SCREENERS FOR DEMENTIA FOR THOSE WITH HEARING LOSS

It is within the scope of practice for you to conduct a cognitive screener. Common screeners include the MMSE or the MoCA. Many clinics have moved to using the MoCA as it is freely available. Several studies have suggested that there those with hearing loss may score lower on these verbally presented tests of cognition given that they cannot correctly hear what is being asked of them.

Recently, the HI-MoCA was developed by Lin et al (2017). This freely-available PowerPoint comes with directions and scoring so you can conduct a cognitive screener on patients with hearing loss that was developed for people with hearing loss. The use of this screener would highly improve the accuracy of your cognitive screener in people with hearing loss.

disorders are unique to the adult population. Many of you, however, will encounter children with hearing loss that is associated with a unique syndrome or disorder that perhaps is not common at all. We would like to close this chapter, therefore, with a summary of these.

Since the early 1990s, we've all enjoyed the many editions of the book *Hearing in Children* by Jerry Northern and Marion Downs. Since the first edition, one of the favorite aspects of this book always has been the extensive review of the different syndromes and disorders associated with pediatric hearing loss. The *Hearing in Children* book is now in its 6th edition, and like good wine, it just keeps getting better with age. We are thankful to Dr. Northern for giving us permission to adapt one of the tables from his recent book that summarizes these important syndromes and disorders that are observed in children—see Table 3–4 (Northern & Downs, 2014). This of course is just a summary—you'll want to check out the 50-page, detailed description of each condition in the book itself.

Table 3–4. Hearing Loss—Syndrome and Condition List for Congenital and Progressive Hearing Loss

	Title	Description	Hearing Loss
A	Achondroplasia	Dwarfism, skeletal ossification disorder	Conductive and sensorineural hearing loss
	Albers-Schonberg disease of osteopetrosis	Brittle, thickened, chalky bones	Conductive and sensorineural hearing loss
	Albinism with blue irides	Pigmentation disorder of the eyes, skin, hair	Sensorineural hearing loss
	Alport's syndrome	Nephritis and cataracts	Progressive sensorineural hearing loss
	Apert syndrome	Craniosynostosis, midface anomalies, middle ear involvement	Conductive hearing loss
	Aplasias (errors during embryonic development)		
	Michel aplasia	Complete absence of inner ear and auditory nerve	Sensorineural hearing loss
	Mondini aplasia	Abnormal development of the structure (turns) of the cochlear membrane	Sensorineural hearing loss
	Scheibe aplasia	Abnormal formation of the cochlear membrane	Sensorineural hearing loss
	Asphyxia at birth / neonatal period	Resuscitation required/ poor APGARs, seizures, neurological involvement	Sensorineural hearing loss, auditory neuropathy
B	Bacterial meningitis	Auditory involvement, can have sudden permanent hearing loss	Sensorineural hearing loss, central effects
	Bjornstad syndrome	Dry, brittle, flat, twisted hair	Sensorineural hearing loss
	Branchio-oto-renal syndrome (BOR)	Renal anomalies, auricular pits, pinnae malformations	Conductive, sensorineural, and mixed hearing losses
C	Carraro syndrome	Absence of the tibia bone	Sensorineural hearing loss
	Camurati-Engelmann disease	Skeletal—enlarged diaphysis of the long bones	Conductive and sensorineural hearing loss

continues

Table 3–4. *continued*

Title	Description	Hearing Loss
Chemotherapy medications (mother and baby)	Cisplatin, carboplatin—inner ear hair cells affected	Sensorineural hearing loss
Cerebral palsy	Hypoxic episode during development or birth asphyxia	Sensorineural hearing loss
Craniofacial abnormalities		
Atresia of the ear canal	Atresia, stenosis of the ear channel	Conductive, sensorineural hearing loss/mixed
Absence or malformed pinna	Atresia, stenosis, malformation of the pinnae	Conductive, sensorineural hearing loss/mixed
Cleft palate	Malformation of the hard palate (exclude cleft lip if only feature present)	Conductive hearing loss
CHARGE syndrome	Coloboma (eyes), heart, atresia of the nares, genital, ear (deafness)	Conductive, sensorineural hearing loss, and mixed; can have auditory neuropathy
Cleidocranial dysostosis	Retarded ossification, narrowed auditory canal	Conductive and sensorineural hearing loss
Cockayne's syndrome	Growth failure and neurologic delay, retinal atrophy	Sensorineural hearing loss
Cornelia de Lange syndrome	Small for gestational age, limb malformations, cardiac defects, cleft palate	Conductive, sensorineural, or mixed hearing losses
Crouzon's syndrome	Craniosynostosis, midface anomalies, outer and middle ear defects	Conductive, sensorineural, or mixed (majority are conductive)
D Dwarfism	Skeletal anomalies, shortness, short fingers	Sensorineural hearing loss
Down syndrome	Middle ear anomalies—ossicles, otitis media infections	Conductive, sensorineural, or mixed hearing losses
E Encephalitis	Infection, auditory involvement	Sudden permanent sensorineural hearing loss
Engelmann's syndrome	Bone dysplasia, increased skeletal density affecting auditory function	
F Fanconi's anemia syndrome	Impaired renal transport, growth delay	Sensorineural hearing loss

Table 3–4. *continued*

	Title	Description	Hearing Loss
	Family history of hearing loss	Permanent hearing loss evident in early infancy >6 years	Conductive or sensorineural
	Fetal alcohol syndrome	Low birth weight, skeletal anomalies, cleft palate, pinnae anomalies	Conductive and sensorineural hearing loss
	Fraser syndrome	Adherent eyelids, external ear malformations, syndactyly	Conductive and sensorineural hearing loss
	Friedreich ataxia	Progressive ataxia, cataracts	Sensorineural hearing loss
G	Goldenhar's syndrome	Eye, ear, and mouth anomalies	Conductive hearing loss or sensorineural hearing loss
H	Hemifacial microsomia	Abnormal development on one side of the face, atresia/stenosis canal	Conductive hearing loss or sensorineural hearing loss
	Hermann's syndrome	Late onset of disease; epilepsy, speech, ataxia, renal disease	Sensorineural hearing loss
	Hyperbilirubinemia	Dampening of the auditory nerve function due to excessive bilirubin	Sensorineural hearing loss, may have auditory neuropathy
	Hypoxic ischaemic encephalopathy (HIE)	Severe aphyxia with neurological sequalae, hypotonic limbs, significant morbidity	Sensorineural hearing loss, may have auditory neuropathy
	Hydrocephalus	Intraventricular hemorrhage (grades 3 and 4), internal cranial anomalies, eighth cranial nerve involvement	Sensorineural hearing loss
	Hunter's and Hurler's syndrome	Progressive manifestation of coarse facial features	Mixed hearing loss
I	**Infections**		
	Cytomegalovirus	Herpes virus 5, microcephaly, hepatosplenomegaly, jaundice, intrauterine growth retardation	Sensorineural hearing loss

continues

Table 3–4. *continued*

	Title	Description	Hearing Loss
	Herpes	Congenital neonatal herpes infection HSV-1 and 2, high mortality	Sensorineural hearing loss
	Rubella	Low birth weight, purpura, jaundice, organ of Corti degeneration	Sensorineural hearing loss
	Toxoplasmosis	Parasitic infection, chorioretinitis, cerebral calcification, convulsions	Sensorineural hearing loss
	Syphilis	Nasal discharge, rash, anemia, jaundice, osteochondritis	Sensorineural hearing loss
	Intraventricular hemorrhage (IVH)	Bleeding within the brain structures causing adverse neurological complications	Sensorineural hearing loss and central effects
J	Jervell and Lange-Nielsen syndrome	Cardiovascular disorder, fainting, sudden death is a feature, auditory involvement	Sensorineural hearing loss
K	Keratopachyderma and digital constrictions nephrosis	Pigment disorder, may include renal disease	Sensorineural hearing loss
	Klippel-Feil syndrome	Craniofacial and skeletal disorder, short neck, cleft, poorly developed inner ear structures	Conductive and sensorineural hearing loss
L	Laurence-Moon-Biedl-Bardet syndromes	Retinitis pigmentosa, polydactyly	Sensorineural hearing loss
	LEOPARD syndrome (multiple lentigines syndrome)	Pigment disorder, café au lait spots, cardiac, ocular, genital, growth delay	Sensorineural hearing loss
	Long QT syndrome	Cardiac condition	
M	Marshall syndrome	Short stature, skeletal defects, cataracts	Sensorineural hearing loss
	Meningitis	Inner hair cells in cochlear damaged by virus	Sensorineural hearing loss
	Mitochondrial disorders	DNA—maternal inheritance pattern	

Table 3–4. *continued*

	Title	Description	Hearing Loss
	Moeibus (Mobius) syndrome	Connective tissue disorder, facial paralysis; cranial nerves 6 and 7, middle ear anomalies	Conductive and sensorineural hearing loss
	Muckle-Wells syndrome	Onset in teens, urticaria, renal failure	Sensorineural hearing loss
N	Neurofibromatosis type II	Intracranial tumors, eighth cranial nerve, acoustic neuroma	Sensorineural hearing loss
	Noonan's syndrome	See Leopard syndrome, café au lait spots	Sensorineural hearing loss
	Norries syndrome	Eye disorder, auditory impairment	Sensorineural hearing loss
O	Oculo-auriculo-vertebralia spectrum (OAV)	Facial asymmetry, anomalies of external, middle ear, cranial nerve	Sensorineural hearing loss and central effects
	Optic atrophy and polyneuropathy	Progressive visual loss, polyneuropathy in childhoods	Sensorineural hearing loss (progressive)
	Ototoxic medication—affecting inner ear hair cells	Neomycin, amikacin, gentamycin, kanamycin, sisomicin, tobramycin, dibekacin, steptomycin	Sensorineural hearing loss
		Furosemide (loop diuretic used in conjunction with antibiotics); quinine—malarial treatment	Sensorineural hearing loss
	Osteogenesis imperfecta	"Brittle bones," stapes malformation	Conductive hearing loss and sensorineural hearing loss
P	Paget's disease	Juvenile skeletal disorder, bone pain, swelling	Progressive mixed hearing loss
	Persistent pulmonary hypertension of the newborn (PPHN)	Ventilation, progressive hypoxia, persistent fetal circulation	Sensorineural hearing loss and central effects
	Pierre Robin syndrome	Craniofacial anomaly, micrognathia, glossoptosis, may have cleft palate	Conductive and sensorineural hearing loss

continues

Table 3–4. *continued*

	Title	Description	Hearing Loss
	Periauricular abnormalities	Periauricular pits, tags, fistulas, ear canal atresia, facial paralysis	Conductive or sensorineural
	Periventricular leukomalacia (PVL)	Ischemic cystic changes in the brain matter predisposing to cerebral palsy	
	Piebaldness	Lack of pigment in hair, ataxia, blue irides	Sensorineural hearing loss
	Pendred's syndrome	Thyroid goiter—iodine imbalance in inner hair cells	Sensorineural hearing loss
	Pyle's syndrome	Enlargement and sclerosis of the facial bones, ribs, clavicles	Sensorineural hearing loss
Q			
R	Refsum's syndrome	Organ of Corti degeneration, inner ear anomalies, eye disorder	Progressive sensorineural hearing loss
	Richards-Rundle syndrome	Central nervous system disorder, ataxia muscle wasting	Progressive sensorineural hearing loss
S	Stickler syndrome	Flattened facial profile, cleft palate, ocular changes	Conductive and sensorineural hearing loss
T	Treacher Collins syndrome	Head and neck anomalies, atresia of canal, abnormal middle ear	Conductive hearing loss
	Trisomy 21 (Down syndrome)	Recurrent middle ear infections	Conductive and sensorineural hearing loss
	Trisomy 13–15 and 18	High mortality rate	Conductive or sensorineural hearing loss
	Turner's syndrome	Gonadal dysgenesis, webbed neck and digits, micrognathia	Conductive and sensorineural hearing loss
U	Usher's syndrome	Retinitis pigmentosa, tunnel vision, vertigo, organ of Corti degeneration	Sensorineural hearing loss

Table 3–4. *continued*

	Title	Description	Hearing Loss
V	Ventilation	Mechanical ventilation for longer than five days, increased neonatal risks	Sensorineural hearing loss
	Van der Hoeve's syndrome	"Brittle bone," stapes malformation	Conductive and sensorineural hearing loss
	Vohwinkel-Nockemann syndrome	See Keratopachyderma reference above	Sensorineural hearing loss (may be progressive)
	Von Reckinghausen's syndrome	Hyperkeratosis of palms, soles, knees, elbows, acoustic neuroma, renal	Sensorineural hearing loss
W	Waardenburg's syndrome (types 1 and 2)	White forelock, iris color different in one eye, prominent mandible, cleft	Sensorineural hearing loss
	Wildervanck's syndrome	Dysmorphic facial features, atresia of ear canals, eyeball retraction	Sensorineural hearing loss or mixed
	Winter syndrome	Renal anomalies, genital malformation, malformed ear and canals	Conductive hearing loss
XYZ			
References		*John Muir Medical Centre, USA, Hearing Loss Indication List 2000; Patricia Gillilan, Audiologist, USA; Northern and Downs Text, Hearing in Children 5th ed., 2002; Newton, Paediatric Audiological Medicine, 2002.*	
Reviewed May 2007; amended March 2012		*Delene Thomas, RBWH, Coordinator HHP; Katrina Roberts, TTH, Coordinator HHP; Kelly Nicholls, RCH, Audiologist; Jackie Moon, MMH, Audiologist; Shree Aithal, TTH, Audiologist.*	
Reviewed August 2013; amended September 2013		*Delene Thomas, Area Coordinator HHP; Rachael Beswick, Audiologist Advanced, HHP.*	

Source: From *Hearing in Children* (6th ed.), by J. L. Northern and M. Downs, 2014, San Diego, CA: Plural Publishing. Reprinted with permission.

4 Hearing Aid Styles and Fitting Applications

In the preceding chapters, we have discussed the different pathologies that might cause hearing loss, provided you a review of the routine audiologic evaluation and how different tests relate to the selection and fitting of hearing aids. It's now time to get down to business, and start talking about the hearing aid itself. When a patient decides that they are ready to try hearing aids, one of the first things we do is sit down and make a few collaborative decisions. Often, the first of these is selecting the best hearing aid style. Although the signal processing of the hearing aid is of utmost concern, packaging this processing in an unacceptable style can lead to rejection of amplification—we'll talk about the signal processing in the next chapter.

Although the most obvious differences in hearing aid styles are cosmetic (size and shape), it is important to understand that style choices also impact hearing aid acoustics, comfort, and ease of use. There are several benefits and limitations that are tied to hearing aid style that are unrelated to cosmetics. It often is the audiologist's job to strike a reasonable balance between *form* and *function*. You might wonder why you have a patient who doesn't have a telecoil. The patient is now asking why they can't use the loop in the local heritage center. It could have been a slip-up by the dispensing audiologist, but it very likely could have been that the patient stated or the audiologist assumed that they wanted the smallest aid possible—hearing aids with telecoils are nearly always a little bigger.

We start by considering the look and physical characteristics of different hearing aid styles. Then, we continue by discussing bilateral versus unilateral fittings, and reviewing fittings aimed at specific special populations and applications. Despite differences in style, hearing aids share several commonalities. At their most basic levels, all hearing aids include three stages that can be generally described as follows:

- The sound pickup stage usually consists of a microphone or telecoil. Most commonly this is located on top of the ear in a behind-the-ear (BTE) instrument.
- The sound processing and amplification stage is where the bulk of the signal processing work is conducted to change the signal into the desired level.
- The sound delivery stage primarily is made up of a tiny loudspeaker (along with supporting processing) referred to as a receiver. Instead of a receiver, the output stage may include a vibrating oscillator that stimulates the cochlea through bone conduction or a variety of other specialized transducers including those associated with middle ear implants (which we talk about later in Chapter 7).

Although there may be multiple goals, which we detail in the next chapter, the primary function of the electronic components and sound processing is to work together to increase the amplitude in a frequency-specific manner. The frequency-specific increase in sound level for a signal at the output of a hearing aid, in comparison with the sound level at the input, is referred to as *gain*. When we fit hearing aids, we apply the amount of gain that provides us with the desired output in the ear canal. In general, the softer the input, the more gain is needed, and hearing aids do this automatically when programmed correctly.

Unilateral Versus Bilateral Amplification

At some point in the hearing aid selection process, a joint decision must be made between the clinician and the patient regarding whether one or two hearing aids will be fitted. This sometimes is dictated by the audiogram (hearing in one ear is either too good or too bad for hearing aid use), but the majority of patients (e.g., 85% to 90%) are potential candidates for bilateral amplification. Although the intuitive notion that two ears are better than one is usually true, there are a few patients with bilateral hearing loss who do not benefit from bilateral amplification, and not all patients who do benefit want to wear two hearing aids.

It might be surprising to you that bilateral fittings have not always been embraced by audiologists, and certainly not by the medical professionals. As recent as the early 1970s, it was common for audiologists to tell patients that a single hearing aid was adequate, and in some cases, when the patient returned from a dispenser (hearing instrument specialist) wearing two hearing aids, the audiologist accused the dispenser of simply trying to double the profit. Contributing to the *unilateral-is-okay* belief was a 1975

ruling by the Federal Trade Commission regarding the hearing aid industry, which stated:

No seller shall prepare, approve, fund, disseminate, or cause the dissemination of any advertisement which makes any representation that the use of two hearing aids, one in each ear, will be beneficial to persons with a hearing loss in both ears, unless it is clearly and conspicuously disclosed that many persons with a hearing loss in both ears will not receive greater benefits from the use of two aids, one in each ear, than the use of one hearing aid.

The importance for children to be fitted bilaterally, however, was beginning to be widely accepted about this time, and the general understanding of bilateral fittings then gradually transferred to adults. It was not until the 1990s, however, that the majority of people in the United States were fitted bilaterally. Current estimates are that 74% of the U.S. fittings are bilateral. This of course does not mean that they are using two hearing aids, or even using *one* hearing aid. However, current data does suggest that most people (72%) who report owning hearing aids use them daily.

Potential Advantages of Bilateral Amplification

There are several benefits of *binaural hearing*, and many of these benefits will be experienced with *bilateral fittings*. These benefits are assuming that the user is an individual who is a reasonable bilateral candidate from an audiometric standpoint. That is, there must be aidable hearing in both ears, adequate speech recognition and central processing ability, and not too much asymmetry. How much is too much asymmetry? A rule of thumb is that we would like to have the *aided* speech signals within 15 dB of each other. We would expect the greatest bilateral benefit when the amplified signals are relatively equal. With that in mind, we'll review the primary bilateral benefits. While it's unlikely that you will be the professional to decide if it should be one versus two hearing aids (unless you're helping out a family member), you may have a patient asking about it, or you might need some ammunition to encourage a patient to use both hearing aids.

KEY CONCEPT: Bilateral Versus Binaural

You may have noticed that in our discussion here and in other chapters that both the words bilateral and binaural have been used in reference to hearing with two ears. There is an important difference, however, between these two terms. When we refer to the auditory system, we use the terms binaural hearing and monaural hearing. The concepts of binaural hearing, and the related advantages, are mostly based on research with normal-hearing individuals. When we are talking about hearing aids, we use the terms bilateral fittings and unilateral fittings. For example, if you presented the same speech signal to both ears (referred to as a diotic presentation), your patient would have *bilateral* processing, but not the same phase and amplitude differences observed in *binaural* processing. In general, you can presume a *bilateral fitting* improves *binaural hearing*, but this is not always the case, which is why we have this differentiation.

KEY CONCEPT: Hearing Aid Versus Hearing Aids (with an "s")

The majority of patients have a bilateral hearing loss, and are best served with a bilateral fitting. You are likely to work with many patients who have hearing loss and are not wearing hearing aids. You might hear questions like, "So, do you think I need a hearing aid?" But rarely do they say, "Do you think I need a pair of hearing aids?" Why is this? Perhaps they have a friend who only uses one? Perhaps they have a mild loss and think two hearing aids are only for people with severe loss? Maybe it is simply wishful thinking (one hearing aid is less hassle, less money). We have found, however, that a common reason is that the patient has been told at one time or another that they only need one hearing aid. Maybe not directly, but they have heard the word *aid* used in the singular rather than the plural form. For example, the family physician said, "Your hearing is getting worse; I think you probably need a hearing *aid.*" So what is our point? Like most things that come in pairs (e.g., eyeglasses, shoes, chopsticks, and turtle doves), using the plural term *hearing aids* or *pair of hearing aids* early on in your discussions with patients might reduce the need for extended counseling down the road.

Elimination of the Head-Shadow Effect

Sounds arriving from one side of the head, particularly high-frequency sounds important for understanding speech, are reduced or attenuated by 10 dB to 15 dB for reception in the opposite ear. In the case of a unilateral fitting, patients may then still lack important audibility if they are not able to turn their head to face the talker when the origin is from their unaided ear. Assuming a relatively symmetrical hearing loss, a bilateral fitting will eliminate the head shadow effect. This will have an impact on speech understanding, as the patient no longer has a bad side.

Loudness Summation

This refers to the auditory system's ability to integrate and fuse sounds from each ear. That is, the sound level has to be reduced to produce the same loudness when listening with two ears in comparison to listening with one. Much of the research on this topic has been conducted with people with normal hearing, but the results for individuals with cochlear hearing loss appear to be similar. In general, summation effects become greater as a function of the degree that the signal occurs above the person's threshold. At threshold, summation effects are 2 dB to 3 dB, but summation may be 6 dB to 8 dB, or even higher at suprathreshold levels (depending on symmetry, individual variances, listening paradigm, and input level).

Improved Auditory Localization

We discuss auditory localization later in this chapter. In brief, localization requires the comparison of phase and amplitude differences between the two ears to determine the location of a sound. Research has clearly shown that this is accomplished more effectively in a bilateral fitting than in a unilateral one. In fact, a person with a mild–moderate symmetrical hearing loss could have worse localization after being *aided unilaterally*, then when they were unaided, especially when they are first fitted. There is evidence to show that it is possible that patients with mild-to-moderate hearing loss who are fitted bilaterally may have localization ability rivaling that of those with normal hearing (Mueller et al, 2017).

Improved Speech Understanding in Noise

Bilateral amplification and binaural processing allows for an improvement in speech understanding in background noise. We expect this advantage to be a 2 dB to 3 dB improvement in the SNR. There are two factors that account for this:

- Binaural redundancy: There is an advantage of hearing the same signal in both ears. The brain essentially has two chances of extracting the correct information.
- Binaural squelch: Through central auditory processing, the brain can compare two individual speech-in-noise signals, and the result will be a fused signal with a better SNR than either of the two.

Clinicians are sometimes tempted to conduct aided speech testing in the clinic to demonstrate the benefits of two versus one hearing aid. While this may sound logical, the findings are not meaningful for the following reasons:

- We would only expect to see the bilateral advantage when noise is present and the listening task is difficult. For a test such as monosyllables in quiet, we would expect the outcome to be no better than that of the best ear.

■ We would only expect the bilateral benefit to be obtained if the person was in a distributed noise field and the noise was uncorrelated (e.g., a typical real-world environment). Most clinics do not have the sound field loudspeaker arrangement or recorded speech and noise material to conduct this type of testing.

■ The bilateral benefit we are observing is small, and may be smaller than the test–retest and critical differences of the speech material used.

The bottom line—if you see a report where bilateral versus unilateral aided speech testing was conducted in the clinic, view any differences between conditions with skepticism.

Improved Sound Quality and Better Spatial Balance

If you have ever compared one versus two earphones while listening to your iPod, we do not have to tell you that bilateral listening provides better sound quality than unilateral. There is a sense of fullness, and the sound seems in your head rather than at the ear. This also applies to the hearing impaired and the use of hearing aids.

It is difficult to measure *spatial balance* in the clinic, but what we mean by this is the general sense of being in sync with your surroundings. A realistic acoustic scene. We frequently hear from bilateral hearing aid users who had to be without one hearing aid because of a repair issue that they felt *unbalanced* by only wearing one hearing aid. Some research has reported that when

individuals compared two versus one hearing aid in the real world, *balance* was the leading reason for preferring the bilateral fitting.

Avoidance of the Unaided Ear Effect

We recall hearing stories from the 1970s of unscrupulous hearing aid dealers telling potential customers that they needed to buy two hearing aids because if they only used one, the other ear would become lazy and their hearing in that ear would get worse. Once viewed as merely a sales tactic, science now tells us that there was some truth to what these salesmen were saying. Research from the 1980s revealed that a sizeable percent of people who once had a symmetrical hearing loss and symmetrical word recognition scores (such as that discussed in Chapter 2), suffered a reduction in word recognition in the unaided ear after being aided unilaterally for several years (with no significant change in pure-tone thresholds). Other studies have shown that this effect occurs for about 25% of unilateral hearing aid users.

This effect often has been referred to as auditory deprivation, or late onset auditory deprivation, although we prefer the term *unaided ear effect*. The reason for this is that it does not seem to happen unless only one ear is aided. People with a bilateral hearing loss who are *not* fitted with a hearing aid in either ear do not experience *deprivation*, even though their hearing loss is the same as the unaided ear of the people who were fitted unilaterally. Why is this? Part of it indeed may be due to deprivation. When people start wearing a hearing aid in one ear, their world generally becomes softer (people do not have to talk to them as loud, the TV is softer, etc.). Hence, there probably is less audibility for the unaided ear than if they were not wearing a hearing aid. But also, the use of amplification in one ear leads to a mismatch in central timing, with the aided ear having the stronger signal. Over time, the brain may become more dominant—some type of plasticity—for the stronger signal and pay less attention to the signal from the weaker ear. Regardless of the cause, the effect rarely occurs in bilateral fittings.

Potential Contraindications for Bilateral Amplification

Although there certainly are many reasons to think of the routine fitting as bilateral, there also are some reasons why a unilateral fitting might be the best choice. We have listed the most common:

- Degree of hearing loss: Simply put, to be a candidate for bilateral hearing aid amplification, the hearing for each ear cannot be too good or too bad.
- Cost: Hearing aids are expensive—the premier models with all the latest technology commonly sell for $6,000/ pair or more. In many clinics, the cost of two entry-level products is about the same as one premier product, so that is an option. But, even two entry-level hearing aids might be more than many people can afford. This of course is what has led to the new over-the-counter hearing aid category. We'll see how that goes.
- Stigma: Some patients believe that two hearing aids make them appear more impaired to their friends and colleagues—"I'm not that bad off, I don't have to wear two" (although the very same patient does not wear a monocle).

- Convenience: Some patients have considerable trouble putting the hearing aids in and taking them out, changing batteries, and making adjustments. Some consider the wearing of a hearing aid uncomfortable or annoying. A bilateral fitting doubles the problems.
- Binaural interference: There is a small portion of the population (approximately 5%–10%) who has a reduction in speech recognition when they experience bilateral amplification, versus using only one hearing aid. Believed to be due to an auditory processing deficit, this is referred to as binaural interference (Note: they would still have all the other benefits of bilateral amplification). Binaural interference is a type of APD that was discussed previously in Chapter 3.

Hearing Aid Styles

Hearing aid styles have been grouped in various ways throughout history. The most common grouping scheme is based on where the amplifier is worn, discussed by Mueller et al. (2017), and our review here parallels their descriptions. Specifically, instruments are categorized as body aids, behind-the-ear (BTE) or over-the-ear (OTE), eyeglass BTE, in-the-ear (ITE), in-the-canal (ITC), and completely-in-the-canal (CIC). The last three types mentioned are also referred to as "custom instruments" (in most cases, the workings of the hearing aid are placed in a custom-made shell for the patient). The most commonly fitted style today is the mini-BTE, which has the receiver placed in the ear canal. This has become known as a RIC (pronounced Rick, not R-I-C), for receiver-in-canal. These of course are BTEs, but they have developed their own category.

This classification scheme is commonly used by organizations such as the Hearing Industries Association (HIA) when they report the percentage of hearing aids sold for each style. Currently, in the United States, BTEs in general account for 80% of all hearing aid sales—the majority of this total are RIC instruments, which alone account for 63%. The other 20% of total sales are custom instruments, with the following breakdown: ITEs = 9%, ITCs = 6%, and CICs = 5%. It is difficult to determine if the popular mini-BTE RICs earned their popularity because they are preferred by audiologists, preferred by patients, or because manufacturers only make much of their advanced technology available in the RIC style.

If we consider the functional differences of today's hearing aids, then they tend to break down into larger classifications such as body hearing aids, traditional BTE, mini-BTE, traditional custom, and smaller custom products such as CIC instruments.

Body Hearing Aids

This style partially is included for historical reasons, although there are still one or two manufacturers that produce it. Body aids, as you might guess from the name, are worn on the body. They are relatively large and include a box-like case (approximately 2 in. high by 2 in. wide by 0.5 in. thick) that contains the microphone and amplification stages, and a receiver that is worn in the ear and is attached to the case by a cord. Access to the hearing aid battery and user controls—including the volume control wheel and the on and off switch—are provided on the case surface, usually on the top and/or bottom. The case can be worn in a variety of positions including on a cord around

the neck, in a shirt pocket, or attached to another part of the user's clothing.

Functionally, body aids are different than all others in that the microphone is worn on the body. The fact that the microphone is not near the position of the ear is not optimal because picking up sound at, or very near, the normal position of the two tympanic membranes is necessary for the brain to process signals binaurally. Binaural processing of sound is necessary for optimal sound localization and also can assist with speech understanding in background noise, as described earlier in this chapter. Partially because of these concerns, the body-aid style is rarely recommended by current practitioners. Inexpensive rechargeable body aids are used, however, in some underdeveloped countries.

Traditional Behind-the-Ear (BTE) Hearing Aids

By the mid-1970s, most people were wearing the BTE style because it offered several advantages over its body-worn counterpart. In BTE hearing aids, all the electronics are inside a plastic case that is fitted behind the ear. Access to the hearing aid battery and user controls are provided on the case surface, usually on the back and/or bottom. Sound is routed from the receiver through an ear hook that also is used to help retention. The sound is then directed to the ear through tubing and a custom-made earmold, shown in Figure 4–1.

An added advantage to the BTE design is that the earmold, tubing, and ear hook all can be used to modify the frequency response of the amplified signal. The microphone port in the BTE is nearer to the position of the tympanic membrane, as it is usually positioned between the case and the ear hook placing it on top of the pinna when

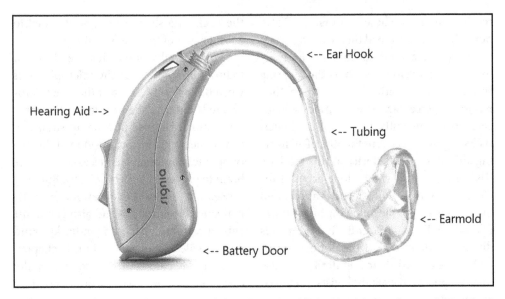

Figure 4–1. External features of a standard BTE hearing aid with tubing and earmold attached. This type of hearing aid is most commonly used for severe losses and with children. Most adults are fitted with a mini-BTE, which also has much thinner tubing to the earmold. *Source*: Photo courtesy of Signia.

worn. This provides the potential for some binaural cues. This design also provides the greatest separation between the sound output (at the end of the tube in the ear) and the hearing aid microphone. Therefore, when used with an appropriate earmold and modern feedback suppression, this style is able to provide adequate amplification without the presence of feedback for most any magnitude of hearing loss for which a listener is expected to benefit from amplification.

The larger size of the traditional BTE case also makes it possible to apply various other technologies. These include strong telecoils and direct auditory input (DAI). Improved miniaturization also has allowed for frequency modulated (FM) receivers to be attached directly to a BTE via a boot, shown in Figure 4–2, or be directly integrated into the BTE case. Because traditional BTEs can provide considerable amplification, are relatively large and easy to manipulate, and have a high degree of flexibility, they are

appropriate for a wide range of hearing losses and populations. Clinically, however, their most common use is for adults with severe or greater hearing loss and in children.

The fact that only the earmold is custom fitted to the ear and it contains no electronics also provides other advantages for the BTE style. Specifically, for children who are still experiencing growth of their ear canals, the earmold can be remade relatively inexpensively without requiring any change to the hearing aid itself—at some ages, this is necessary every three months or so. In addition, the separation of the electronic components from the warm, moist, cerumen-producing environment of the ear canal can lead to improved durability. This is important because cerumen clogging the receiver continues to be the number one cause of hearing aid repairs for ITE, ITC, RIC, and CIC styles. The BTE tubing can still become clogged with moisture and debris, but it can be cleaned out or changed without approach-

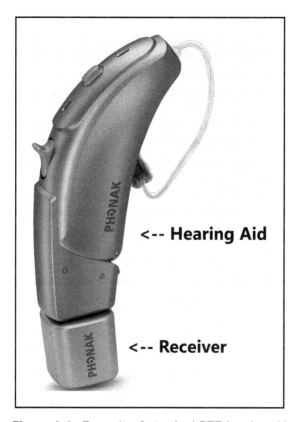

Figure 4–2. Example of standard BTE hearing aid with FM receiver. Note boot attached that is designed to snap onto the bottom of the hearing aid for reception of FM signals. *Source*: Image © Sonova AG. Reproduced here with permission. All rights reserved.

ing any of the electronic components. Finally, an advantage of the BTE style over custom instruments is that they can be stocked in the clinic. This means that if necessary (or desired), a stock ear piece can be used, and the patient can be fitted with a pair of hearing aids on the same day he or she walked in the door for a diagnostic exam.

Although traditional BTEs are among the largest of the hearing aid styles, it should be pointed out that they are not necessarily the least cosmetically appealing. The right hair style, especially those styles that cover the top of the pinna, in conjunction with the use of a clear earmold and tubing can result in an instrument that is actually much less

visible than some of the custom styles such as the ITE, which completely fill the concha with colored plastic. Moreover, as we discuss later, it is now common to use barely noticeable thin tubing with mini-BTEs, and there are adaptors that allow the use of this thin tubing with the larger BTEs, making the overall fitting even less noticeable.

Eyeglass BTEs

Functionally, most *eyeglass* hearing aids also fall into the category of traditional BTEs. What are often termed eyeglass hearing aids are simply a BTE that is integrated into the temple (or bow) of eyeglasses. This style reached the height of its popularity in the 1960s, particularly in the VA/Military health-care system. In some respects, the notion was logical—most people who used hearing aids also used eyeglasses, so why not have an all-in-one product? Some even saw this as a cosmetic advantage, as it was more accepted to wear glasses than hearing aids. There were problems with this style from the beginning, however. These products were heavy and uncomfortable, and did not stay adjusted. Many people needed to keep their glasses on to see well enough to change the battery. Maintenance also was a big problem, as patients would be missing their eyeglasses while their hearing aids were repaired—people did not own several pairs of glasses in the 1960s as they do now. The bottom line—the idea did not go over as well as combining a camera with a cell phone!

The BTE/eyeglass style is rarely recommended today. Reduced use of eyeglasses because of increases in contact lenses and vision surgery, changes in popular eyeglass styles leading to very thin temples, and the general miniaturization of other styles of hearing aids have further contributed to the decline of the eyeglass style. A few models of eyeglass hearing aids are still available, however. Miniaturization has led to modern eyeglass hearing aids that are much more compact than their counterparts of the 1960s.

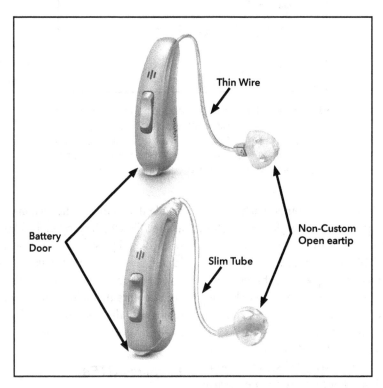

Figure 4–3. Two examples of mini-BTE hearing aids. The upper instrument is the most popular of the two, a receiver-in-canal (RIC). The lower instrument is slightly larger, as it has the receiver in the hearing aid. Both types utilize very thin tubing going to the earmold, which in this case is a modular open ear tip. *Source*: Photo courtesy of Sivantos GmbH or its affiliates © 2019. All rights reserved.

Mini-BTEs

A more recent incarnation of the traditional BTE instrument is the mini-BTE hearing aid. As the name suggests, these hearing aids are significantly smaller than traditional BTEs but do fit behind the ear. Some have the receiver in the hearing aid, but nearly all of these have the receiver in the canal (RIC). As the name indicates, this is a small BTE case, which is coupled to a thin wire that attaches to a small external receiver that is placed in the ear canal. This receiver is then coupled to the ear using a custom or non-custom eartip. The advantage of the RIC is that because the receiver is removed from the case, the case can be made somewhat smaller, and more unique designs can be implemented. Also, larger receivers can be coupled to the hearing aid to provide more power. Examples of a RIC product are shown in the top portion of Figure 4–3. While indeed the hearing aid itself is smaller, another factor that has led to cosmetic acceptance is the use of the very thin wire (encased in a tube) leading from the hearing aid to the ear (Figure 4–4). The mini-BTE RIC style accounts for 63% of all hearing aid sold, and about 80% of the BTE market.

Although we usually think that with hearing aids, small is good, some patients have trouble handling these mini-BTEs. The small

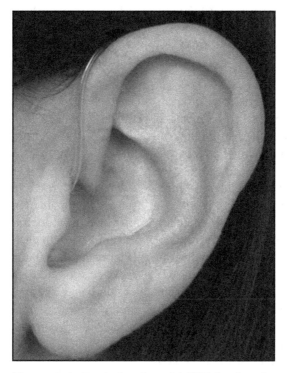

Figure 4–4. Example of a mini-BTE fitted to the ear. Notice that because of the thin tubing utilized, it is difficult to even determine that the hearing aid is in place. This is considerably more cosmetically appealing than the once popular ITE, which filled much of the concha. *Source*: Photo courtesy of Unitron. All rights reserved.

CLINICAL TIP: Oh No . . . Another Plugged Receiver!

If you talk to an audiologist who fits a lot of hearing aids, and you ask him or her what drives them "nuts," there is a good chance they will say *plugged receivers*. They also might add that the patients with this problem tend to bring in their nonfunctioning hearing aid at 4:30 p.m. on Friday afternoon. As we've reviewed, RIC hearing aids are very popular, and are becoming more popular each year. You don't need a PhD in electronics or chemistry to figure out that it's not a good idea to place a miniature finely-tuned electrical component (the hearing aid receiver) in a damp, gooey place (the ear canal).

So, to no one's surprise, with the RIC product, there is a tendency for the receivers to become plugged with cerumen. If you are working with a patient who wears the RIC product, and they tell you that their hearing aid is "dead," you can bet that the receiver is plugged. We say plugged, but this isn't something that you can just clean, it requires a replacement receiver. So what is the solution? Some audiologists give their patients replacement receivers, and if the patient is savvy enough, they can replace them themselves. In most cases, however, this problem prompts a clinic visit—most audiologists have spare receivers and sometimes can do the replacement while the patient waits. In other instances, the aid needs to be sent back to the manufacturer.

---

size of the case also presents some problems regarding what controls can be included. Many products do not have a volume control. Also, there is not room for a strong telecoil, or for some, any telecoil. If the RIC style is used, there sometimes are additional problems related to placing a large receiver in patients with small ear canals (particularly when high levels of amplification are required). Finally, an emerging trend is for hearing aids to be rechargeable (>50% of mini-BTE market). In general, these rechargeable mini-BTEs are slightly larger than the mini-BTEs that use very small batteries. Maybe we should call the later mini-mini-BTEs.

When first introduced, marketing experts believed these mini-BTE products would attract a younger hearing aid user, and this appears to be somewhat true. Given the same degree of hearing loss, market penetration for younger individuals is only about one-quarter of what it is for older individuals.

There is a general movement to make these smaller hearing aids more fun and less old looking. To assist in attracting the younger generation (e.g., baby boomers), these hearing aids come in a wide range of designs and colors. A design introduced recently makes the product a little longer and much slimmer, making it look more like some kind of cool Bluetooth device than a hearing aid (Figure 4–5). Some manufacturers have replaced the traditional BTE color names of tan, beige, and brown with names like crème brûlée, champagne, granite, snow blade, flower power, and pinot noir!

Traditional Custom Instruments

As advances in electronic circuitry continued, manufacturers were able to reduce further the size of the hearing aid and began developing custom hearing aids such as the

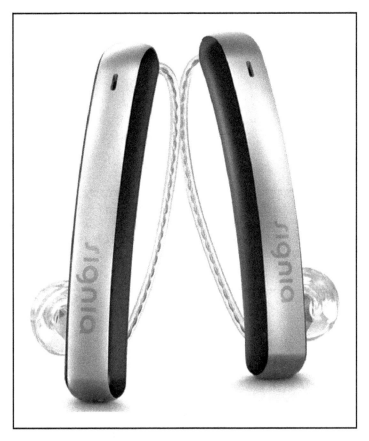

Figure 4–5. Example of a unique mini-BTE design, where the hearing aid resembles a Bluetooth device. Rather than the traditional hearing aid shades of brown/beige, these instruments come in black, cobalt blue, and white gold. *Source*: Photo courtesy of Sivantos GmbH or its affiliates © 2019. All rights reserved.

ITE and a more recessed version called the ITC. For simplicity, we are going to call them traditional customs (TC). The TC actually includes several sizes between and including ITE and ITC, as shown in Figure 4–6. Functionally, most ITE and ITC styles are similar enough for our purposes, to fit into the TC category, although there are clear size and cosmetic differences. Although ITEs were developed in the 1960s, these early instruments were generally of poor quality. As a result of improved miniaturization, however, the quality of these instruments is now essentially identical to their larger siblings, and currently, many of the physical components and processing used in BTEs and TCs are the same.

During the 1980s, the percentage of people purchasing all styles of custom hearing aids, including TC and those described in the following sections, quickly grew from 34% in 1980 to approximately 80% of total hearing aid sales by 1990. Improved cosmetics in comparison with the BTE style is the most often cited reason for this rapid increase in popularity. It was not just cosmetics, however, but rather, the custom product was considered to be the *modern*

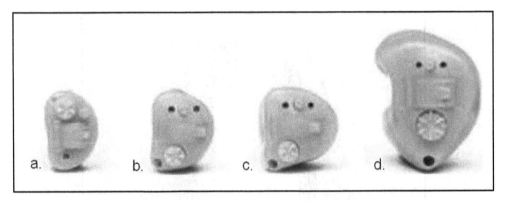

Figure 4–6. Example of four different custom instruments, ranging from the smallest CIC to the largest full-concha ITE. *Source*: From *Essentials of Modern Hearing Aids: Selection, Fitting, and Verification* (p. 248), by T. A. Ricketts, R. Bentler, and H. G. Mueller, 2019, San Diego, CA: Plural Publishing. Reprinted with permission.

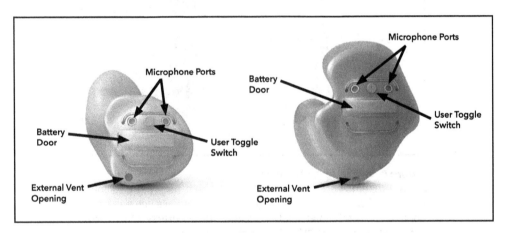

Figure 4–7. External features and controls of a full-concha hearing aid. *Source*: Photo courtesy of Sivantos GmbH or its affiliates © 2019. All rights reserved.

hearing aid, and anything behind the ear was old-fashioned. In recent times, however, the dominance of custom hearing aids has eroded with the introduction and increasing popularity of mini-BTE products, which we just discussed in the preceding section— strangely enough, the standard custom product is now considered old-fashioned.

Like the BTE style, all the TC hearing aid electronics are contained within a plastic case. However, with TC instruments, the plastic case is small enough that it can be placed in the ear, usually within an earshell

that is fabricated from an impression made of the individual patient's ear and covered with a faceplate that provides access to the battery and any user controls, as shown in Figure 4–7. With traditional custom hearing aids, the microphone port opening is on the instrument's faceplate near the position of the natural ear canal opening. This placement gives the user the additional benefits over the BTE style related to the normal acoustics provided by the pinna, including increased high frequency gain. Pinna acoustics are also important in providing sound localization

THINGS TO REMEMBER: What Is the Occlusion Effect?

We mentioned that with the full-concha ITE hearing aids, one common downside is that the patient will experience the occlusion effect. What is the occlusion effect, you might ask? Notice that we are using the term *occlusion effect*, not simply occlusion. You can have occlusion without the occlusion effect. The occlusion effect may increase the level of sounds in the lower frequencies (e.g., 200 to 500 Hz) by up to 20 dB to 30 dB in the occluded ear canal when compared with the level in the open ear canal. The occlusion effect causes the hearing aid user to report, "My head sounds like it is in a barrel when I talk" or that their own voice sounds hollow or booming. In addition, this problem can make chewing food sound very noisy and unpleasant. You can experience this sensation yourself tonight at the dinner table. Simply, tightly plug your ears with your fingers and then speak, or better yet, chew a raw carrot or eat a few kettle-cooked potato chips.

So what causes the occlusion effect? The process goes like this:

■ When we talk, certain sounds, especially vowels, reach 120 dB SPL to 130 dB SPL or more in the back of the throat.
■ The high intensity sounds travel via the mandible (bone conduction) to the condyle, which is positioned adjacent to the ear canal.
■ This bone conducted signal then becomes an air-conducted signal by setting up vibrations (primarily low frequency) in the cartilaginous portion of the ear canal.
■ In normal situations, this low-frequency energy escapes out the open ear canal and does not contribute significantly to our perception of our own voice.
■ If the lateral portion of the ear canal is plugged with a hearing aid or earmold, this signal cannot escape, and the resulting trapped energy in the residual ear canal volume is reflected back to the eardrum and transmitted to the cochlea in the typical air-conducted manner.
■ These sounds will then change the perception of our own voice and can also enhance sounds of chewing and even breathing.

Note that the occlusion effect process is not related to the signal going through the hearing aid. In fact, the occlusion effect will be the same whether the hearing aid is turned on or off. To fix the problem, you need to open up the ear canal to allow the loud sounds to leak out. This then goes back to our original point—with many custom instruments, once you package all the necessary electronics, there isn't much room left to open things up.

cues and some natural directional effect as discussed in detail in the next section. Most full-concha instruments employ, or at least allow for, the option of using directional technology by using two omnidirectional microphones, and as a result, there are two microphone ports, as shown on Figure 4–7.

The receiver output terminates in a short tube in the end of the case within the listener's ear canal. This termination is similar to the position provided by the earmold of BTE instruments. As is the case for BTE earmolds, TC instruments can be manufactured with varying canal lengths; however, the canal portion generally extends no more than 10 mm to 15 mm into the cartilaginous portion of the ear canal. Longer canal portions usually are avoided because this can lead to discomfort when wearing the hearing aid as well as increase the difficulty a patient has with insertion and removal.

ITCs in this TC category differentiate from ITEs in that they are smaller and generally fill little of the concha bowl. The larger ITE fits entirely in the outer ear, filling the concha. The smaller ITC model fits mostly in the ear canal and generally does not extend beyond the tragus. The technology for manufacturing ITE shells continues to improve as does miniaturization and sound processing technology. For these reasons, current TC hearing aids are appropriate for patients with hearing loss ranging from mild through severe. When combined with modern feedback suppression technologies, in some cases, ITEs may even be appropriate for some listeners with severe-to-profound hearing loss. The maximum hearing loss that is appropriate, however, depends somewhat on ear geometry. In addition, the maximum severity of loss that can be appropriately fit decreases with progressively smaller instruments (i.e., ITE to ITC) because higher power instruments require larger batteries and larger receivers.

Given that these styles do not extend deeply into the canal portion, one potential problem with the TC style is that a tighter fit may lead to more problems with the occlusion effect (see related Things to Rember). Although the occlusion effect can be reduced or eliminated by increased venting, this will also increase the hearing aid's susceptibility to feedback. Because of the close proximity of the microphone and receiver, the traditional ITC is usually not appropriate for patients with severe hearing loss, unless the product's digital feedback suppression (DFS) is particularly effective. Even then, power is limited in half-shell ITEs and ITCs because of the use of smaller receivers and smaller batteries.

Although smaller than the BTE, the ITE and ITC styles are still large enough to accommodate directional microphones, wireless streaming technologies, and telecoils; however, DAI usually is not possible. This may be a problem for people wanting to use assistive technology as will be discussed in depth in Chapter 8. Further, because of size constraints, the telecoils in these smaller instruments are often weaker than those in BTEs, or not positioned to maximize effectiveness. Because of their smaller size, patients with dexterity problems may have more difficulty changing batteries and operating the controls on ITEs—especially ITCs, when compared with traditional BTEs. These products also are not typically rechargeable, a feature that is requested by more and more patients.

Completely-in-Canal (CIC) Products

With the CIC instruments, the microphone opening as well as the entire hearing aid case will be recessed into the ear canal (CIC

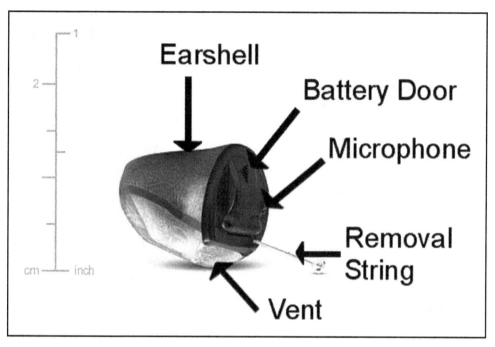

Figure 4–8. Latest generation of small CIC, designed so that the faceplate is recessed in the ear canal. *Source*: From *Essentials of Modern Hearing Aids: Selection, Fitting, and Verification* (p. 249), by T. A. Ricketts, R. Bentler, and H. G. Mueller, 2019, San Diego, CA: Plural Publishing. Reprinted with permission.

example is shown in Figure 4–8). In fact, by definition, to be a CIC, the faceplate must be recessed in the ear canal, or at the least, equal to the opening of the ear canal. Depending on the specific manufacturer, the recessed ITC or the CIC are the physically smallest instruments made. In some cases, the CICs are actually slightly larger (when viewed in your hand, not in the patient's ear) because they may be made to extend deeper into the ear canal. Some manufacturers may try to achieve a marketing edge by calling their CICs something like I-CICs (which we think means invisible), but really, they all are visible from some angles (there are a couple notable exceptions of products, usually inserted in the canal by an otolaryngologist, which truly are invisible—they are rare and we won't be discussing them here).

The popularity of the CIC product grew rapidly in the early 1990s as more and more manufacturers offered this model. Many of the potential benefits were directly linked to the deepness and tightness of the fit; something that seemed ideal from a theoretical aspect, but was not well received by most patients. In the early days, it generally was assumed that a CIC would be deeply fitted, but manufacturers soon became proficient at producing smaller hearing aids that indeed were recessed in the ear canal but were not fitted much deeper than the standard ITE.

Regardless of whether the tip of the CIC is made to extend deep into the canal or not, the fact that the faceplate is intended to be recessed inside the ear canal or at the opening of the ear canal can make the CIC the most cosmetically appealing of all the styles. Because of this, there is some debate as to whether the faceplate of the CIC should be skin-colored to blend in with the concha, or colored to blend with the shadow of the ear canal. On the downside, the close proximity of the microphone to receiver has negative connotations with regards to feedback. Therefore, the smallest of the recessed faceplate instruments are usually not appropriate for patients with hearing loss falling above the moderately severe range unless highly effective digital feedback suppression is used.

Other than cosmetic appeal, the primary functional advantage provided by the ITC/CIC style relates to the more natural listening position of the microphone. Why might this provide an advantage? Actually, there are a couple of reasons, namely advantages related to localization and natural directional sensitivity. The filtering properties related to microphone position, commonly referred to as microphone location effects (MLE), can act to change the frequency shape of sounds entering the hearing aid. Simplistically, we can think of the MLE of instruments with recessed faceplates as providing *free gain*. That is, the greater the boost provided by the pinna, the less that is needed by the hearing aid amplifier. For the open ear, the average concha effect is around 5 dB at 3000 Hz with a peak at 4250 Hz of around 10 dB— these same effects are therefore present for a CIC fitting.

In addition to being important for localization, the natural filtering for this style has the (usually) desirable property of providing less sensitivity to sounds arriving from behind the user in comparison with sounds arriving in front (especially in the high frequencies). This natural directional sensitivity can help us in noisy situations like restaurants by essentially turning down the level of noise and other sounds behind us a little bit relative to the level of sounds arriving from in front of us.

KEY CONCEPT: Choosing a Style

So how does an audiologist recommend a style of aid? There are many ways to present options. When considering devices the first thing that the audiologist considers is physical characteristics of the patient that would limit his or her ability to use or manipulate a hearing aid. The audiologist considers the audiogram and what would be appropriate for a patient based on their degree of hearing loss, the configuration, and the power needed to provide them appropriate amplification. Whether the patient admits it or not, cosmetics usually do matter. For example, for a woman with longer hair covering her ears, a full-shell ITE might be just fine. But if she had a short hair style, this product would be very noticeable. Features also tend to be very important. If a patient walks in the door requesting rechargeable hearing aids, many styles already have been eliminated. After the inappropriate styles have been ruled out, the audiologist presents the options to the patient for their preference. Most audiologists will try to sway patients to a particular style based on several factors, but in the end, it is what the patient will wear that mattes.

KEY CONCEPT: Open Is "In"

To this point, we've been talking about hearing aid styles, which revolve around form factors (e.g., BTE, ITE, CIC). There is another way to classify a fitting, however, and that has to do with the "openness" of the ear canal. Over the past decade, it has become popular to do open-canal fitting, or what might simply be called an "open" fitting. As the name suggests, this means that the patient is fitted with an earmold (eartip) or a revised custom instrument that leaves the ear canal open. There are several reasons why this might be beneficial:

- There is little or no occlusion effect.
- The low-frequency components of speech are allowed to pass directly to the ear, which might sound more natural than amplified signals (Note: in theory, open-canal fittings would not be used with patients who need significant gain in the low frequencies).
- Annoying low-frequency noises will not be amplified.
- The open fitting mold/tip is more comfortable than the closed version.

While the above all sounds good, there are some potential negative consequences:

- It's not possible to deliver significant low-frequency gain (it leaks out).
- The hearing aid is more prone to feedback.
- Directional processing and noise reduction are not as effective (there is a direct path for noise to go to the eardrum).
- The open fitting tip is a poor anchor for keeping the hearing aid on the ear.

In addition to these directional sensitivity and localization advantages, the deep faceplate placement can lead to a reduction in wind noise. The wind noise advantage varies considerably depending on the origin of the wind, but can be a 15 dB to 20 dB advantage compared to a BTE (Mueller et al, 2017). Finally, if CIC instruments are fitted tightly enough and with low enough gain settings (and/or a strong digital feedback suppression algorithm is activated), effective acoustic telephone use without feedback may be possible. Telephone use typically exacerbates feedback because bringing any surface close to the hearing aid microphone can cause sound leaking out of the ear canal to reflect back toward the microphone. This increased sound reflection—also common in many of situations such as hugging, scratching your ear, and so forth—greatly increases the likelihood of feedback.

Despite the positives, there are also a few potential disadvantages of the CIC style for some patients. Most notable are problems for patients without good dexterity as the instruments become smaller and insertion depth increases. Changing the smaller batteries can be quite challenging both for those with limited dexterity or poor vision. In addition, the instruments can be more difficult to insert and remove, although this difficulty is somewhat alleviated in the CIC style through the use of a plastic filament removal string shown in Figure 4–8. These

---

TECHNICAL TIP: Wax Guards or Wax Traps?

■ Most manufacturers have a variety of wax guards, and because there is no magical wax guard, designs continually change. The goal of these devices is to protect the receiver from being impacted with wax. Instead, the wax guard will become clogged and it can be changed, rather than requiring a receiver repair or replacement. You can think of it as a trap, as well as a guard. In some cases, the patient is instructed to replace wax guards at home, which works fine for those patients with good vision, dexterity, and diligence.

■ Wax guards differ in how effective they are. If we consider wax guards from a single manufacturer, those that protect the receiver very well tend to clog more easily and, therefore, require more frequent changing. Those that provide less protection also tend to clog less often. This of course also interacts with the consistency of the individual patient's cerumen.

■ Earlier, we talked about plugged receivers for RIC hearing aids, where the hearing aid is "dead" and the entire receiver needs to be replaced. If you encounter a patient with a dead hearing aid, but it is not a RIC, you might be able to bring it back to life by cleaning the wax guard.

---

handles also can be ordered for ITC products or custom earmolds if necessary.

The very small size of this style and their rounded shape can also be confusing to many patients. It is not unusual for patients to try to force them into their ears sideways or upside-down or even confuse the right and left instruments before they have enough training and practice. We even know of a situation when a CIC that had been laid on a table during an intense card game was mistaken for a peanut, which then required both hearing aid and dental repair. Differentiating between instruments made for the right and left ears can be made easier through the use of colored ink or other markers that are often added during the manufacturing process. Some manufacturers make the entire earshells different colors (commonly red and blue) while matching the faceplate to the user's skin color and tone.

CICs are generally not large enough and/or are in the wrong position to implement directional microphone technology. This technology requires that sounds arriving from the front and the back can be differentiated. This is very difficult if the microphone ports are recessed inside the ear, as sound will hit the ports after bouncing around on the surface of the pinna and ear canal. Space limitations also prevent the effective use of telecoils, FM coupling, or DAI.

Hearing Aid Style: Mini-Summary

■ Selection of hearing aid style is a complex process. Although some styles can be ruled out based on the degree of hearing loss alone, many styles often are appropriate for a single hearing loss configuration.

■ Style decisions can be highly impacted by cosmetics; however, the cosmetics in the hand do not always relate to the cosmetics on the head. Hair style, choice of color and material, and the exact instrument chosen can all affect the final cosmetics on the head. Patients who walk in the door with a preference for one style, may walk out the door with a preference for another.

■ In addition to cosmetics and degree of hearing loss, the desired features should always be an important consideration because not all features are available in all styles. Size and movement of the ear canal should also be considered, especially when considering a tight and/or deep fit.

Fitting Applications

The styles we have talked about so far are all quite common in clinical use. Although the distinction is somewhat artificial, we will now talk about some applications that are designed for specific cases. For many patients, the same application could be accomplished with different styles of products.

Contralateral Routing of Signal (CROS)

The CROS (for contralateral routing of signal) hearing aid is designed for patients with no usable hearing in one ear and normal hearing or a minimal hearing loss in the other ear. This configuration of hearing loss is commonly referred to as *single-sided deafness*. The goal is to give the patient two-sided hearing, when true bilateral hearing is not possible. Recall that one of the requirements

for bilateral amplification is aidable hearing in both ears; the CROS is an alternative to a traditional unilateral fitting for these patients.

In the traditional CROS system, the microphone and amplification stages are contained within either a BTE or TC case that is located on the impaired side. The receiver is located on the side with better (normal) hearing within a BTE or TC case. Early versions of the CROS often used a wire, sometimes routed through eyeglasses or a headband. Current CROS fittings are achieved through the use of wireless transmission that is in a mini-BTE or TC cases— the appearance is more or less the same as we discussed earlier for these styles. Currently, it is common for wireless streaming from one hearing aid to the other to be completed by near field induction or one of a number of radio wave protocols. An example of the CROS (and BiCROS) configuration is shown in Figure 4–9.

The clearest advantage for the CROS fitting is that the user can use the good ear to hear signals from the impaired side that are otherwise attenuated by head shadow. This of course can be very helpful for children with unilateral loss to assist them in difficult classroom situations. For all of these type of fittings, when there is normal hearing in the better ear, sound from the receiver is usually directed into the ear using as much venting as possible, so that the normal sound pathway for the better ear is not blocked. As a result of the large amount of venting, it is typical for only higher frequency signals to reach the ear with normal hearing. By convention, it is usual to refer to the device as a left CROS when the aided signal is routed to the left ear and a right CROS when the aided signal is routed to the right ear.

Clearly, CROS hearing aids are more successful for some patients than others. Consider that they do have one normal

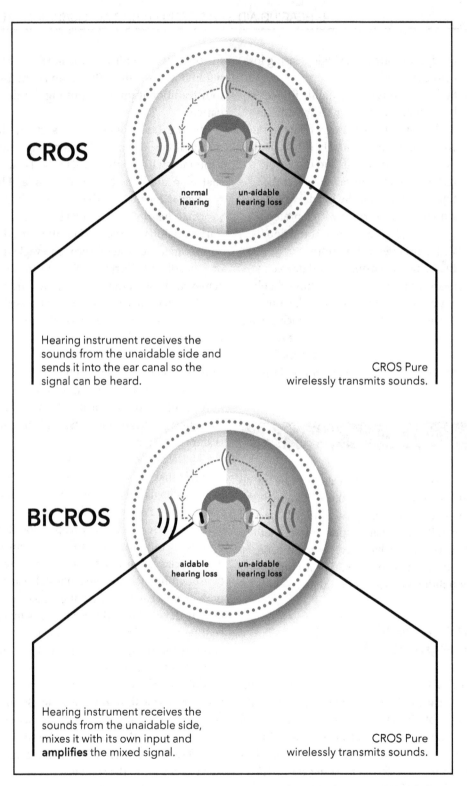

Figure 4–9. Illustration of the amplification design of the CROS and BiCROS fitting application. *Source*: Photo courtesy of Sivantos GmbH or its affiliates © 2019. All rights reserved.

hearing ear. The inconvenience of using two hearing aids for what is viewed as a "minor" problem, with the added cosmetic issue, is often cited as reasons for rejection of CROS amplification. Successful users often report a critical communication need in an environment in which they are surrounded by important speakers, and are highly motivated to hear sounds arriving from both sides equally. Acceptance also might depend on the recency of the hearing loss. Someone who has had a unilateral loss for years is less likely to report advantages for the CROS fitting than someone who has just had a sudden hearing loss. Most of today's products have the option of switching off the transmission. In this case, the patients actually have an advantage over normal hearing—we can't switch off noise coming from one side or another.

BiCROS Applications

Patients with single-sided deafness (SSD) who also have some hearing impairment in the better ear are more successful CROS candidates than those with normal hearing in the fitted ear, partly because they entered the fitting with more communication problems. In cases in which amplification is provided to the better ear in addition to the contralateral routing of signals, the instruments are referred to as BiCROS, for Bilateral-CROS (e.g., there also is a microphone for the instrument on the side of the "better" ear; two microphones sending signals to one amplifier/receiver). The success rate for BiCROS users is much greater, these patients are going to be wearing a hearing aid anyway (probably a mini-BTE), so adding a second aid (microphone on bad ear) is not viewed as much of a difference. The general rule of thumb is that if you look at the good ear in isolation and you

consider that ear in need of amplification, then the BiCROS rather than the CROS would be selected. These products are also switchable, so that the patient can turn on or off either microphone for specific listening situations—if noise is present from the side of the bad ear, this microphone could be turned off; if noise is from the good ear, this microphone can be turned off. In some modern instruments, there is also preprocessing, such as directional technology, on the transmitter side.

Less Common CROS and BiCROS Solutions

As we mentioned, CROS and BiCROS fittings usually involve mini-BTEs, the same as for traditional fittings. There are some other amplification methods that accomplish the fitting goal of moving the acoustic signal from one side of the head to the other. One method is the use of an implantable bone conduction device. We describe this application in Chapter 7. Two other less common methods are as follows:

- Transcranial CROS: As the name indicates, in this type of fitting we are referring to sending the signal through the skull (via bone conduction). The goal of this type of CROS fitting is to place an air conducted signal in the bad ear that is loud enough that it crosses over via bone conduction to the good ear. This intervention usually implements a single deep canal instrument (usually a CIC or BTE style with deep-fitted earmold), which is fitted to the ear without hearing.
- TransEar: With this device, the microphone and processing are contained within a BTE case that connects to a piece in the ear using a small wire. The configuration of

this part of the device is essentially identical to that used in the receiver in the ear mini-BTE devices, so we could call this a RIC hearing aid. The difference, however, is that with the TransEar, the wire terminates in a small bone conduction vibrator encased in an earmold placed in the ear canal of the poorer ear, rather than in a typical receiver. As with other transcranial approaches, the patient must be willing to accept a hard shell that is fitted fairly deeply into the ear canal.

Knobs, Switches, Buttons, and Remote Controls

Another decision that must be considered in concert with hearing aids style is the selection of user controls. Some styles will be physically limited in size to such a degree that few user controls are possible. Some hearing aids in fact have no user controls on the hearing aid itself. The need for user control of the hearing aid primarily depends on five factors:

- How well the audiologist programmed the hearing aids. If both the gain and output are set appropriately for a large variety of input signals at the time of the fitting, the patient will not need to make as many changes during use.
- How well the patient *trained* the hearing aids. If the hearing aids are trainable and the patient actively adjusts gain for different settings during the first few weeks of use, there should be less need for a volume control once training is completed (see the section on trainable hearing aids in Chapter 5).
- The quality of the signal classification system and automatic functions

of the hearing aids. For example, if the classifier correctly identifies speech in noise and switches to appropriate directional and noise reduction characteristics, there is less need for the patient to change gain or programs.

- Lifestyle of the patient. If the patient has a very active lifestyle and different telephone and wireless streaming applications are included in the fitting, this will require more active program changes by the patient.
- The patient's interest in controlling the acoustic environment. Some patients like to fiddle and make discrete volume control adjustments as the listening environment changes.

Common user controls contained on the hearing aid include volume control (VC) wheels (volume, turn instrument on/off) and button/toggle/rocker switches (used in many styles to change volume or to switch between programs and/or features by repeatedly pushing either the same button or two different buttons). For bilateral fittings, hearing aids often are paired using wireless communication. This allows for simultaneous volume control changes on both hearing aids by only pushing the button on one of them. As an alternative, hearing aids may be fitted so the button on one side changes the gain, and the button on the other side changes programs (memories).

User controls including volume control also can be placed on a separate remote control. Remote controls range from the extremely simple to quite sophisticated (individual controls for on and off, volume and hearing aid user memories, frequency response, and special features). Today, the most common "remote control" is simply an app for the patient's cell phone, which links wirelessly to the hearing aid.

In the past, patient demand for remote controls has been fairly low since they were introduced in the 1980s. The low demand likely relates to complaints or concerns about keeping track of another device as well as cost, and/or the patient does not see any potential benefit. Today, given that most patients already own a smartphone and carry it with them, these reasons are less relevant. An example of how a cell phone app might be used is shown in the screenshots pictured in Figure 4–10. The left panel shows the simple adjustment of volume for the right and left hearing aids. More advanced adjustments are shown in the panel on the right. As we discuss in Chap-

ter 5, today's hearing aids have the capability to focus in a given direction, providing less gain for sounds coming from other azimuths—presumably sounds that the patient is not interested in hearing. If you look at the five icons on the bottom of the screen (dark gray is what the patient wants to hear), you can see that they can change from hearing everything equally from all around (good when outside or general household communication), to the far right icon, which is a very focused beam to the front (good for when trying to hear an individual talker in background noise). Other options (not on this screen) include a focus to the back (good for when driving a car and

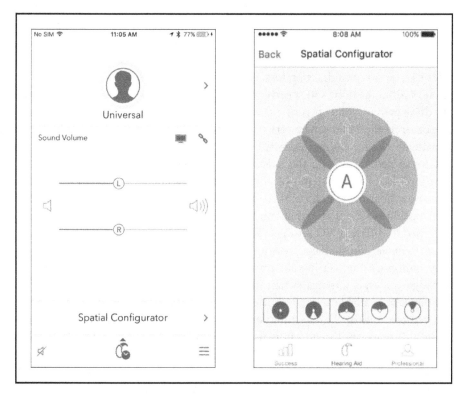

Figure 4–10. Illustration of smartphone app for controlling the hearing aids. The left panel illustrates the basic volume control, whereas the right panel shows how the focus of the microphone can be adjusted—ranging from all-around sound, to a narrow beam, to the front (i.e., the dark gray part of the circle is the focus of the sound). *Source*: Photo courtesy of Sivantos GmbH or its affiliates © 2019. All rights reserved.

talking to someone in the backseat). These directional functions do change automatically, but some patients prefer to override this with the app.

Fortunately, modern hearing aids have greatly enhanced the old-fashioned hearing aid VC. These enhancements might include the ability to link the VC of two hearing aids together (changing the volume on one hearing aid changes both), clinician control of the volume range, and/or step size (e.g., volume range could be as small as +/− 4–6 dB or as large as 16 dB, or can be turned off completely). Finally, for small children or others who may not be able to appropriately adjust desired loudness level, but for which a VC is still desired, a screw-set VC may be used. This is simply a VC that must be set with a small screwdriver (as we describe in Chapter 5, while the VC is set at one position, the amplifier of the hearing aid automatically delivers different gain for different input levels—for a typical hearing loss, we might see 30 dB of gain for soft speech, but only 10 dB of gain for loud speech).

One other method that can be very useful for patients who have poor dexterity but who desire some control over the hearing aid gain level is to use a program switch. That is, most hearing aids have three or four (or more) user memories that can be programmed to different VC settings. The level can then be adjusted by pressing a memory button on the hearing aid (most often a single button or a rocker switch that toggles between available user memories) or on a remote control. This technique is most useful if there are three to four user memories available. Two levels may not give the patient enough control (although this is fine for a few patients), and more than four levels can become confusing and/or difficult to manipulate. The audiologist will need to work with the patient to determine exactly what gain alterations are programmed, but often, one memory might have gain 3 dB to 5 dB louder, another 3 dB to 5 dB softer, and if the patient has considerable low frequency gain for the primary fitting, maybe a program that cuts some of the gain in this region. This technique, however, may not be possible if the user memories are already being used to activate other features (e.g., telecoil, wireless connectivity).

Hearing Assistive Technology

One very important, but unfortunately often overlooked, portion of hearing aid selection and assessment for the purpose of (re)habilitation is consideration of hearing assistive technology (HAT). This category includes any and all devices other than the primary interventions of hearing aids and cochlear implants that are specifically used to assist patients with hearing difficulties. HATs differ from traditional hearing aids and cochlear implants in that they usually are aimed at addressing a small range of needs, rather than general hearing problems. Therefore, HATs often fill a useful supplementary roll to hearing aids, and in some cases, more than one different type of HAT may be appropriate for the same patient. That is, some patients may benefit from two, three, or even several HAT devices. For other patients, however, the benefit provided by a HAT may not be large enough to warrant the cost and/or inconvenience. We describe HATs more completely in Chapter 8, but listed below is a summary of some of the HAT applications:

- Near-sound personal listening devices aimed at increasing the level of sounds near the listener (e.g., personal amplifiers, amplified stethoscopes, etc.).

- Far-sound personal listening devices aimed at bringing sounds far from the listener effectively *nearer* (e.g., note-takers, speech-to-text systems, FM systems, room loops, infrared systems, wireless routing from microphones [e.g., spouse microphone], and other devices that route signals of interest to the hearing aid or listener).
- Alerting and warning devices (e.g., flashing and vibrating alarm clocks, smoke alarms, door bells, telephone ringers, and amplified telephone ringers and smoke alarms).
- Telephone assistance (e.g., amplified telephones, teletypewriters, instant messaging translation services).
- Television and radio assistance (e.g., closed captioning, television amplifiers—many personal listening devices can assist with television and radio listening).

Earmolds and Associated Plumbing

We've discussed how the choice of hearing aid style not only affects cosmetics and available features, but also can have important acoustic implications. More specifically, we know that hearing aid style can have considerable implications for amount of gain, potential feedback problems, and issues related to the occlusion effect. Although the general choice of hearing aid style will impact these factors, how tightly and deeply an instrument is fitted in the ear canal also can have a significant effect. That is, two different products that are both full-concha ITEs can have very different fit properties.

The physical fit matters in no small part because it can affect the amount of venting (sound leakage), as well as the overall wearing comfort for the patient. If the hearing aids are not comfortable, it is unlikely the patient will wear them. For the majority of hearing aid styles, other than the open-canal mini-BTEs, which are often fitted with noncustom coupling systems, the quality of the ear impression greatly affects how well a hearing aid shell or earmold physically fits an individual patient's ear. The sound delivered to the patient's ear(s) from the hearing aid can be significantly altered by the sound delivery system in a number of ways. We generally refer to this delivery system and the resulting physical changes as hearing aid plumbing, a term we think fits well.

When BTEs are fitted, the choice of earmold will depend on several factors, some of which are similar to the factors considered when choosing a hearing aid style. They include the degree of hearing loss, how open you want the fit to be (based on hearing loss configuration and quality of the feedback suppression algorithm you are ordering), shape and size of the external ear, texture and sensitivity of the patient's skin, stiffness of the patient's external ear, and potentially other factors. Because all of these factors are important, how the choice of earmold material and earmold style might interact with the patient and the fit must be considered at every step in this process.

There are three primary families of earmold materials including acrylic/Lucite, polyvinyl chloride (vinyl/PVC), and silicone—each of which has potential benefits and limitations. Polyethylene, a fourth material type, is used less often. It is similar in advantages and disadvantages to acrylic; however, it is slightly more prone to feedback, but the most hypoallergenic of all the materials. It is also sometimes criticized for its plastic-like

KEY CONCEPT: From Impression to Finished Product

The beginning of a good earmold is a good ear impression. Taking a good impression is a learned skill, hopefully mastered by most audiologists working with hearing aids. After it has been determined that the impression is adequate, it is commonly mailed to an earmold or hearing aid manufacturer so that an earmold or custom product can be ordered. There is some concern that the important fine details of the impression can be altered through this mailing process (e.g., shrinkage, damage from excessive heat, squashing, etc.). For this reason, technologies that can perform three-dimensional scans of earmolds in the clinician's office and store the earmold as a digital image have been introduced. This technique of creating a virtual earmold has the benefits of avoiding any shipping-related deformation of the ear impression and providing a nonshrinking, permanent impression that can be easily stored and used for making additional earshells or earmolds. The scanning devices that are commonly used are about the size of a computer printer and use three-dimensional technology with color-coded triangulation. The ear impression is affixed to a rotating platform where a projector illuminates it with colored light stripes from different angles. The light stripes conform to the object's surface in line with its geometry. This is simultaneously captured with a camera. The process takes about two min. Changes, markings, or comments to assist in the fabrication can be made by the audiologist directly on the digital scan.

The method described above has been available for several years, but has not been readily adopted. What has been introduced recently is equipment that takes a direct scan of the ear/earcanal itself. That is, no physical impression is taken—everything is digital. We expect this procedure to become the standard in the upcoming years.

For either scanning method, the resulting scan can then be e-mailed to the earmold lab or the manufacturer. The benefits of using the scanner include the following:

- Reduced shrinkage and damage during shipping
- Digital record of impression is available, which can be used for remakes (e.g., lost or damaged earmolds/hearing aids), or the making of other products (e.g., custom earplugs, swim plugs, etc.).
- Provides electronic method to indicate where changes need to be made on remakes (the audiologist can draw and write on the scan)
- Reduced turnaround time
- Reduced cost of impression material and shipping expenses
- Convenience: impressions do not have to be boxed up and orders can be placed at any time, night or day

appearance. A summary of the types is as follows:

Acrylic/Lucite: This material may be regular or body temperature reactive, which gets slightly softer when warm.

- Positives: Because it is very hard, it is possible to make thin ridges, keeps its shape without shrinking, is very durable, and is easy to modify. The hard, slick surface also makes earmolds made of this material easier to insert and remove. It is fairly hypoallergenic and the best material for many older patients.
- Negatives: Because of the hardness, it will not bend or compress to get past narrow openings on insertion, and it may be more prone to feedback. However, studies suggest a good seal can be obtained with this material as well as softer materials. Not usually recommended for children for fear of ear injury if struck in the earmold.

Polyvinyl chloride: This material is often available in softer (recommended for children) and harder varieties.

- Positives: Softer and more comfortable than acrylic. Softness makes it appropriate for children and for hearing losses in the moderate to severe range. Although not as slick as acrylic, it is also not as tacky (sticky) as silicone, making it reasonably easy to remove and insert.
- Negatives: Not very durable, lasting from 4 months to 2 years depending on body chemistry. Soft nature makes them much more difficult to modify than acrylic. More prone to discolor after time. Problematic for patients with vinyl allergies.

Silicone: This material is often available in tacky/low pressure cured (recommended for greater hearing loss) and high pressure cured varieties.

- Positives: Soft and tacky nature makes this material appropriate for children and ideal for severe to profound hearing loss, and it is fairly hypoallergenic.
- Negatives: Soft nature makes it much more difficult to modify than acrylic. Soft and tacky nature makes it the

---

TAKE FIVE: Decisions, Decisions

Just in case you think audiologists working with hearing aids have an easy life, consider what they might have to go through when simply ordering one earmold. The following is the list of the 20 material options for just one earmold style from just one of the major manufacturers: Acrylic, Acrylic with Flex Canal, Acrylic with hard or soft e-Compound canal, Acrylic DisappEar, FIT, Formula II, Formula II Clear, Rx, Superflex, Neon Colors, Vinyl Marble, Mediflex, Mediflex with e-Compound, Frosted Flex, Frosted Flex with e-Compound, OtoBlast, OtoBlast DisappEar, and Cat Eyes. That's almost as confusing as ordering a coffee from Starbucks.

most difficult to insert and remove (especially difficult for floppy ears) and can cause skin abrasions in patients with fragile skin. Tubing adhesive does not bond well with some versions, leading to the need for a mechanical tubing lock.

Earmold Styles

Now that we have considered earmold materials, let us discuss earmold styles. One of the things that makes selection challenging is that there are so many different styles, and many manufacturers use different naming schemes. Even within the same manufacturer, naming schemes are often either nondescriptive (e.g., based on numbers or letters) or inconsistent (e.g., depending on the earmold, descriptive names, inventor names, application names, and function names are used). The general rule for all earmolds is the more severe the hearing loss, the more the earmold should fill the ear canal and concha, and the greater importance that it extends into the ear canal a reasonable distance. Common earmold styles are summarized in Figure 4–11.

Modular Earmold Tips

Today's mini-BTE products come with an assortment of modular/semi-disposable earmold fittings. These tips/domes come in a large variety of sizes, for large to small ear canals and for very closed to very open fittings. Some audiologists fit more than 50% of their patients with this type of "instant" earmold. Manufacturers provide kits that include all the tips and tubing that are used for these modular fittings. The fitting kits also often include tube shapers, measuring gauges, wax guards, and cleaning wires. Consider that from just one manufacturer for a RIC product there are three different

receiver power choices, four different wire length choices, and eight different dome choices—96 different combinations! There are both pros and cons of using these modular tips and domes.

Reasons Why Modular Tips Could Be a Good Choice

■ Openness: The open fitting tips are indeed open. Not only does this eliminate the occlusion effect, but it provides some free gain, as the ear canal resonance is still in play.

■ Efficiency: The modular tips allow for same-day service. The patient can walk in the door with an appointment for a diagnostic and leave a couple hours later owning a pair of hearing aids.

■ Reduced procrastination: Related to efficiency, there is the old adage, "strike while the iron is hot." Although not blacksmiths, audiologists dispensing hearing aids know well that when a patient says, "You know, I think I'll go home, talk to my wife about this, and get back to you," you very well might not see that patient again for five years, if ever. Or, the patient goes home, starts price shopping, and returns a week later with a bulging folder of competitive offers and Internet printouts.

■ Comfort: Most of the modular tips and domes, especially the open ones, fit rather loosely and are more comfortable than a custom earmold.

■ Cosmetics: The modular tip is typically less noticeable than a custom earmold.

■ Cost: There is a $50 or more extra cost for the custom earmold. Many manufacturers provide the tips and domes free of charge to the audiologists.

■ Maintenance: If the patient has good dexterity and is attentive, they can replace the tips when they become

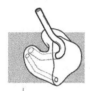

Full Shell

- Often used for more severe to profound hearing losses and younger children
- Canal portion can be made thicker (better seal), thinner (for better cosmetics), fitted with a snap ring instead of tubing (for body aid, powered stethoscopes, etc.), or the top portion of the canal can be removed (half shell).
- Can be difficult to insert if tight fitting.

Skeleton

- One of the more common styles used with traditional BTE hearing aids.
- Can be used with a wide range of hearing loss.
- Sometimes modified to remove the middle portion of the "ring" that fills the concha bowl (semi-skeleton).

Canal

- Not usually fit as tight, so it is more suitable for mild-moderate loss. Appropriate for some patients with severe hearing loss using soft materials. Retention can be a problem, though easier insertion than many styles.
- Can be modified with a "concha lock" or by hollowing out the canal (sometimes combined with soft material for a comfort fit for patients with large changes in earcanal size with jaw movement).

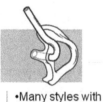

Custom Open

- Many styles with various combinations and configurations of the heel, concha, and helix lock portions.
- Can be used for CROS style, open fits with BTE style or with the OC style for better retention than non-custom open.

Non-Custom Mini-BTE

- Usually manufacturer specific and using tubing with a very narrow inner diameter.
- Both RITA (tube) and RIC styles available.
- Can have some problems with retention for which a custom solution is suggested.

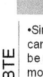

Custom Mini-BTE

- Similar to the standard canal, but intended to be used with specific models of deep canal (occluding) RIC fittings. Manufacturers often supply non-custom versions, but custom versions are often available from earmold companies when better retention is desired.
- Usually made using soft materials.

Figure 4–11. Advantages and limitations to a few common earmolds. This information is particularly useful when deciding on an earmold style within the constraints of individual patient differences, cosmetics, and gain requirements. *Source*: From *Essentials of Modern Hearing Aids: Selection, Fitting, and Verification* (p. 285), by T. A. Ricketts, R. Bentler, and H. G. Mueller, 2019, San Diego, CA: Plural Publishing. Reprinted with permission.

plugged or discolored. Audiologists often give their patients a handful of replacement eartips.

Reasons Why Modular Tips May Not Be a Good Choice

- Feedback: If a patient needs considerable gain, it is difficult to find a noncustom tip or dome that will fit tight enough.
- Ear geography: If the patient has a sharp turn in their ear canal, there may be problems with the tip bumping against the canal wall. There is not the flexibility of going deeper or shallower, like one would have with custom earmolds.
- Dexterity: For some people, putting in a dome can be difficult to feel it if is in the "right place." By using a custom tip, the patient can often feel when the mold is in correctly.
- Retention: It is fairly common for modular tips to work out of the ear canal, or partly out of the canal, when the person talks or chews. Because they are light and fit loosely, the patient sometimes does not even know that the tip is not in the ear canal.
- Anchoring: Related to retention—mini-BTEs are very light and easily can fall off the ear when a person bends over. A custom earmold will serve as an anchor, keeping the hearing aid suspended at the ear. A loose fitting tip will not.
- Maintenance: In general, the tips need more maintenance (changing) than a standard custom earmold. A common problem is the plugging of the RIC receiver. This occurs more frequently when a modular tip is used, than when the receiver is cased in a custom earmold.
- Overall product impression: A pair of hearing aids is the most expensive electronic devices most people purchase. Fitting them to the ear with a 50 cent, disposable eartip may not seem consistent with the purported high level of technology.

Venting Effects

Venting is a term that simply refers to opening up an air/sound transmission pathway from the tympanic membrane to the environment outside the head. Venting is the most common alteration made to earmold plumbing. It's possible to obtain the effects of venting by simply having a loose fitting ear tip. In other cases, a channel is placed in the earmold to accomplish the venting— four different types of this are illustrated in Figure 4–12. The effects of venting can make a substantial change to low frequency gain and output.

Venting is used with hearing aid fittings for several reasons, including the following (from Mueller & Hall, 1998):

- To allow amplified low-frequency signals to escape: In some cases, the gain of the instrument in the lower frequencies is greater than necessary, or what is desired by the patient.
- To allow low-frequency signals generated in the ear canal to escape: When a person talks, his or her voice is transmitted from the throat via bone conduction along the mandible to the condyle, which is adjacent to the ear canal. This vibrates the cartilaginous portion of the ear canal, which creates low-frequency, air-conducted energy within the cavity. The most effective treatment of the occlusion effect is venting—allowing the low-frequency energy to escape.

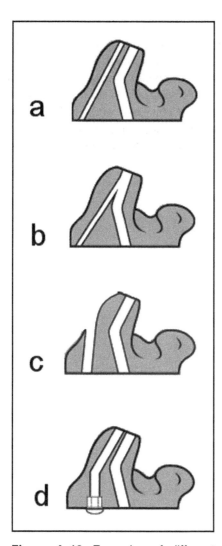

Figure 4–12. Examples of different types of drilled vents that could be placed in a custom earmold. *Source*: Reproduced with permission from Westone Laboratories.

▢ To allow unamplified signals to pass unobstructed to the eardrum: When a person has normal hearing for a given frequency range (usually the lows), it often is desirable to allow speech and environmental sounds to pass naturally to the eardrum and not be attenuated by an earmold/hearing aid shell. This may improve localization, give sounds a more natural perception, and improve the overall quality of the signal.

▢ To allow pressure relief: When earmolds or hearing aid shells are fitted tightly, there can be a buildup of pressure in the residual open canal, and the patient will report a sensation of fullness. Some patients can sense this pressure increasing as the daily hearing aid use continues. A small vent can relieve this pressure, and in fact, these small vents often are called pressure vents.

▢ To allow aerations of the ear canal and/or middle ear: In some cases, when external or middle ear pathology exists, the pathology is aggravated when the normal ventilation of the ear is altered. For these patients, venting is used for medical rather than acoustic reasons, and there may need to be some compromise in the applied low frequency gain (e.g., less than desired) to allow for the necessary aeration.

In Closing

You will encounter patients using a wide variety of hearing aid styles. Why is one wearing something behind the ear, but another has a product that is all in the ear? Why are some larger than others? Hopefully, our review helps categorize why these differences are observed. In some cases, as we discuss, it may simply be patient preference with no clear audiologic theory behind it. While 20 years ago about 80% of hearing aids dispensed were custom, the pendulum has swung a long way in the other direction, and today, 80% of the fittings are BTEs. This means that once again, the earmold is part of the selection process. We have taken a look at earmold plumbing, and we hope you have gained some insight regarding how this can impact the success of the fitting. You'll notice patients wearing small, modular, semidisposable ear tips, which are popular today. They may be comfortable, but often are not the best acoustic solution—look for a return to more custom earmolds.

A hearing aid with the best technology on the market may be rejected if the plumbing is not right. Finally, remember some of the special applications, such as CROS and BiCROS fittings. These devices have become extremely efficient, and might be a reasonable solution for your pediatric patients with severe unilateral hearing loss.

5 Hearing Aids: How They Work!

Anyone who has driven a car for the past 25 years knows how much automobiles have changed over that period of time. Just about every aspect of the driving experience today is computerized and automated. You can even start your car remotely on a cold January morning from the warmth of your home, which is a very positive technology advancement if you live in North or South Dakota (and we do!). There are warning signals relative to your speed, tire pressure, nearby objects, drivers in your blind spot, driving lane alignment, and most every other car-related thing you can think of. Even though cars have become more automated, many of the basic parts have not changed over the years. You still have to put gas in it and change the oil and spark plugs every so often. For the majority of cars, you still need a very basic battery. In many ways, hearing aids are like cars in the sense that many of the internal operations have become computerized, there are many external gadgets to facilitate use, but the basic components have remained unchanged.

You already know that a hearing aid is an electronic sound amplifier. Simply stated, it is designed to take sounds that are too soft for those with a hearing loss to hear appropriately and make them louder. Basically, we usually want the hearing aid to make soft sounds audible, average sounds comfortable, and loud sounds loud—but not too loud. To do that, you have to apply different amounts of amplification to different inputs—we'll get to how that works shortly. A modern hearing aid accomplishes amplification through the use of a microphone, amplifier, receiver, and a series of electronic calculations. All of this then needs to be programmed correctly—the way in which you program (fine tune) them makes a tremendous difference in how they work for the patient—the best hearing aid on the market will be of little benefit if programmed incorrectly (we'll talk about that next in Chapter 6).

What Is Amplification?

A hearing aid performs an electronic sleight of hand. It takes sounds that occur naturally in the real world, borrows energy from an outside source (a battery), changes it into an electrical current (microphone), makes it a digital signal, digitally manipulates the signal (processing algorithms), boosts it up (amplifier), changes it back to an acoustic signal (receiver), and sends the sound to the person's ear canal. And it does all this in a few milliseconds, often while immersed in a hot and humid environment (behind the ear or in the ear canal). Figure 5–1 shows the manner in which sounds travel through a simple electronic hearing aid. While we have been in the "digital era" with hearing aids for the past 20 years, digital hearing aids continue to use microphones and receivers that are very similar to what is used with analog instruments.

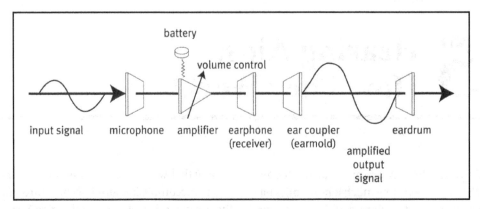

Figure 5–1. Basic components of a hearing aid. *Source*: From *The Hearing Aid: Its Operation and Development*, by K. Berger, 1974, National Hearing Aid Society.

DID YOU KNOW: A Little Hearing Aid History

The electronic era of hearing aids began with inventions initially appearing in other innovations of the day. An era sometime called the "carbon era" began around 1900, and is characterized by the use of carbon material behind the diaphragm of the carbon-style microphone. The carbon-style era hearing aid was capable of providing about 20 dB to 30 dB of amplification (also with a limited frequency bandwidth). This era lasted into the 1940s. When the vacuum tube triode amplifier was invented in 1907, the "vacuum tube" era was born. Vacuum tubes appeared in some hearing aids during the 1920s, and emerged more fully during the 1930s. They were very large, requiring multiple tubes and batteries. Power, however, did increase substantially to near 70 dB gain and 130 dB output. This would be appropriate for much more severe losses. During this era, filtering, shaping, and limiting were electronically possible. The first one-piece hearing aid was not introduced until around 1944. The wearable body aid was born. The vacuum tube era ended in the 1950s with the acceptance of the transistor style hearing aid.

The "transistor era" began in 1947, and hearing aids began to use the technology in the early 1950s. In the transistor era, hearing aid components became smaller, yet more efficient. Hearing aids could now be worn on the head via eyeglass or BTE aids. Eventually (1964), transistors became small enough to be put on a small integrated circuit chip, allowing for in-the-ear custom hearing aids. As recent as 1960, body aids accounted for approximately 25% of sales; eyeglass aids, 45%; and BTEs, 30%. In-the-ear sales were reported as 2% in 1961, and did not reach 10% until 1967, not 30% until 1977.

Programmable analog hearing aids become commercially available in the mid-to-late 1980s. In the mid-1990s, digital hearing aids were introduced. Digital signal processing (DSP) enables sound to be shaped by the hearing aid in an infinite number of ways. Today, in the United States, digital hearing aids comprise essentially 100% of the market.

Basic Components

As we mentioned earlier, all hearing aids have some basic components in common. While "digital" is the word today, there are some things like microphones and receivers that while improved, are similar to hearing aids of decades ago. We'll review some of the basic features.

Hearing Aid Batteries

Hearing aids are electronic devices. They need energy to work. This energy comes from a dry cell battery. Batteries come in a variety of sizes. Commonly used battery sizes include the #675 for power BTEs and some cochlear implants, #13 for smaller BTEs and ITE aids, #312 for canal aids, #10 for small canal and CIC aids, and the #5 for very small CICs. The size of the battery determines its life; that is, hours of use. Figure 5–2 shows the most common size hearing aid batteries on the market today.

The composition material for most all hearing aid batteries is zinc/air. Although batteries need to be disposed of in an environmental-conscious way, zinc-air batteries are considered nontoxic. These batteries are not activated until a tab is removed, exposing the "air holes." For convenience, these tabs or background of the battery packet are color coded to help identify the size of the battery—all manufacturers use the same coloring system (why can't the manufacturers of AA and AAA batteries be like this?). The associated colors are as follows:

Blue Tab	Size 675
Orange Tab	Size 13
Brown Tab	Size 312
Yellow Tab	Size 10 (or 230)
Red Tab	Size 5

How long does the typical hearing aid battery last? If you are asking this question, you are no different than most every hearing aid user. The answer is—it depends. The milliamp hours are usually listed on the battery package, and vary by battery size: 675 = 600 mah, 13 = 260 mah, 312 = 130 mah, 10A:70 mah, and 5A = 35 mah. With those number in mind, we need to know two more things: battery drain of a given hearing aid (listed on hearing aid spec sheet), and how many hours a day the patient uses the hearing aid. Let's say a patient you are working with says that his batteries just aren't lasting very long. He is using a pair of mini-BTEs with 312 batteries (capacity of 130 mah and a drain of .75 ma). A little math tells you that the battery should last for about 170 hrs (130 × .75). If he tells you that he is using the hearing aid for about 12 hours a day, then again, a little math tells you that the battery should last for about 14 days (170 ÷ 12 hrs). More math than you like? We do have to add that the drain is dependent on the features being used or if the aid is streaming

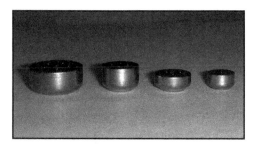

Figure 5–2. The four most common battery sizes from left to right: 675, 13, 312, and 10A/ 230. *Source*: From *Fitting and Dispensing Hearing Aids* (2nd ed., p. 232), by B. Taylor and H. G. Mueller, 2017, San Diego, CA: Plural Publishing. Reprinted with permission.

signals such as music, or like the CROS application described previously in Chapter 4. If feedback reduction of some other algorithm is continually running, the batteries may only last half as long. If the patient does a lot of wireless streaming, the battery will be depleted even faster.

Rechargeable Batteries

Considering how often hearing aid batteries need to be changed relative to many other electronic devices, it's not surprising that rechargeable batteries are rapidly gaining in popularity. Like most things in our environment, when it comes to batteries, it's good to "go green," as 1.4 billion disposable hearing aid batteries go into landfills each year; that is more than 3 million pounds of waste. All of today's major manufacturers offer rechargeable hearing aids, and this tends to be favored by most patients (even older patients are now used to charging their phone, so charging their hearing aids doesn't sound that odd). Chargers continue to be smaller and more versatile. Figure 5–3 is an example. This charger is about the size of a deck of cards, and doubles as the carrying case for the hearing aids. It easily fits in a pocket or purse. For some manufacturers, it also holds its own power supply, so the hearing aids can be charged while on-the-go, or when away from a power source. Rechargeable hearing aids are good for patients with poor dexterity where changing a battery may be difficult

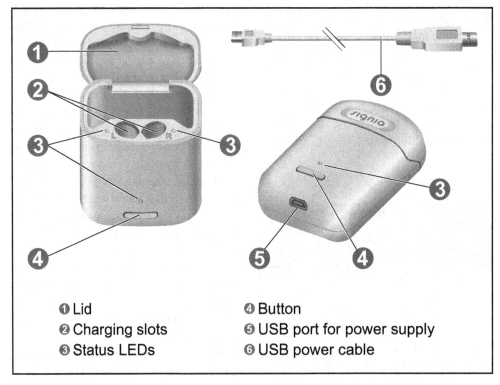

❶ Lid
❷ Charging slots
❸ Status LEDs
❹ Button
❺ USB port for power supply
❻ USB power cable

Figure 5–3. Example of a small portable charger that also serves as the carrying case (about the size of a deck of cards). The charger also has storage capability, so charging on-the-go also is possible. *Source*: Photo courtesy of Sivantos GmbH or its affiliates © 2019. All rights reserved.

or children so we don't have to worry about them swallowing the battery. However, they may not be the choice for people who are doing a lot of streaming or who cannot consistently charge the aids. Like many other current devices, you cannot "overcharge" a rechargeable hearing aid battery, so leaving the hearing aids to charge overnight is the most common time for charging.

There also are some manufactures who allow many hearing aids in their portfolio to be retrofitted with a rechargeable battery. Zpower Electronics makes a "battery pack" that can be swapped for the regular battery + door in many of the most popular hearing aids. Once the Zpower battery is placed into the hearing aid, the device can be recharged in a portable station that sits on a tabletop. An overnight charge allows the Zpowered hearing aid to operate all day until another charge is needed.

Microphone

The first electrical component in a hearing aid is an input transducer, most commonly, the microphone. Its duty is to pick up the acoustical sound in the wearer's environment and change it into an electrical form that the amplifier can use. The microphone changes the acoustic input into an analog electrical waveform, similar to a sine wave, of greater and lesser electrical voltages. These changes in voltage eventually are transformed into changes in sound coming out the hearing aid into the wearer's ear. Most of today's products have two omnidirectional microphones, which can be used to accomplish "directional processing" through the use of digital algorithms. We will talk about that later in this chapter.

The following are a few more things about microphones:

- Microphones used in hearing aids today are quite small and range in size from around 5 mm × 4 mm × 2 mm, to a cylinder microphone that is 2.5 (diam) × 2.5.
- Microphones have different frequency responses and are "tuned" for different applications.
- Microphones have a resonant frequency that can be shifted during their production.
- Microphones have internal noise because of the resistances and semiconductors of the electrical circuit. Expansion circuits assist in reducing microphone noise (more on that later in this chapter).
- When wind strikes, the hearing aid microphone noise results. This tends to be worse with BTE instruments (hearing aids have special wind-noise reduction circuits that try to minimize this).
- Like receivers, microphones are easily damaged by debris. Even a small amount of debris in the microphone port can alter the frequency response, or turn a good directional instrument into an omnidirectional one.

Telecoil

Another type of input transducer is a telecoil, which certainly is worthy of special mention. As the name suggests, this transducer was originally designed for use with the telephone. Many hearing-impaired people have trouble talking on the phone while using their hearing aids. This is either because the telephone signal is not loud enough to be audible because there is too much background noise, or because placing the phone by the ear causes acoustic feedback.

A telecoil uses the electromagnetic energy present around all phones and turns it into an electrical signal the hearing aid can amplify. The magnetic field, which is picked up by the telecoil, is generated by an electrical current that has the same waveform as the audio signal. The effectiveness of a telecoil is determined by the size of the magnetic field that is generated. The strength of the magnetic field is directly related to the ferrite rod size and the number of coil turns. By increasing the size of the ferrite rod, the telecoil becomes more sensitive, thus more effective. Many devices such as loudspeakers, telephones, and other common electrical gadgets produce a magnetic field. The process of an electrical current inducing a voltage in the coil some distance away is called induction. An induction loop system is intentionally generated by looping a wire around a room or a small area. Importantly, many cell phones do not work effectively with the hearing aid telecoil—most have a published T-rating regarding this. A telecoil switch is often placed on the hearing aid, or this could be a separate memory, accessed with a memory button or remote control. With some hearing aids, the switching is triggered automatically when the telephone receiver nears the ear.

A telecoil is not always a standard option on hearing aids today. In fact, most often there is *not* a telecoil. This is because most patients want smaller hearing aids, and these products simply are not the size requirement needed to accommodate the coil. Also, when manufacturers introduce new technology, it is usually introduced in one of these smaller products. Of course, most products have direct streaming, which for some patients reduces the need for the telecoil (for listening on the telephone at least—see next paragraph).

In addition to use on the telephone, the telecoil can be used to pick up electromagnetic fields generated by electric currents traveling through wires, such as induction loop systems used in public facilities (e.g., auditoriums, museums, places of worship, etc.). With a properly functioning telecoil, patients can take advantage of "looped rooms" by switching the regular microphone setting over to the telecoil setting. A "looped room" or induction loop allows the patient to listen at a much more favorable signal-to-noise ratio when their hearing aids are on the telecoil setting. In some noisy areas, they may do better than someone with normal hearing. There is a concerted effort to increase the looping of public facilities in America, which is far behind many other countries in this regard. Unfortunately, many patients, even those who have a telecoil, are not aware of this great feature. You may want to remind your hearing aid patients to look for the symbol shown in Figure 5–4 when they are in public facilities. You can also refer them to the website: http://www.loopamerica.com/.

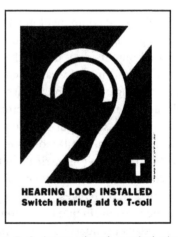

Figure 5–4. International symbol showing that a hearing loop is installed. *Source*: From *Fitting and Dispensing Hearing Aids* (2nd ed., p. 236), by B. Taylor and H. G. Mueller, 2017, San Diego, CA: Plural Publishing. Reprinted with permission.

KEY CONCEPT: Background Noise and Phone Communication

As we have discussed, telecoils are a good thing, and in general are under-utilized. Today, we also have wireless streaming as an option for telephone communication. And of course, there is the time-honored approach of simply holding the phone to the hearing aid and using the acoustic pathway. Which one of the three is best if you have an open-earmold fitting? Well, interestingly, for patients with mild-to-moderate hearing loss and open fittings, what actually works the best for listening on the phone when background noise is present is the simple approach of hold-ing the phone to the ear. Why is this true when such sophisticated alterna-tive technology is available? Con-sider that for both the telecoil and the streaming, when the fitting is open, all the important low-frequency com-ponents of the speech signal will leak out of the ear. With the phone at the ear, however, they will travel directly to the tympanic membrane (TM), as they do with normal conversation. Also, when the phone is at the ear and held tightly, it provides a little extra attenuation of the background noise.

Receivers

If you are on your back deck listening to a lit-tle Tom Petty from your sound system, your receivers are called loudspeakers. In hear-ing aids, we call them receivers. What they do is the same: they change the amplified electrical signal from the amplifier back into an acoustic form. The wearer then hears an amplified "sound" once again. The term for what comes out of the receiver is "output" or "acoustic output." As the receiver transduces electrical information into acoustical infor-mation (or vibratory, in some cases when a bone conducted signal is used—more on that later), the receiver is called the "output transducer." Most hearing aid companies use receivers from Knowles Electronics, and in case you think it's a simple process, this company alone produces around 20 differ-ent receivers that can be used with hearing instruments.

The following are a few things about receivers:

- The size of the receiver determines its output: larger parts can carry a greater magnetic field.
- Most RIC hearing aids allow you change receivers to have different amounts of power depending on the hearing loss. That is, the hearing aid doesn't have to get bigger, just the receiver, which sits in the ear canal.
- The receiver is a major consumer of the hearing aid battery, ranging from around 40% to 50% for a low-power instrument, to as much as 80% to 90% in a high-power instrument that is normally operating at a high output.
- There is an increased interest in extended high-frequency amplification, which means that receivers will have to be designed for this, but the net

effect will only be as effective as the accompanying amplifier gain.

■ Receivers are easily plugged, and this is the number one hearing aid repair problem. For decades, the industry has looked for workable solutions—wax traps, wax guards, and wax screens—yet, the problem continues.

Digital Amplification

Since essentially any hearing aid that you will encounter today is digital, it is a good idea for us to take a closer look at what makes digital, well, digital. Figure 5–5 is a block diagram of a digital hearing aid. It can be contrasted with the block diagram of an analog hearing aid shown in Figure 5–1. Note that all of the differences between analog and digital rest between the microphone and receiver. It is the digital signal processor between the mic and receiver, which is often referred to as the "black box," that warrants our attention for a few paragraphs.

Digital amplifiers have an analog-to-digital converter that digitizes the electrical waveforms into strings of mathematical bits. A digital amplifier can manipulate bits of information at great speed, allowing for less internal noise and distortion, great shaping flexibility of the incoming sound, and the ability to perform changes in the frequency response (e.g., noise suppression, feedback management). DSP must convert the digital waveform back into an analog output via a digital-to-analog converter. The purpose of the digital signal processor is to generate an output signal based on the incoming signal. It performs this feat by performing a series of breathtakingly fast calculations. The incoming acoustic signal to the hearing aid is converted to a series of numbers for these calculations to be performed. This series of calculations is called an algorithm.

You've probably heard reference to "chip technology." When we are talking about hearing aid chips, we are referring to all the electronics that sit on one extremely tiny integrated circuit board. Hearing aid chips have gotten progressively smaller and, inversely,

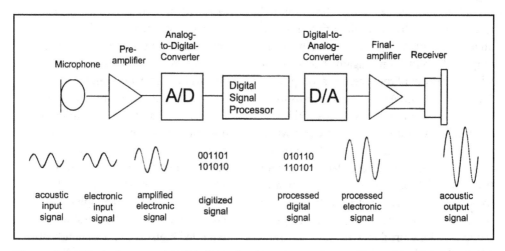

Figure 5–5. Block diagram of a digital hearing instrument. *Source*: From *Sandlin's Handbook of Hearing Aid Amplification* (3rd ed., p. 223), by M. J. Metz, 2014, San Diego, CA: Plural Publishing. Reprinted with permission.

more "stuff" can be placed on the chip. And, it is these electronic components that perform all of the necessary functions of a modern hearing aid. Unlike their old analog cousins, digital hearing aids have some significant advantages, including the ability to allow for extremely complex processing on a tiny circuit chip. It is because of DSP processing and microchip improvements that hearing aid manufacturers are able to bring to market faster and smarter algorithms nearly every year. Over the past 20+ years, major hearing aid manufacturers have brought a new "chip" to market about every two to three years. During the lifespan of the chip, several sound processing algorithms can be created and etched onto the chip. It's common for hearing aid manufacturers to update their sound processing algorithms, adding and discarding various combinations of algorithms that comprise various hearing aid modes during the life of a single chip. A hearing aid often becomes obsolete in 5 to 6 years.

Today, all major hearing aid manufacturers use one chip for an entire line of products. In case you're not aware, manufacturers typically have an entry-level product, an intermediate product, and a premier product. They vary in cost, and audiologists then also tend to sell these products in incremental cost increases. For example, a pair of entry-level hearing aids may sell for $4,000; midlevel $5,000; and a pair of premier for $6,000. The point we are making here is that it's typically the same chip for all products—the difference is that extra features have been added or simply opened up on the chip. A more sophisticated algorithm does not necessarily translate into a better hearing aid for a given individual patient. A patient who is not interested in direct streaming from his smartphone, doesn't want rechargeable batteries, and lives a fairly quiet lifestyle, could very likely do just as well with the entry level as the premier

level. Some manufacturers have even given control to the clinician, as they allow the fitter to turn a hearing aid into an entry, midlevel, or premium product in the office with their computer. And, chances are good that in the near future, patients will be able to make these changes on their own. At the core of hearing aid chips and algorithms, however, are some essential functions that we discuss next.

Basic Descriptors of Hearing Aid Performance

As you recall from our discussion of audiometry, two core components in audiology are intensity and frequency. "Audiologists do it with frequency and intensity" is a cheesy slogan you can find on a T-shirt in the closet of most any AuD student! Intensity relates to how much energy a sound possesses. In the hearing aid world, the terms gain and output quantify the intensity level of amplified sound. On the other hand, frequency is related to pitch and timbre of sound. Frequency response is the term used to describe this concept in hearing aids, and indeed, hearing aids have a "frequency response," an essential component in the fitting process.

Gain

Gain is the amount of sound pressure difference between the input of sound as it enters the hearing aid and the amplified sound as it leaves the hearing aid receiver. Gain is always expressed in dB (note that the plural for dB is dB, not dBs). For example, if the input signal is 50 dB SPL and the final output is 80 dB SPL, the gain is simply the difference between the input and output, or 30 dB. Even though this example was in SPL, *gain* is not expressed using any reference, as it is a relative measure.

If we want a given signal to be audible to the hearing aid user, then the gain, added to the level of the input signal, must exceed the users threshold (in ear canal SPL). For example, let's say that a patient had a 60 dB HL hearing loss at 2000 Hz. We need to convert that to ear canal SPL, which is a correction of around 10 dB; so for simple math, we'll say that his hearing loss is 70 dB SPL (i.e., the SPL in the ear canal). If a soft speech signal at 2000 Hz is around 40 dB SPL (which is very possible), this patient would then need 30 dB of gain to make that signal just barely audible (70–40 = 30 dB). We just worked through some of the basic fundamentals of a "prescriptive fitting," but let's save that discussion for Chapter 6.

Because the input of speech is different for different frequencies and the patient's hearing loss usually is different for different frequencies, it shouldn't surprise you that the programmed gain of the hearing aid also will be different at different frequencies. As the input signal becomes louder, the gain that is necessary usually goes down, as most patients have a nonlinear loudness growth function. The exact amount of gain that is necessary for different inputs for various frequencies is related to the degree and slope of the hearing loss.

As gain does vary for the different frequencies, we often measure average maximum gain to describe the overall gain of the hearing aid using a single number. Peak gain (sometimes called full-on gain) is the maximum amount of gain when the volume control of the hearing aid is fully on. We also need to remember that we usually will want some "reserve" gain, as most individuals hearing loss becomes worse over time. Or, they may develop a mild temporary conductive hearing loss. Also, there may be some listening situations where greater gain is needed. So, if we're thinking that a patient probably will "use" around 25 to 30 dB gain, we'd want an instrument that had a maximum of 35 dB to 40 dB of gain.

Output

Although gain is simply a difference measure (output minus the input), output is an expression of the overall sound power. Output is expressed in dB SPL and is referred to as maximum power output (MPO) or saturation sound pressure level (SSPL) or output sound pressure level (OSPL). For some measures (e.g., 2-cc coupler), a 90 dB input is used, and the term would then be "OSPL90; previously called SSPL90." When probe-mic measures are used, the maximum output can be measured in the real ear. In this case, it is referred to as the real-ear aided response (REAR) for a specific input, such as the REAR85 or REAR90 (previously called the real-ear saturation response, or RESR).

Nearly all of today's hearing aids allow the fitter to select the maximum output (within a 15–20 dB range), by adjusting the output limiting compression. Using compression to set the MPO correctly on a hearing aid is important because this keeps loud sounds from becoming uncomfortably or painfully loud. With children, there may also be a safety issue—it is not common, but it is possible to observe a threshold shift from excessive hearing aid amplification.

If loud sounds are too loud, the patient will turn down gain and not obtain benefit for conversational speech. And again, from a safety standpoint, it may not be wise to allow the patient to determine how loud sounds should be. Patients with severe–profound hearing losses are not always a good judge of when things are dangerously loud, especially if they have become accustomed to listening to very high-level outputs.

On the other hand, if the MPO is too low, and the louder components of speech are unnecessarily reduced, the dynamics of speech will be altered, which can result in poor speech quality and reduced speech understanding ability. An MPO setting that is too low will also make music sound dull, and it won't have the necessary dynamics. In other words, the MPO can't be too low or too high; it has to be "just right." (Think Goldilocks and the bears' porridge.) As we discuss in the next chapter, audiologists conduct a test using high-level pure tones at different frequencies, which results in determining the patient's loudness discomfort level (LDL). The findings of this test are then used to individualize the hearing aid output for each patient.

It's easy to confuse gain and output. In Figure 5–6 we show an example of both of these measures for the same hearing aid

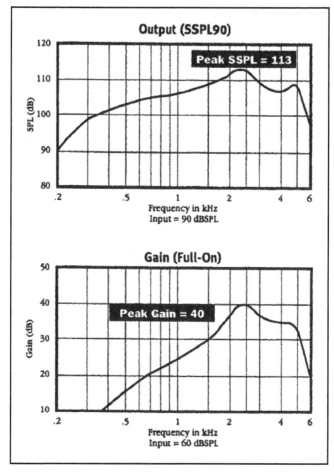

Figure 5–6. The top graph shows the output for a hearing aid, whereas the bottom graph shows the full-on gain for the same hearing aid. Notice that the vertical axis is different for the two graphs: the top being absolute (in SPL) and the bottom is relative (gain). *Source*: From *Fitting and Dispensing Hearing Aids* (2nd ed., p. 245), by B. Taylor and H. G. Mueller, 2017, San Diego, CA: Plural Publishing. Reprinted with permission.

using an input signal of 60 dB SPL. Note that in the upper curve (output), the dB values are absolute. In contrast, the lower curve represents a difference value (the input of 60 dB has been subtracted from the output). There is a point where an increase in input does not result in an increase in output. This is when we know that we have reached the hearing aid's maximum power output (MPO).

Frequency Response

A curve depicting the relative gain of the hearing aid over the entire range of amplified frequencies is called a frequency response curve. A hearing aid does not amplify all frequencies uniformly, and hence, the frequency response of a hearing is not "flat" like you might expect from a high-end stereo system. It is not intended to be.

The frequency response on a modern hearing aid can be altered significantly by using the programming software (i.e., adjusting amplifier gain). Just like output and gain, the fine tuning of the hearing aid's frequency response is determined by several factors, including the patient's audiometric thresholds and their LDLs. Most hearing aids provide significant low-frequency gain down to 200 Hz or so, although this only is possible with a relatively tight fitting in the ear canal (remember that low frequencies easily leak out of the ear canal if there is venting). High-frequency gain usually extends out to 5000 Hz to 6000 Hz or so, and then rolls off. In recent years, there have been efforts to extend this high-frequency gain. This has been shown to have some benefit for children learning speech sounds. For adults, the true benefit of extended high frequencies has yet to be determined, and depends on the slope of the audiogram and the degree of the high-frequency hearing loss. Does input + gain = audibility? For most older adults obtaining hearing aids, for frequencies at 6000 Hz and above, the answer is "no."

Hearing Aid Compression

A final component that we will find on nearly all hearing aids today is something called "compression." Compression can be classified into two major categories: input compression and output compression—also referred to as automatic gain control-input (AGCi), and automatic gain control-output (AGCo), respectively. Hearing aids have both as they serve different purposes for the hearing aid user. Audiologists program both so that the loudness sensations are individualized for a given patient. The two circuits can operate simultaneously, although usually AGCo just sits back and waits for something loud to happen. Both types of compression are programmed for each channel (frequency band) of the hearing aid. A hearing aid with 16 channels could have 16 different compression settings. Because the dynamic range and LDLs for most hearing losses change as a function of frequency, programming different compression characteristics is one of the main benefits of multichannel processing.

AGCo is used to limit the maximum output of loud sounds. Think of it as a "stop sign," setting the ceiling for loud sounds—ensuring that those loud sounds fall below the patient's LDL. If the patient's LDL is 105, then the audiologist will set the AGCo kneepoint (dB level of compression activation) just below this value—maybe at 102 dB or so. Input compression, on the other hand, is commonly used for mild to moderate hearing losses to manage the incoming speech signal. That is, AGCi is used to

---

KEY CONCEPT: Quick Reference for Major Components

- Microphone: An auditory transducer, which converts the acoustic signal from the sound field into an electrical signal that goes to the amplifier. Nearly all hearing aids today have two microphones, which allows for special directional processing.
- Digital conversion: The electrical signal is converted into digital information to allow for computerized signal manipulation and application of different processing algorithms. The digital signal is subsequently reconverted to an electrical signal that is sent to the receiver.
- Amplifier: The heart of the hearing aid circuitry where the input signal is increased in level and filtered in frequency, and then sent to the digital converter. This chip also includes algorithms for all special signal processing features of the hearing aid.
- Receiver: An auditory transducer (speaker), which converts the amplified signal from the hearing aid into an acoustical signal that is delivered to the patient's ear.

- Battery: Provides the power source for the hearing aid. Batteries come in different sizes to match the size and power requirements of the hearing aid. Many models have rechargeable batteries.
- Volume control: Many hearing aids have a volume control that can be a wheel or button on the aid itself or could be a function part of a remote control device that also can be used to change the programmed settings. Volume also can be controlled with smartphone apps. In some cases, the volume control can be deactivated or the volume control range can be limited.
- Button/rocker: The button on a hearing aid can have several functions including changing programs, activating assistive technology or even can be used as a volume control. It can also be deactivated so that it does nothing at all.
- Telecoil: An alternative input source that converts the electromagnetic signal from a telephone or an assistive listening device and delivers it to the amplifier; available on all but the smallest hearing aids.

---

restore loudness (or nearly restore loudness) for soft, average, and loud inputs. By "restore loudness" we mean that when the hearing aids are programmed correctly, the person with a hearing loss (mild to moderate) should hear soft sounds soft, average sounds average, and loud sounds loud (but not too loud), just like someone with normal hearing hears them. Because AGCi starts its compression at a low level, it is usually referred to as wide dynamic range compression (WDRC).

A Few Tidbits About WDRC

- This is a specific type of input compression. It is associated with low-threshold kneepoints—the starting point of compression (less than 55 dB SPL; as low as ~25 to 30 dB SPL on some instruments).
- It has low compression ratios (less than 4:1, most commonly around 2:1). Think of the ratio as the "squash effect." If something is squash by 2:1, it is made only half as big—if 40 dB of an 80 dB signal is compressed, that 40 dB turns into only 20 dB. This is how we accomplish loudness normalization.
- Because of the low kneepoints and relatively small ratios, compression takes place over a wide range of input levels, including nearly the entire average speech signal.
- The simple rule to remember is that as input goes up, gain goes down.
- People with mild–moderate cochlear pathology have LDLs similar to people with normal hearing. An advantage, then, of WDRC is that little or no gain can be applied for loud inputs, but significant gain can be applied to soft inputs, making them audible.

ACGo Compression

- Output limiting compression (shutting things down on the top end) is typically associated with output compression (AGCo).
- Output limiting compression is associated with high compression kneepoints (just below the LDL) and high compression ratios (very serious squash effect).
- The kneepoints used for output limiting are usually around 100 dB to 115 dB (i.e., for 2-cc coupler). Why? Because this corresponds to the LDL of the average hearing-impaired patient (when converted to 2-cc coupler values).
- The compression ratio of an output-limiting compressor is usually around 10 to 1, which means that there is only a 1 dB corresponding increase in output for a 10 dB change in input, once the signal is above the kneepoint.
- Our final point: Consider that output-limiting compression is used as a partner with WDRC. WDRC takes care of the soft to loud speech sounds; output limiting takes care of the very loud sounds. When they are programmed correctly, the patient might not ever need to adjust their volume for any listening condition.

Hearing Aid Features

Today's hearing aids have many, many features. So many that after we talk about a dozen or so in the new few pages, there still might be a few minor ones that we have left out. And, different manufacturers add more all the time. The ones we'll cover definitely do address all the important factors related to speech understanding and listening in background noise. Many of these features and algorithms are designed to improve the amplified signal and to provide added audibility in different environments. Some features are designed for increased listening comfort and easier operation for the patient. And what we've seen in the past few years is the marriage between hearing aids and other health-related wearable devices, and increased communication between the hearing aids and the patient's smartphone.

Multiple Channels

Depending on the model, digital hearing aids have between 4 and 48 frequency channels (frequency processing regions), allowing for adjustments in gain and output to be made in individual frequency regions that can compensate for a hearing loss. Although one might think that "more is better," and this is generally true, the differences are not as striking as they may seem. We usually see 8 or so channels, even in the entry-level products, and for some patients, this is probably enough.

Real-world example of benefit: Patti often sits in her office at work at Rush University writing book chapters. Occasionally, students come in to talk. The air conditioning system in the building is quite loud; it's predominately low frequencies. Her hearing aids detect this as noise, but only for the lower frequencies, and they automatically reduce gain in the low frequency channels. She can still hear the higher frequency speech sounds, as gain was left untouched in this region.

Multiple Memory Programs

A pushbutton, remote control, or smartphone allows changes to different programed settings. A "program" is a "memory" that can be programmed totally different than other memories. For example, a patient may have special programs for listening to music or listening in a car. For most situations, the hearing aid automatically selects the most optimum programing for a given listening situation, as determined by the signal classification system, and this happens all in one program, often labelled "universal." There are times, however, when the patient might want to override this, or has listening needs different from the default programming.

Real-world example of benefit: In the summer, Butch likes to sit on his back deck sipping a beer, looking at the Missouri river flow by, and listening to his favorite musical artist, John Prine. He had his audiologist give him a special program for music that had considerably more gain in the lows, no compression, and raised the output of the hearing aids up to 110 dB (his LDLs for most things are around 100 dB, but for music it's 110 dB). When he heads to the deck, he simply takes out his smartphone and taps on "Butch's deck music" (custom-named by his audiologist).

Signal Classification

This can be considered the "coach" or "manager" of the hearing aid processing. It decides who plays in the game when or where, as well as what features sit on the bench for some listening conditions. It operates automatically and continually measures the input signal to determine overall level, spectrum of the signal (speech, noise, music, etc.), and also the azimuth of the signal. Armed with this information, the algorithm controls features to automatically switch on or off to optimize processing for a given input signal. This classification process is used to control gain and output, and to trigger different types of noise reduction, directional microphones, or beam forming technologies.

Real-world example of benefit: Ben works as a waiter at the House of Prime Rib in San

Francisco. The job creates a unique listening experience in that the dining room is fairly quiet (mostly older customers, a carpeted floor in one area), but the kitchen is very noisy (people talking, pots clanging, music blaring, etc.). He spends all evening going back and forth from the quiet to the noise. Fortunately, his hearing aids easily detect this and automatically change (within a few seconds) from omnidirectional when in the dining area (to hear his customers from all around) to directional processing (focused listening with noise attenuation in the kitchen).

Expansion

Some manufacturers label this feature "microphone noise reduction," some call it "soft squelch," and others call it "low level noise reduction." Some don't call it anything at all, but it is still there. Expansion compresses signals *below the kneepoint* and is used to minimize annoyance from amplified microphone noise and low-level environmental sounds. Expansion often allows the patient to use the gain necessary to make soft speech audible without the negative side effects of excessive amplification of ambient noise. You can think of expansion as compression in reverse: when sound is *below* the kneepoint, it is squashed. It has no effect whenever the signal is *above* the kneepoint. The relationship between expansion and compression is shown in Figure 5–7.

Real-world example of benefit: Herman has a relatively flat bilateral hearing loss and needs considerable gain in the low frequencies to hear soft speech. He frequently sits in the kitchen talking to his wife, who talks fairly softly—he needs considerable gain to make her speech audible and his

hearing aids are programmed accordingly. But, he doesn't need to have the hum of the refrigerator motor amplified. Fortunately, his expansion kneepoint is adjusted so that it is *above* the sound of the refrigerator (which then attenuates this signal), but *below* the level of his wife's voice (which means that this soft speech will receive maximum gain).

Digital Noise Reduction (Basic)

Based on the signal classification, different types of noise reduction are implemented, often simultaneously. Modulation-based is the most fundamental, and tends to reduce overall gain for a given channel when noise is the dominant signal in that channel. The modulations of speech (4–6/s) are much different of those of noise, and even a low-level hearing aid can detect the difference. This specific type of DNR does not improve the SNR directly, as gain is reduced for everything (including speech), but it reduces annoyance and creates more relaxed listening, making daylong listening less fatiguing.

Real-world example of benefit: Lee is always out fishing, looking to catch the biggest walleye. He's often with his wife or a friend, trolling the various lakes of central Minnesota—a big part of the day is the fun conversations and the fish stories. He's lucky because the modulation-based noise reduction in his hearing aids is very effective in cutting down the noise of the boat motor (low-frequencies), yet not changing gain for 1000 Hz and above, where the important speech frequencies are located. Currently his DNR is set to "mid," but an option would be to have a special "Lee's Boat" program with it set to "max."

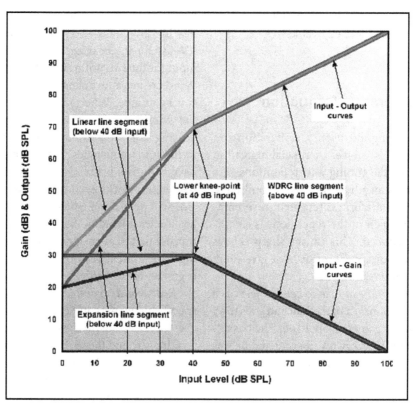

Figure 5–7. Input/output and input/gain curves for compression and expansion. The top two curves are input/output curves, and the bottom set are input/gain curves. Note the compression kneepoint (CK) is 40 dB SPL. The lower line on the chart illustrates the effects of expansion for inputs below the 40 dB SPL kneepoint. The kneepoints of compression and expansion are not always the same, as shown here, but do tend to be similar. The SPL setting of these kneepoints changes throughout the speech range to mimic the spectrum of soft speech—kneepoints higher in the low frequencies than in the high frequencies. *Source*: From *Fitting and Dispensing Hearing Aids* (2nd ed., p. 261), by B. Taylor and H. G. Mueller, 2017, San Diego, CA: Plural Publishing. Reprinted with permission.

Impulse Noise Reduction

All incoming signals are analyzed, searching for any spectrum that has a very rapid rise time. When this is detected, the signal is dampened. The DNR in this case acting much like AGCi with a very fast attack and release. The effect to the user is a less harsh, smoother signal.

Real-world example of benefit: One of Caitlin's favorite restaurants is The Kitchen in Sacramento. She really enjoys sitting at the counter by the open kitchen, but with her old hearing aids, the constant clinking and clanging of the dishes and pots and pans was more than she could tolerate. Her new hearing aids, however, have "sound smoothing." With this feature, these sounds are still audible, but not as harsh, making her 3-hr dinner much more enjoyable.

Reverberation Reduction

To a hearing aid user, reverberation can be as bad as "noise." A special algorithm examines the timing and repetitions of a given waveform within a few seconds, and when the waveform is repeated (reverberation), the gain of the repetitions is significantly reduced. This causes sharp echoes to almost disappear, or at least give them some dullness.

Real-world example of benefit: Jerry is a big fan of Gonzaga basketball and goes to all their home games in Spokane. The basketball stadium is very reverberant and he was having trouble understanding conversation, not to mention that all the reverberation and noise was annoying. He was considering simply not wearing his hearing aids—making it tough to talk to his son during the games. His new hearing aids, however, have a feature called "EchoShield," and his audiologist programmed them to "max effect" and stored this in Program 2 of his hearing aids (and simply labeled the program "Zags" so he could remember). Now, when he enters "The New Kennel," he simply pulls out his cell phone and taps on the Zags program. He notes that everything sounds mellower, and he thinks he can even understand better than with his conventional program.

Wind Noise Reduction

If you've handled a microphone at all, at one time or another, you've probably blown on it to see if it was working—the result is a nasty low-frequency noise. Recall that nearly all hearing aids have two microphone ports. It's easy for the hearing aid to compare the input for the two ports and made decisions. Wind creates a turbulence at the ports that is very unique. When this is detected, and the wind noise feature is activated, the hearing aids will automatically reduce gain in the low frequencies. If the hearing aids have complete bilateral full-audio sharing, the feature works even better. The hearing aids will determine which side of the head has the least wind noise, and automatically transfer that cleaner signal to the other hearing aid—a great feature if the wind noise is greater for one side.

Real-world example of benefit: Kirby spends his winters in Scottsdale, and most every day he's out on the golf course. While standing around the tee box or on the green, it's common that he and his buddies share a few jokes or sports stories. Kirby is in good shape to hear the punch lines, as his hearing aids have the automatic wind noise reduction feature and also full-audio sharing between hearing aids. He has learned to position himself so that the wind is mostly striking one side of his head (his worse hearing ear), which means he obtains the bilateral reduction in gain, with the cleaner signal from the off-wind side delivered to both ears.

Adaptive Feedback Reduction

This feature first detects any *acoustic feedback* or "whistling" and then reduces or eliminates the problem through phase cancellation. This is accomplished by introducing an out-of-phase signal, the same frequency as the feedback. Some products also add frequency shifting and narrow notches to enhance the effect. In most products,

---

DID YOU KNOW: Modern Feedback Reduction Is So Good That . . .

1. For many years, patients determined if their hearing aids were turned on and the battery was working by cupping the aids in their hand before putting them on the ear. If they were working, there was feedback. Many of today's systems are so good at reducing feedback that no feedback is present when this technique is used.

2. For many years, to effectively adjust the gain of their hearing aids, patients would turn the volume control louder and louder until they heard feedback, and then turn it down just a little below this level. Many of today's systems are so good at reducing feedback that even on the ear, you can turn the gain to "max" and no feedback is present.

3. For many years, stand-up comics and cartoonists enjoyed making fun of people wearing whistling hearing aids. A recent Google search revealed 10 or more cartoons related to this problem. In 20 years, no one will get the intended humor.

---

this allows the user an additional 5 dB to 15 dB of gain without feedback and is one of the most beneficial features introduced in hearing aids in recent years. Most hearing aid users rarely or ever experience feedback during routine use (see related "Did You Know.")

Real-world example of benefit: Bernice is 80 and has used hearing aids for 20 years—she has a bilateral moderate–severe hearing loss. She lives alone and enjoys talking on the phone with her friends. But, she can't understand without her hearing aids, and because she has started to use more gain, when she places the phone to her ear, she has acoustic feedback. As a result, Bernice has stopped calling her friends. Last week, Bernice got new hearing aids with modern feedback technology—her audiologist fit her with the product that has the best technology (not all manufacturers are the same). Bernice now has plenty of gain, and no feedback on the phone. She was up until 10:00 p.m. calling everyone she knows!

Directional Microphone Technology (General)

Directional microphone technology reduces the output of the hearing aids for sounds from specific azimuth origins by using two omnidirectional microphones and creating phase delays between the output from them. Sounds (noise) coming from the sides and back can be reduced without changing the output for sounds from the desired listening direction. For example, if the desired talker is in front, noise from the sides and back are reduced. Most of today's hearing aids automatically will switch to directional processing when certain noise conditions are detected.

Real-world example of benefit: Ryan has a favorite Atlanta micro-brewery, where he likes to go with his Army buddies—during Happy Hour it tends to be very noisy. He's convinced his friends that they all sit in a specific corner of the pub, and Ryan sits with his back to the crowd. The directional

---

CASE STUDY: A Real Fish Story

Not all hearing aid patients are satisfied customers, but one of the most glowing letters from a patient that we've seen supporting adaptive directional technology came from a fellow who worked at the famous Pike Place Fish Market in Seattle. While meeting with the public in the open market area, there was a constant stream of forklifts traveling behind him unloading fresh fish. He was a long-time user of directional technology, but noticed a significant improvement in his ability to understand his customers when he switched to the new adaptive directional hearing aids. The reasons should be obvious: the customers were in front, the noise was from behind—the noise was loud enough to trigger directional processing, the noise was a true broadband noise (not other speech signals), the adaptive technology could track the noise, and there was little reverberation. A fish story that doesn't even need any exaggeration!

---

technology serves to reduce the overall background babble (behind) and allows for maximum gain for his friends (in the front hemisphere of his listening circle), making his Peachtree IPA even more enjoyable.

Directional Microphone Technology (Spatial Focus)

This is an advancement of directional technology, which allows the focus of amplification to be placed at the right or left side, or the back, rather than always toward the front. Signals from other azimuths (presumed to be unwanted) are reduced in output, improving the SNR for the desired speech signal—if the hearing aid detects a talker from the back and noise is present, it will reduce the noise from the front. Unlike traditional directional, the patient does not have to look at the talker to obtain the desired benefit. The hearing aid can be set so that this happens automatically, or it can be manually selected by using a smartphone app (Figure 5–8).

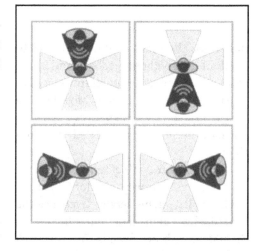

Figure 5–8. Screenshot of the spatial configuration feature from the smartphone app. The patient can override the automatic function of the hearing aids by tapping on any one of the four squares. The darkened triangle on each square indicates the focus for speech. *Source*: Photo courtesy of Sivantos GmbH or its affiliates © 2019. All rights reserved.

Real-world example of benefit: Elaine is a doting grandmother, and likes to take her two young grandchildren with her on shopping trips. They always sit in their car seats in the back seat of her car. Elaine's hearing aids have directional spatial focus. Normally for driving the car, her hearing aids will be in omnidirectional for listening to music. But with spatial focus, when one of the children is talking, the hearing aids will detect the presence and location of the speech, and the polar plot (speech focus) of the hearing aids will automatically provide maximum amplification for sounds coming from the back, and reduce gain for sounds from other azimuths (bothersome car noise). This feature is also helpful when Elaine is a passenger, riding in the car with her husband, as now the algorithm will automatically focus to the left whenever he is talking.

Directional Microphone Technology (Bilateral Beamforming/Narrow Focus)

Bilateral hearing aids can share full-audio information from the four microphones (two on each side), which allows for creating "beams of focus" for different azimuths.

THINGS TO REMEMBER: Important Directional Hearing Aid Terms

Nearly all hearing aids are directional (or can be) and therefore it's important to understand some of the terms and functions of these instruments.

- Directivity Index (DI): It is a ratio that compares the output of a hearing aid for a signal presented at 0 degrees versus signals presented at all other azimuths around the hearing. In theory, the DI of an omnidirectional microphone would be 0 dB (equal for all azimuths). A good directional hearing aid system will have a DI of 4 dB to 6 dB or so, depending on the style of the hearing aid and the test method. The DI loosely relates to the expected SNR advantage in a diffuse noise field.
- Automatic directional: A hearing aid that automatically switches between directional and omnidirectional depending on the classification of the input signal.
- Adaptive directional: The polar plot null (point of maximum attenuation) automatically changes as the detection algorithm locates noise at different sources behind the user. Ability to track a single noise source such as a moving car.
- Bilateral beamforming: Input for microphones on right hearing aid communicates with the microphones for the left hearing aid, which allows for forming a narrow beam of focus, and enhances forming beams to azimuths other than the front.
- Spatial focus: Through detection of the dominant speech signal, the focus of amplification can be placed toward other azimuths than the front (even though the patient is looking to the front), such as the right or left side, or to the back.
- Strange but true: At one time (1970s–1980s), directional hearing aids had directional microphones. Not so today. Directional technology is accomplished by manipulating the phase of the input from two *omnidirectional* microphones.

This is referred to as bilateral beam forming. This gives a much narrower beam to the front than can be obtained with traditional directional technology. The focus of the narrow beam will be in the "look direction" of the user, meaning that it is most useful when there is single target speaker, or when it's easy to look at the speaker of interest (sitting at a table in noisy restaurant).

Real-world example of benefit: Karen has two grandchildren (twins), and last week she went to their kindergarten class play. It was on a stage in an old gymnasium which had terrible acoustics. To make it worse, there were some people standing in back talking. There was enough noise in the room to prompt her hearing aids to automatically switch to directional, but not enough to cause them to switch to narrow directivity. Understanding the little girls was difficult. Karen used her smartphone app to select the narrow-beam function, as she knew she'd be looking directly at the girls. Also, unknown to Karen, the hearing aids are designed to add an extra 5 dB of gain within the focus of the beam (the logic is that you are looking at what you want to hear, and there is noise in the room, so making the desired signal 5 dB louder makes sense).

All was better, and in fact, at one point she had to tell her friend sitting next to her, who had normal hearing, what was said on the stage!

Own Voice Processing

A common problem, especially for a new hearing aid user, is that when the hearing aids are programmed so that the speech of others is audible and comfortably loud, the patient's own voice is too loud. The own-voice feature automatically detects when the person is talking (after a minute of one-time training), and then instantaneously reduces gain whenever the person's own voice is detected. As soon as the user's voice stops, gain instantly returns to programmed settings.

Real-world example of benefit: Sienna is 10 and, unfortunately, her hearing loss has gotten worse the last couple years. She was just re-fitted with new closed earmolds so that the necessary low-frequency gain could be obtained (she had been wearing open earmolds). Initially, she was very disturbed regarding how her own voice sounded, but

---

CLINICAL TIP: The Latest on Frequency Lowering

Frequency lowering is an intriguing topic, and we could write an entire section on it, rather than only provide one clinical example. The research results for patients using this technology are mixed, but it is available from all major hearing aid manufacturers. In general, research findings have been more favorable for children than adults. If this is a topic that you are interested in, or you have clients using frequency lowering, we suggest you review the work of Susan Scollie, Danielle Glista, and colleagues at Western University in Ontario, who have conducted many of the pioneering studies in the area, and have presented detailed protocols for verification. Figures 5–10 and 5–11 shown here are from their work.

once the hearing aids were trained for her voice and the own-voice algorithm was activated, her voice sounded the same as it had with her previous open fittings.

Frequency Lowering

This technology is accomplished using frequency compression or linear frequency transposition (Figure 5–9 is an illustration of frequency compression). Patient benefit appears to be the same regardless of what technology is used. The algorithm takes the spectral speech energy available at higher frequencies and lowers it to a frequency region where the listener has better thresholds, increasing the likelihood that the speech signal (e.g., such as /s/ or /sh/) will be audible, albeit at a different frequency. The /s/ and /sh/ frequency range is shown in Figure 5–10. Frequency lowering usually is applied when there is mild to moderate hearing loss in the low to mid frequencies, and a severe to profound loss in the high frequencies that is not usable for speech recognition with traditional amplification.

Real-world example of benefit: After initially using standard amplification, at age 3, Cori was fitted with hearing aids that had frequency lowering. Probe-mic testing clearly showed that her hearing loss was so severe in the high frequencies, that traditional gain adjustments were not making high-frequency speech sounds audible, even at maximum settings. Frequency lowering was carefully adjusted using probe-mic verification to ensure that the higher frequencies had indeed been made audible at the target frequency range (Figure 5–11). Initial testing indicated benefit with frequency lowering. It's now a year later and her parents state that she is doing much better hearing and understanding speech. And—

there was a bonus dividend; her speech quality also has improved significantly.

Linked Hearing Aids

Earlier we talked about hearing aids with *full-audio* data sharing. Most products do not have this feature, but the hearing aids still are linked for other communication. This allows bilateral hearing aids to "talk to each other" and share information through a type of near-field magnetic induction transmission. This linking allows the patient to change a feature on one hearing aid and the other aid will automatically equally change—the feature can be selected during programming. In some cases, one hearing aid can control one function and the other hearing aid a different function.

Real-world example of benefit: Don is now 70, and all the years of being a baseball pitcher in his younger days have caught up to him. He can only lift his right arm up to midchest, certainly not to ear level. Not good for throwing a baseball, but things with his hearing aids aren't that bad. His audiologist programmed them so that he only has to touch the toggle on the left hearing aid to make both hearing aids louder or softer (she gave him a +/– 8 dB range). Now, you're maybe saying, why doesn't he just use his cell phone app? Don doesn't own a smartphone, and has no intention of ever owning one!

Data Logging

The hearing aids keep a record of the daily environments experienced by the patient—such as the overall input level and the SNR for all listening situations—as well as the attributes of the hearing aid function—such

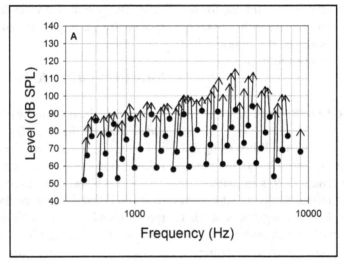

A

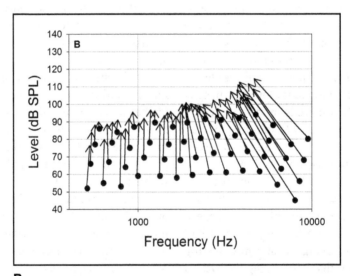

B

Figure 5–9. Illustration of frequency lowering using frequency compression. The top panel (**A**) illustrates how the soft, average, and loud components of average speech are amplified in a traditional fitting (e.g., the end of the arrow is the destination frequency, and the vertical length of the arrow represents the amount of gain applied). The bottom panel (**B**) represents how this would be altered with frequency lowering using frequency compression. Note that for approximately 2000 Hz and above, the destination frequency is lower than the input frequency, and the higher the frequency, the greater the lowering. *Source*: Adapted from Kokx-Ryan, et al., 2015. From *Essentials of Modern Hearing Aids: Selection, Fitting, and Verification* (p. 463), by T. A. Ricketts, R. Bentler, and H. G. Mueller, 2019, San Diego, CA: Plural Publishing. Reprinted with permission.

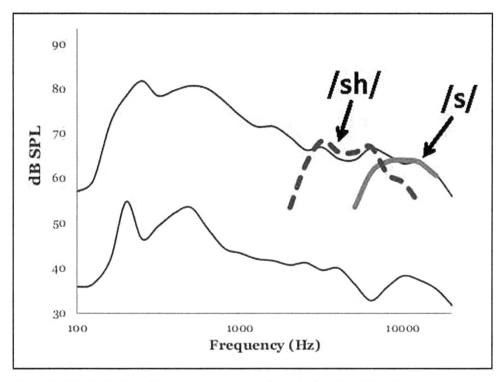

Figure 5–10. Illustration of the speech sounds /s/ and /sh/ as they fall in the average speech spectrum (displayed here in SPL). (Adapted from Scollie et al, 2014)

as volume control position and the listening program/memory setting. For example, after the patient has used the hearing aid for a period of time, the audiologist can read out (in the fitting software) the amount of time the aid (presumably on the patient's ear) was in different environments (based on the data from the signal classification system).

Real-world example of benefit: Sloan is a teenager who likes to listen to music after school in her bedroom while doing homework. From her iPhone, she streams Pandora to her portable Bose speaker. She just obtained new hearing aids, and her audiologist gave her a special program for listening to music (Program #3) and also gave her a dedicated program for the telephone (Program #2), which she can select with

her iPhone app. When she returned for her postfitting follow-up, she mentioned that the music at home doesn't sound as good as it did in the clinic demo a few weeks earlier. The audiologist reads out the data logging, and finds that Sloan has not used the music program. She had thought that the music program was Program 2, which had been used for nearly 50 hours. Some repeat counseling was in order (thanks to data logging).

Patient-Driven Training

This is the ability for the patient to train the gain and output through hearing aid adjustments for different listening conditions. The hearing aid "remembers" the pairing of the patient's selection, the input

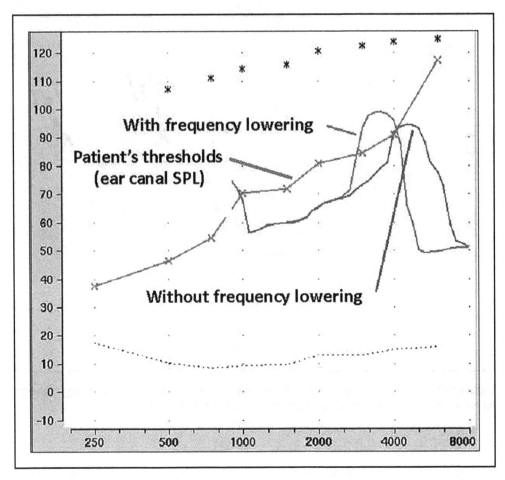

Figure 5–11. Real-ear values showing the effects of frequency compression for on versus off. The upward sloping line (X—X) represents the patient's threshold converted to ear canal SPL. Note that before lowering, the /sh/ sound was not audible, but following frequency lowering, the signal is now above the threshold values. (Adapted from Scollie at al, 2014)

level, and the listening setting (e.g., speech in quiet, speech in noise, noise, music, etc.). While the audiologist is indeed in charge of the initial programming, the notion is that giving the patient some control allows them to become more vested in his or her hearing rehabilitation—getting the "best" fitting becomes a shared task between the patient and the audiologist.

Real-world example of benefit: When an audiologist programs a hearing aid to pre-scriptive targets, using an WDRC instrument, it is assumed that when the patient goes out into the real world, soft sounds will be soft, average sounds will be "average," and loud sounds will be loud (but not too loud). The fitting algorithm is based on the assumption that the patient has a linear loudness growth function. Not all patients do, and Robin was one of those who fell into this category. He was a long-time hearing aid user, but was just fitted with a new pair, programmed to prescriptive targets. Once he started using them around the house, he immediately found that he could hear soft sounds that he had not heard for many years—he was okay with that. He also noted that loud sounds were not as annoying as they had been with his old hearing aids—he was really okay with that. But there was one problem. Whenever he was talking to his wife or listening to TV (at the level that his wife had it adjusted to), speech was just not loud enough. He always had to turn up the hearing aids. But interestingly, he noticed after a week or so that he no longer had to change the hearing aid volume. It was just right. Trainable hearing aids can be an amazing thing!

Audiologist-Driven Training

Audiologist-driven trainable hearing aids can be used to "auto-acclimatize" the patient to the prescribed settings over the first several months of hearing aid usage. The feature is commonly used when desired audibility is not met on the day of the fitting. The audiologist can program the hearing aids to increase gain by a fixed amount (e.g., 1–2 dB/week) over several weeks or months. Gain for the patient is then slowly, automatically increased over time, with the thought that the gradual change will be acceptable to the patient.

Real-world example of benefit: Sharon has a moderately severe hearing loss, and has been putting off getting hearing aids for many years. She's gotten used to her "quiet" world, and wonders if maybe she should just keep it that way. Her audiologist programed her hearing aids to the desired prescriptive values for Sharon's hearing loss. Sharon immediately cringes, and states it's just too loud. Not uncomfortably loud, but annoy-

ing loud. The audiologist would like to keep the settings where they are, as she knows this is the settings where Sharon will do the best. But on the other hand, the hearing aids have to be programmed so that Sharon will wear them during this initial adjustment period. Through some adjustments, the audiologist finds that what Sharon says is "okay," is about 8 dB below prescribed values. The audiologist then sets the automatic gain increase feature to increase by 1 dB/week for the next 8 weeks. Hopefully, at the end of two months, both the audiologist and Sharon will be happy!

Wireless (Bluetooth) Connectivity

Wireless electromagnetic induction allows for bilateral beamformers with full-audio transfer and linked hearing aids. Bluetooth also can be used to connect directly with smartphones, computers, personal audio players, and even navigation systems.

Real-world example of benefit: Brad dabbles in real estate, mostly selling farm properties. In the spring, when people are looking to buy or rent land, he spends a lot of time in his pickup driving around with a client. While driving, he tends to receive a few phone calls, some of which are too important not to answer. When by himself, he links his phone to the speaker system of his pickup, and he does okay understanding. But this isn't so good when someone else is in the vehicle, as some of his conversations need to be private. Fortunately, with his new hearing aids, he can link to his iPhone directly. Now when a call comes in, he easily can take calls in private. Moreover, the intelligibility is much better, as the majority of road noise is eliminated with the direct link.

KEY CONCEPT: *Tele-Audiology for Hearing Aid Fittings*

Tele-audiology is not a new concept. The first transatlantic tele-audiology test was performed in April 2009, when audiologist Jay Hall tested a patient in South Africa from Dallas at the AAA conference. It has been only in the past few years, however, that hearing aid fitting has found its way under the tele-audiology umbrella. The following are just some of the areas that tele-audiology can be helpful in assisting patients using hearing aids:

■ Ability to deliver at-home patient care by solving issues after the initial fitting through remote programming: changes to the gain, output, frequency response, feedback reduction, noise reduction, and other algorithms.

■ The ability to remotely monitor indicators such as wearing time, program use, and situation classification to determine when intervention might be necessary.

■ Ability to track the patient's satisfaction for different real-world listening conditions to determine if programming changes or additional counseling is warranted. (Note: the patient's app allows for real-time ratings of different listening situations. The hearing aid simultaneously records the acoustic characteristics of the situation.)

■ Real-time video calls as well as text and voice chat capabilities, which enable easy and direct communication between the audiologist and the patient.

Tele-Audiology

From a hearing testing standpoint, tele-audiology has been around since 2000, but only recently has this Internet-assisted tool been used for the fitting of hearing aids. Through a portal and a smartphone app, audiologists can adjust hearing aids in the patient's home from their office. This feature also allows for easy messaging with patients, or video chats if necessary.

Real-world example of benefit: Otto is 84 and has dementia. He recently was fitted with his first pair of hearing aids. Getting him to and from the clinic requires a fair amount of effort from his caregiver, his wife Bertha. Fortunately, Bertha is a big Facebook user, and as a result, is reasonably facile at using a smartphone. During the initial fitting, the tele-audiology app was installed on her smartphone, and she was instructed regarding the use. The audiologist messaged Bertha a day after the fitting, and the report was that all was well with the hearing aids. A couple days later, however, Bertha texted that there was a whistling problem when Otto sat in his favorite recliner watching TV. He always had a pillow propped behind his head, which was probably causing the feedback issue. Through coordination with Bertha, while Otto was sitting in the chair at home, the audiologist made a couple minor changes in programming, and the problem was solved! No clinic visit needed.

Movement Detection

A miniature accelerometer is placed on the chip of the hearing aid, which interfaces with the signal classification system. Depending on if the user is still or moving, the processing of the hearing aid can be programmed to change accordingly.

Real-world example of benefit: Like most female teenagers, Messina likes to go to the mall on Saturday with her girlfriends. The mall is pretty noisy on Saturdays, and her hearing aids default to directional. This is good when she stops to talk to a clerk, or when ordering her favorite drink, an Orange Julius. While walking and talking to her friends at her side, however, directional isn't the best setting, as it is attenuating their voices. Fortunately, the motion detector notes that she is moving, and already has made an agreement with the signal classifier—whenever movement occurs, switch processing to omnidirectional. Problem solved.

Geotagging

All smartphones have geotagging, which helps us track if our Uber driver is making progress, or direct us to our favorite restaurant when driving or on foot. Through wireless communication with the smartphone, the patient's hearing aids also know where he or she is located geographically.

Real-world example of benefit: Ervin lives a pretty quiet life, but during the winter, every Wednesday night he goes to the Ryder Bar for the pool league. It's noisy in there, and for a while, he simply didn't use his hearing aids. Fortunately, his brother is an audiologist and took Ervin on as project. For a couple weeks, Ervin had four different

---

CASE STUDY: A Pastoral Story

Related to the geotagging feature of hearing aids that we discussed, using his or her smartphone, the hearing aid user also can find a misplaced hearing aid. Now, you might think that this is simply to track it down in the patient's home, but there are other applications. We couldn't make the following story up. A western North Dakota rancher bought a pair of new hearing aids with this feature and, fortunately, his audiologist had trained him regarding the use. A couple days after the purchase of the hearing aids, he decided to walk the fence line of his 160 acre pasture—a common thing for ranchers to do, checking for possible breaks in the fence caused by the cattle, known to always think that the grass on the *other side* of the fence is greener. He decided to wear his new hearing aids on his walk, thinking that maybe he could hear the call of the meadowlarks occupying the pasture, a beautiful sound that he had been missing for many years. He indeed found some places needing repair, and stopped a few times to do mends. When he returned to his pickup, he realized that one of his hearing aids was missing. He activated his "find hearing aid app" and repeated his walk around the pasture. He found his lost hearing aid. No report on whether he heard the call of the meadowlarks.

"noise" programs in his hearing aids, and would switch between them (using his smartphone) to see if one was better than the rest. Indeed, there was one program where he did fairly well. His brother saved that as the "Bar" program, and linked it to the location of the bar. And so now, whenever Ervin parks in front of the Ryder Bar, he doesn't have to think about hearing aid adjustments, only sinking the 8-ball on a tough bank shot!

In Closing

While you most likely won't be fitting hearing aids, knowing a little regarding how they work will still come in handy when working with patients who are wearing them. Simple things, like knowing to switch to telecoil in a looped church, can be life changing. Hearing aid features change every year, and it's difficult for even audiologists to keep up. Most patients are not really familiar with many of the features that they have, and are totally unaware of most features that they could have, but don't. Not all features are on all products, so if an audiologist only sells their "favorite" brand, some features may never be mentioned during the familiarization process. We'll admit, the examples we gave for all the special features, although fairly typical, were selected for specific listening conditions where the possibility for success is high. Patients who don't experience those conditions wouldn't benefit from the feature, and probably don't need it in their hearing aids. But all in all, it's an exciting time in the world of hearing aids—they are not your father's Oldsmobile anymore!

6 The Hearing Aid Fitting A to Z

It was Vincent Van Gogh who said, "Great things are done by a series of small things brought together." We are not certain if he was talking about the fitting of hearing aids, but the comment is appropriate for this venture. We've heard a lot about OTC hearing aids lately and, indeed, they will serve a group of consumers who might not otherwise obtain hearing aids. But we want to make it clear: the successful fitting of hearing aids is a lot more than simply grabbing a box off a shelf. In this chapter, we'll review how the prudent audiologist fits hearing aids, and by "fit," we don't mean simply placing them on the ear, we mean the complete process. The following is a quick review of hearing aid fitting A to Z. This is all after a complete diagnostic has been completed:

- Assessment of listening needs
- Questionnaires assessing unaided handicap, real-world performance, and aided goals
- Speech-in-noise testing
- Assessment of unaided loudness discomfort level
- Development of prescriptive fitting goals
- Verification with real-ear measures
- Validation with aided speech testing
- Postfitting follow-up counseling and adjustment
- Validation using validated self-assessment outcome measures
- Rehabilitation plan, which may include auditory training

In this chapter we'll give you a glimpse into the fitting process, so that when you talk to your patients about obtaining hearing aids (from an audiologist), you'll have some idea of what they are experiencing (Portions of the following section were adapted from Mueller, Ricketts, and Bentler, 2017, and Ricketts, Bentler, and Mueller, 2019).

Before the Hearing Aid Fitting

Prefitting tools are used to assess the patient, the patient's hearing handicap, and his or her communication needs in order to begin making decisions regarding hearing aid candidacy and selection. Given the time limitations in a typical clinic setting, it is necessary that an appropriately small number of measures are selected that provide the most important information for each specific patient in an efficient manner. Because every patient is different and there is not time to gather exhaustive clinical data, this handful of assessment tools must be selected individually for each patient's situation out of the large group of possible assessment measures available. This is often an iterative process, during which the clinician uses information gathered earlier (e.g., general case history, type and degree of hearing loss, general patient goals, and problems) to determine what additional information is most critical to gather for the individual patient via additional assessments.

Understanding the Speech Signal

A big part of the success of the overall fitting relates to making speech audible, with the caveat that it also must have the appropriate loudness, minimal distortion, and a reasonable sound quality. This is why we include a soft real-speech input signal when we conduct our real-ear verification—to verify that, indeed, soft speech is appropriately audible. It is helpful during the prefitting appointment to ensure that the patient understands this fitting goal. For the new hearing aid user who still might be questioning the need for hearing aids, it might be necessary to illustrate how much of the average speech signal is *not* audible. For the experienced hearing aid user obtaining a new pair of hearing aids, it might be helpful to explain why the new

hearing aids will sound different from the old ones. These demonstrations can also be very helpful for family members who might be wondering why Mom can "hear but not understand."

For all these reasons, it's important to understand the speech signal. Unfortunately, because the audiogram is what we see and think about the most, we (and we are including audiologists in this "we") sometimes forget the representation of the speech signal in the real world, which is what is important for the patient. Most often, speech is described in static terms (overall level, overall frequency shape, etc.). By static we mean that a single number representing an average value over time is used rather than representing the signal moment by moment. For example, even though the level of speech naturally fluctuates over time, it is common to examine the level across frequency (spectrum of speech) after averaging it over some predefined segment (e.g., an entire passage). Graphic plots of these data are referred to as a Long-Term Average Speech Spectrum (LTASS). The LTASS representation is particularly useful because it can be used to quantify the relationship between speech levels and hearing thresholds, giving us a specific indication of audibility for a given patient. By comparing audibility with and without a hearing aid, we can directly demonstrate the degree that a specific hearing aid fitting changes audibility for an individual listener. We think of the typical LTASS as having a dynamic range of 30 dB. The "average" of the LTASS is not the middle, but rather it is 12 dB below the louder levels and 18 dB above the softer levels (Figure 6–1).

There has been considerable work examining the average overall speech levels. Data from one study are shown in Table 6–1. There is not total agreement among studies, but in general the values are as follows:

> **DID YOU KNOW: Classic Quote**
>
> The most common reason patients seek help and purchase hearing aids is because of difficulties in hearing and recognizing speech. Much of this is related to simple audibility. There are many variables to consider for speech recognition, but Pascoe (1980) eloquently states:
>
> > "Although it is true that the mere detection of sound does not insure its recognition, it is even more true that without detection the probabilities of recognition are greatly diminished."

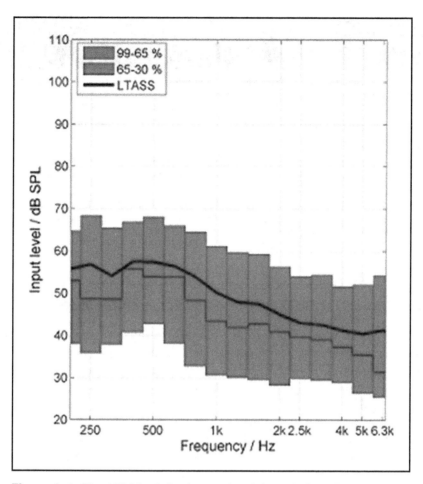

Figure 6–1. The LTASS of the International Speech Test Signal (ISTS), designed as an international speech spectrum. The ISTS was created by segmenting (into 500 ms units) and then splicing back together the recordings of female speakers reading the internationally known passage, "The North Wind and the Sun" in six different languages (American English, Arabic, Chinese, French, German, and Spanish). Because of splicing and segmentation, the ISTS is largely unintelligible. The final reassembled signal was then filtered to match the average female LTASS as described by Byrne et al. (1994). The resulting ISTS has been lauded for its speechlike characteristics including a realistic 20 dB to 30 dB dynamic range, as well as having relatively natural combinations of voiced and voiceless speech segments.

- Soft vocal effort: an overall level of approximately 50 dB SPL to 53 dB SPL
- Conversational vocal effort: overall level of approximately 58 dB SPL to 62 dB SPL
- Raised vocal effect: overall level of approximately 64 dB SPL to 66 dB SPL
- Shouted vocal effort results in speech that has an overall level of approximately 82 dB SPL to 86 dB SPL
- **Importantly:** These all are *SPL values*. On the audiometric dial, soft speech is around 35 dB HL, and average speech is around 45 dB HL.

Table 6–1. Mean Speech Levels in dBA and Unweighted Sound Pressure Levels for Casual, Normal, Raised, Loud, and Shouted Speech by Males, Females, and Children in an Anechoic Chamber

	Casual	Normal	Raised	Loud	Shouted
Females	50[54] (4)	55[58] (4)	63[65] (4)	71[72] (6)	82[82] (7)
Males	52[56] (4)	58[61] (4)	65[68] (5)	76[77] (6)	89[89] (7)
Children	53[56] (5)	58[61] (5)	65[67] (7)	74[75] (9)	82[82] (9)

Note. All values are rounded to the nearest dB; Unweighted sound pressure levels are in [ ]; Standard deviations are in ( ).

Source: From Table 1 and Figures 16, 17, and 18 in Pearsons et al. (1977). From *Essentials of Modern Hearing Aids: Selection, Fitting, and Verification* (p. 76), by T. A. Ricketts, R. Bentler, and H. G. Mueller, 2019, San Diego, CA: Plural Publishing. Reprinted with permission.

KEY CONCEPT: LTASS and Probe-Microphone Verification

Let us go to the clinic for a moment. Later in this chapter we'll talk about probe-microphone verification. The importance of the LTASS becomes clear during this process—a technique often referred to as *speech mapping*. This testing approach has increased the awareness of the LTASS and the effects of LTASS amplification (or lack of it) among clinicians. Early probe-microphone systems used swept pure tones or noise that was shaped (filtered) to mimic an LTASS. This often led to measured attributes of the hearing aids that did not completely reflect how the hearing aids performed when real speech was the input signal. Today we have several real speech LTASSs that can be used for testing. The most notable LTASS used today is one that is spliced together from a variety of speech signals that differ in terms of talker and language (six females), which is the International Speech Test Signal (ISTS). An example of the ISTS LTASS is shown in Figure 6–1.

The AI and the SII

It is possible to calculate the audibility of speech under conditions of hearing loss and/or masking by a noise signal with a fairly high degree of accuracy. However, rather than just knowing audibility, it is of interest to know how frequency-specific audibility translates into importance for speech recognition performance. Calculation of not just audibility, but importance-weighted audibility is the explicit goal of what is referred to as the Articulation Index, or simply AI. These procedures, in one way or another, have been employed since the early 1900s. A couple decades ago, the standards changed slightly, and what we once called

THINGS TO REMEMBER: A Rainbow and a Shoe Bench

Over the years, it has been popular to use phonetically balanced passages, both in research and in clinical testing. What we have here are the longest and the shortest passages that we can find:

■ **Rainbow Passage:** When the sunlight strikes raindrops in the air, they act as a prism and form a rainbow. The rainbow is a division of white light into many beautiful colors. These take the shape of a long round arch, with its path high above, and its two ends apparently beyond the horizon. There is, according to legend, a boiling pot of gold at one end. People look, but no one ever finds it. When a man looks for something beyond his reach, his friends say he is looking for the pot of gold at the end of the rainbow. Throughout the centuries, people have explained the rainbow in various ways. Some have accepted it as a miracle without physical explanation. To the Hebrews, it was a token that there would be no more universal floods. The Greeks used to imagine that it was a sign from the gods to foretell war or heavy rain. The Norsemen considered the rainbow as a bridge over which the gods passed from earth to their home in the sky. Others have tried to explain the phenomenon physically. Aristotle thought that the rainbow was caused by reflection of the sun's rays by the rain. Since then, physicists have found that it is not reflection, but refraction by the raindrops which causes the rainbows. Many complicated ideas about the rainbow have been formed. The difference in the rainbow depends considerably on the size of the drops, and the width of the colored band increases as the size of the drops increases. The actual primary rainbow observed is said to be the effect of superimposition of a number of bows. If the red of the second bow falls upon the green of the first, the result is to give a bow with an abnormally wide yellow band, since red and green light, when mixed, form yellow. This is a very common type of bow, one showing mainly red and yellow, with little or no green or blue.

So that was the longest, here is the shortest. Use of this passage goes back to Bell Labs in the 1920s, although no one is sure who invented it. The most notable scientist from the group was Harvey Fletcher. While we are not sure about his shoe bench, we do know that in 1907, he designed a 320 × 120 foot Y on the mountain overlooking Provo, Utah, home of BYU.

■ **Shortest Balanced Passage:** "Joe took father's shoe bench out; she was waiting at my lawn."

DID YOU KNOW: Are You a "Yanny" or a "Laurel?"

As you might recall, in May of 2018, a short audio clip was completely puzzling the world, and creating an online debate among millions. What was the voice saying—was it Yanny or was it Laurel? You can listen to the sound sample in question here at http://www.tinyurl.com/yannylaurel.

In a Twitter poll of more than 500,000 people, 53% heard the original word "Laurel," while 47% reported hearing a voice saying the name "Yanny." Spectral analysis of the recorded speech signal confirmed that both sets of sounds were present in the recording, but some users focused on the higher frequency sounds in "Yanny" and could not seem to hear the lower sounds of the word "Laurel." The debate resulted in many of our colleagues in speech and hearing to be called into action by their local media outlets. Hearing science professors were quick to show that you could easily shift the pitch of the speech, and if lowered, people who previously had heard the word Yanny, now heard Laurel.

So what does this have to do with our chapter? A lot. First, priming can contribute to speech understanding. Before listening, you are expecting to hear one of these two words, not a third word. Other factors that might contribute to the Laurel versus Yanny decision that are directly related to hearing aid processing, involve the quality of the signal recorded (the talker) and the quality of the loudspeaker used to listen to the recording (receiver of a hearing aid). And of course, the person's hearing status can influence the outcome. All these Laurel versus Yanny factors also play a part when our patients are attempting to understand speech using their hearing aids.

All in all, Laurel versus Yanny was the most perplexing Internet phenomenon since the great dress color debate of 2015 (white/gold vs. blue/black), but we can't think of a good reason to talk much about dress colors in a speech acoustics section.

the AI, is now usually referred to as the Speech Intelligibility Index (SII). We won't get into detail, but the way this calculation works is to divide the entire speech dynamic range into small segments and precisely quantify the relative importance of the speech signal in each frequency band (importance weightings), and can be plotted as frequency importance functions or band importance functions. These are usually plotted so that the total importance for all bands adds up to 1.00 (i.e., 100%).

The SII computations we mention above sound complicated (and they are), but these calculations are conducted automatically on all probe-microphone equipment for the patient's unaided thresholds and for the output obtained with the hearing aids. For this reason, it's probable that you will see SII values mentioned more and more in reports, especially for pediatric patients where audibility is critical. While there is not a precise one-to-one prediction, it is possible to obtain an estimate of speech recognition based on SII data—this is assuming that audibility is the primary issue (this would not account for a processing problem unrelated to audibility). A chart that can be used for that purpose is shown in Figure 6–2.

Looking at Figure 6–2, you see on the bottom the AI (SII) in percent. This represents the percent of the important speech signals that are audible. Shown on the graph are the functions for different speech materials (in percent correct). Let's review a couple examples for understanding monosyallble words (lowest curve on chart). If a patient had an SII of 40%, we predict that he or she would understand about 58% of

monosyllables (presented at the level of average speech). If the SII were 60%, then we'd predict that he or she would understand about 80% of the words. Note that performance would be better for words in sentences, and in fact, it's not necessary to have an SII of 100% to do very well for this type of speech task. It should also be noted that these percentages are based on test-booth testing in quiet, not the real-world ability of a patient; it is likely they would need a much better SII to hear what is being said on a daily basis in normal conversation. Additionally, the tests used here are clear speech, not the conversation co-articulated speech we use every day.

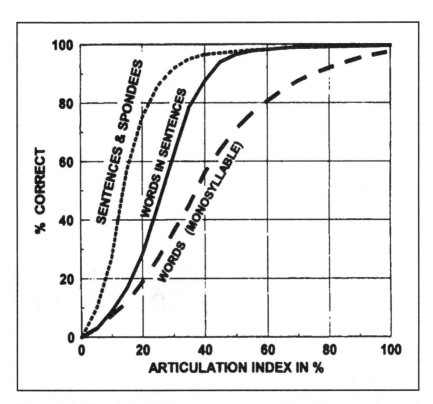

Figure 6–2. The relationship between an average SII and the percent correct for three different speech materials. *Source*: Adapted from the original work of Davis and Silverman, 1960. From *Essentials of Modern Hearing Aids: Selection, Fitting, and Verification* (p. 87), by T. A. Ricketts, R. Bentler, and H. G. Mueller, 2019, San Diego, CA: Plural Publishing. Reprinted with permission.

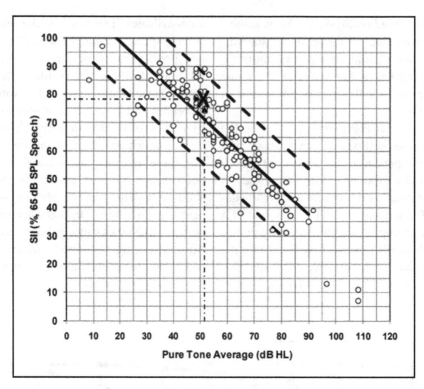

Figure 6–3. Data from acceptable pediatric hearing aid fittings, showing the relationship between the pure-tone average and the aided SII. The dark diagonal line represents the median of the data, with the dashed lines indicating the general range of acceptability. The X is for a sample patient with a pure-tone average of 52, and an acceptable aided SII of 78%.

A common question regarding the aided SII is, "How good is good enough?" This is especially important for infants and toddlers. Fortunately, the folks at Western University in Ontario (Formerly UWO) have helped us answer this question. They have collected data for a large number of pediatric patients fitted successfully to the DSL5 fitting algorithm (more on this later in the chapter). They then have plotted the aided SII as a function of the pure-tone average (as hearing loss becomes worse, it simply isn't possible to have an SII in the 80% range or higher—realistic expectations are needed). Their findings are displayed in Figure 6–3. A sample case is shown with the "X" on the chart. Note that this patient had a pure-tone average

of 52 dB, and an aided SII of 78%. According to the Western University data, this would be considered an acceptable fitting.

The Audiogram and the Speech Signal

There are several methods of using the patient's pure-tone audiogram for prefitting counseling—we just talked about the SII, which is derived from the audiogram. Some methods are more detailed than others, and the method selected often relates to the sophistication of the patient, the level of interest in learning about hearing loss, and how the loss might impact speech understanding. When we plot the LTASS of average speech (see Figure 6–1) on the HL scale, it more or less resembles a banana—so much so, that even many lay people know what the *speech banana* is. This is commonly used for counseling patients regarding their hearing loss. Some audiologists have only the banana shaded on the audiogram, other forms have symbols for common environmental sounds or have the various speech consonants or vowels printed on the audiogram—this is a common option in the software of computer-based audiometers. Usually this is not the audiogram placed in the patient's records or sent out to referral sources, but rather simply something unofficial that can be used for counseling, and that the patient can take home for review.

An example of using the "banana" for counseling is shown in Figure 6–4. This is the audiogram of a 71-year-old male, who reported he was having increased problems understanding speech in background noise, mostly at his favorite brew pubs during happy hour. What you see is an automated optional view of his audiogram using a computer-based audiometer. There is the option of using no banana, using the banana, displaying speech sounds, or displaying typical environment sounds. What you see here is reprinted in black and white, but in the clinic, it's displayed

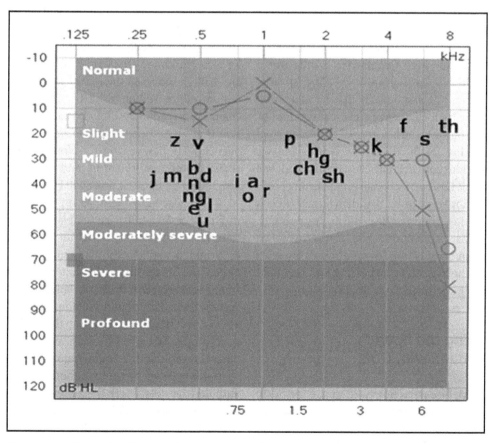

Figure 6–4. Example of the results of air conduction testing, illustrating how placing the intensity of different speech sounds on the audiogram can be used for patient counseling.

CLINICAL TIP: A Banana or a Bean?

A few times in this chapter we have referenced the "speech banana." You probably have heard of the term even before reading the chapter. Some audiologists, however, suggest that when we are thinking about amplification for children, we should be thinking of a string bean, rather than a banana (Madell & Flexer, 2017). Their point is understandable. If we look at the banana when graphed correctly on the audiogram (often it isn't), the range is from 20 dB to 50 dB. The point made by Madell and Flexer is that for young children, especially if they are developing speech and language, it's critical to make soft speech audible. That would be the part of the banana in the 20 dB to 30 dB range. So if you highlight this upper portion of the banana, you really have something that looks more like a string bean than a banana!

---

on a large monitor in bright colors, which enhances the informational counseling.

Our patient must have led a fairly "clean" life, as for age 71, his hearing isn't too bad. Note that presbyacusis is starting to take its toll in the high frequencies, a little worse in the left ear than the right. The "speech-sounds" display reveals that he is missing a few high-frequency consonants. More or less, however, he has normal or near-normal hearing for 3000 Hz and below, and we wouldn't consider him a hearing aid candidate at this time, partly because his listening needs do not seem to be that demanding (unless he's doing business deals during happy hour). If this was a young school teacher who was having trouble understanding his students and he had this same hearing loss, we might recommend bilateral amplification.

Using the Speech Banana with Dots

We've discussed how we can use the SII to roughly assess the "goodness" of the amplified signal—something that is calculated automatically on most probe-microphone systems. These calculations also can be used during the prefitting process. One handy paper-and-pencil complement to the automated procedures is the count-the-dots audiogram, originally introduced by Mueller and Killion in 1990. In 2010, Mueller and Killion modified their 1990 count-the-dot procedure (Killion & Mueller, 2010); the change provided a new SII importance function that gives more weight to higher frequencies. The new version, therefore, slightly redistributed the 100 dots and includes weightings for 6000 Hz and 8000 Hz.

The revised 2010 audiogram is shown in Figure 6–5 (a full-page template can be found in Appendix D—this form is not copyrighted, so photocopy away and enjoy!). Note that the density of the dots varies by frequency, related to the importance of that specific frequency for understanding speech, as we discussed earlier relative to the AI. We have plotted a typical hearing aid candidate's thresholds on the audiogram. Observe that this person has only about 20 dots audible (the dots *under* the audiogram)— an estimated SII of .20 (20%). If we go back to Figure 6–2, we can predict his speech understanding.

We have found the count-the-dot audiogram to be particularly helpful when counseling patients who are in denial regarding the degree of handicap that they might have. Using a percentage to make the point is something that everyone can relate to. Graphically showing someone that they are missing 80% of average speech, when they have just said they hear everything, can be a convincing message. Patients often forget much of what we tell them during the prefitting counseling process, but they usually remember the percentage of dots they could hear!

Although the audibility calculations that we have been discussing can easily be computerized (and they have been), there is something to be said about using the paper-and-pencil version. Sitting at a desk with a patient, plotting the audiogram, having the patient help you count the audible dots, showing what happens when the low-frequency dots are covered up because they are masked by noise, all tends to have a memorable counseling impact. The patient takes the sheets home with them, and in general, they seem to get it. We've had patients call back months later and say, "I'd like to come

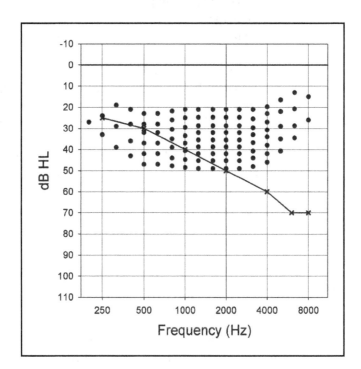

Figure 6–5. Typical downward sloping hearing loss plotted on an audiogram displaying the 2010 Killion and Mueller count-the-dots SII speech spectrum. The audibility index (AI) can be calculated by counting the dots that fall below the audiogram. *Source:* From *Speech Mapping and Probe Microphone Measurements* (p. 199), by H. G. Mueller, T. A. Ricketts, and R. Bentler, 2017, San Diego, CA: Plural Publishing. Reprinted with permission.

TAKE FIVE: Pick Your Banana Carefully!

As we have mentioned, it is common to place the speech banana (average LTASS with percentiles) on the audiogram and use this for counseling. There have been several studies of defining average speech over the years, and LTASS findings do vary somewhat from study to study, but they are more or less in fairly good general agreement. So why is it then, that if we would do a Google image search on *Speech Banana* today, we find audiograms (apparently used in offices and clinics somewhere) with the 1000 Hz to 2000 Hz frequency region of the LTASS ranging anywhere from 15 dB to 45 dB for the upper boundary and 40 dB to 70 dB for the lower boundary, with everything in between also used. A 25 dB difference! Since this is a fundamental concept of audiology, wouldn't it be nice if we all could get it right?

Imagine if you took your 3-year-old son in for testing and the audiometric results revealed that he had a 35 dB loss (or is it really a loss?). If he were tested at Clinic A, where they use the 15 dB to 45 dB banana, you would be told that your son was missing about two-thirds of the important sounds of average speech. On the other hand, if he were tested at Clinic B, where the audiologists use the 40 dB to 70 dB speech banana, you would be told that all is well—he is hearing 100% of average speech! In our opinion, this borders on malpractice, as a child suffering from middle ear effusion, which often results in a hearing loss of 30 dB to 35 dB, might go untreated for months or years, simply because the parents were given the wrong counseling based on the wrong banana. For the record, hearing screenings are conducted on kids at 20 dB because that is the upper range of soft speech—but back to hearing aids.

In general, we recommend using a spectrum that has the soft components for the midfrequencies around 20 dB HL to 25 dB HL, with the loud components of the LTASS at 50 dB HL to 55 dB HL, similar to what is shown in Figure 6–5.

CLINICAL CONCEPT: Hearing, Not Understanding

Although we believe that using the AI/SII *percent audibility* of average speech can be effective for patient counseling, we do need to mention a fine point that often needs to be clarified. It is important to clearly state that this is the percentage of speech that the patient *hears*, not the percentage of speech that he or she *understands*. Patients sometimes want to think of it as percentage understanding, or even percentage hearing loss. It is neither.

back in and try hearing aids. I only heard 18 dots when you tested me."

A "Real-Speech" Banana

Another way that an audiologist might illustrate how the patient's hearing loss relates to the average speech signal is to use their probe-microphone equipment. The advantage of this is that we now have converted everything to ear canal SPL, and we are using an SPL-O-gram, a display method where loud sounds actually fall appropriately above soft sounds, unlike the standard audiogram. And, we are using the patient's ear for the demo! One way to use this display is to plot the patient's hearing threshold, and conduct an open ear unaided measure for a 65 dB SPL speech signal (this replicates what happens in the real world). In general, this is more intuitive for patient counseling than the standard audiogram, as we see that what is *not audible* falls *below* the patient's thresholds, and what *is* audible falls *above* (Figure 6–6). What you see here are the same hearing thresholds as used before with the dots (see Figure 6–5), but now they are converted to ear canal SPL, and compared with the measured real-ear output of the

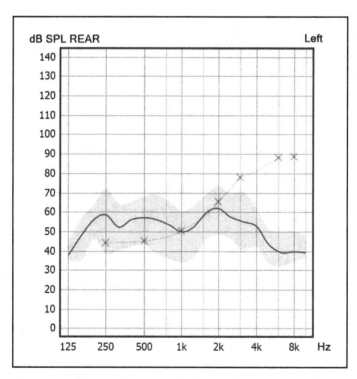

Figure 6–6. Typical downward sloping hearing loss plotted in the SPL-O-Gram format (reference = ear canal SPL). Rather than displaying the average speech spectrum, the spectrum shown was obtained from a real-speech signal (65 dB SPL) delivered to the patient's open ear with the probe-microphone tip at the patient's eardrum. *Source*: From *Speech Mapping and Probe Microphone Measurements* (p. 201), by H. G. Mueller, T. A. Ricketts, and R. Bentler, 2017, San Diego, CA: Plural Publishing. Reprinted with permission.

calibrated real-speech input signal. Most probe-microphone systems will calculate an SII for this measure. The Killion-Mueller spectrum was based on a 60 dB SPL overall level, and what was used here was a 65 dB SPL input, so the SII should be slightly better. Indeed, the probe-microphone system calculated an SII of 28%, slightly better than what was obtained using the count-the-dots method. Depending on the time that is available, this counseling and demonstration can be expanded by presenting speech of different input levels (soft, average, loud), or even using the live speech of family members to illustrate to the patient what he or she is missing.

Loudness Discomfort Level Testing

Now that we've reviewed the speech spectrum and how it relates to the fitting, let's talk about some prefitting tests that need to be conducted following the routine diagnostic exam. The most critical aspect of the hearing aid verification process is ensuring that the gain and the maximum output are adjusted correctly for a given patient. Although these two adjustments are not totally independent (one could not achieve high gain levels for average inputs without a moderately high output setting), for the average patient, it is usually possible to vary the gain by 40 dB to 50 dB and the MPO (for maximum power output) by at least 20 dB. Gain prescriptions are typically based on audiometric thresholds, but how do we determine the best MPO setting? The logical approach, which also has been specified in best practice guidelines for the past 30 years, is to conduct frequency-specific loudness discomfort level (LDL) measures, and use these values to set the hearing aid MPO (often by manipulating the output compression limiting kneepoint) so that loud sounds are loud, but not too loud.

CLINICAL CONCEPT: UCL, LDL, or TD?

There are many terms used to denote the point at which loud sounds become uncomfortable—ones that you might encounter on an audiogram or in a report include: UL, UCL, ULL, TD, and LDL. Does it matter what term is used? Probably not. For reasons unknown, many clinicians prefer the term "UCL"—an interesting selection, as the "UC" stands for uncomfortable, which is all one word! We review many of the terms that have been used relative to loudness and hearing aid output in Table 6–2. It has been suggested by some that TD is the most appropriate term, as dimensions other than the *loudness* of a perceptually abusive sound play a part in what is considered uncomfortable—it is not determined by the RMS level of the signal alone. Factors that tend to cause LDLs to be rated lower include annoyance, peakiness, high-frequency content, and the subjective perception of tinniness. In this chapter, we will use the more common LDL (loudness discomfort level) term to describe this loudness perception.

Table 6–2. Terminology Associated with the Measurement of Loudness Discomfort

■ Uncomfortable Loudness (UCL): This is perhaps the most commonly used term among clinicians to describe the point at which loud sounds become uncomfortable. The common use of the letter "C" in the abbreviation is somewhat puzzling and, indeed, some simply use the abbreviation UL. The abbreviation ULL also is used, with the final "L" referring to *level*.

■ Loudness Discomfort Level (LDL): This is the term that we prefer. It is used interchangeably with UCL/ULL.

■ Threshold of Discomfort (TD): This is another term for the same measure. For the most part, it can be used interchangeably with LDL, UCL, and ULL.

■ Upper Level of Comfort (ULC): This is the category of loudness falling just below the LDL. When using the 7-point Cox Contour Anchors, this is the #6 Loud, but an okay rating. In general, we want the output of the hearing aid to fall at this level; the DSL prescriptive software has used ULC values for this purpose.

■ Highest Comfortable Level (HCL): This is the same as the ULC.

■ OSPL90: This is the broadest, most powerful output of a hearing aid with the gain control "full on" measured in a 2-cc coupler using 90 dB swept pure tones. This is a component of ANSI Standard S3.22 and used for hearing aid specification, documentation, and quality control.

■ Maximum Power Output (MPO): In some cases, the term MPO is used synonymously with OSPL90. More commonly, however, in the clinic, MPO refers to the maximum output of the hearing aid when specific settings have been made (e.g., settings of gain, input, and output compression), and not the *potential* maximum output of the instrument (the OSPL90). The MPO, therefore, cannot be higher than the OSPL90, and it is often significantly lower. For example, lowering the AGCo compression kneepoint for a given patient would lower the hearing aid's MPO.

■ Real-Ear Saturation Response (RESR; REAR 85/90): This is an MPO measure obtained with the hearing aid fitted to the patient's ear, rather than in a 2-cc coupler. Typically, this measure is made with the hearing aid's gain and compression parameters set to approximate use conditions using an 85 dB to 90 dB swept pure tone.

■ Real-Ear Coupler Difference (RECD): This is a measure that compares the output of a hearing aid in the real ear to the output in a 2-cc coupler with identical settings. If the RECD is known, it can be added to the hearing aid coupler MPO (*not* the OSPL90) to predict the maximum output in the ear canal.

■ Reference Equivalent Thresholds in SPL (RETSPL): This is the difference between the HL dial setting and output in a 2-cc or 6-cc coupler. Because insert earphones (which are calibrated in a 2-cc coupler) are typically used for HL LDL testing, RETSPL values can be used to convert HL LDLs to 2-cc coupler values (so you can speak the same language as your fitting software).

■ Real-Ear Dial Difference (REDD): This is the addition of the RETSPL and the RECD (or it can be measured directly); using this you can convert from HL LDL to ear canal SPL. This provides the RESR output targets you see on the probe-mic fitting screen.

■ Automatic Gain Control-input (AGCi): This is input compression, typically having a low activation kneepoint (in which case it is referred to as WDRC). It can be used to control the hearing aid's MPO if kneepoints are low enough and the ratios are big enough.

■ Automatic Gain Control-output (AGCo): This is output compression, typically having a high activation kneepoint and high compression ratios (in which case it is referred to as compression limiting)—the most common method to control the MPO.

Source: From *Speech Mapping and Probe Microphone Measurements* (p. 203), by H. G. Mueller, T. A. Ricketts, and R. Bentler, 2017, San Diego, CA: Plural Publishing. Reprinted with permission.

A busy clinician might be tempted to simply use the "average" LDL based on the patient's hearing loss. This can be very risky, as shown in the finding from the most extensive study of LDLs that was reported by Bentler and Cooley (2001). They determined LDLs for a total of 433 subjects (710 ears), with presumed cochlear pathologies. Their data (averaged for five test frequencies) are displayed in Figure 6–7.

Several important teaching points are evident:

1. From 20 dB to 60 dB hearing loss, there is no average change in LDLs.
2. Above 60 dB, average LDLs go up roughly 5 dB for each 10 dB increase in hearing loss.
3. The range of LDLs for different individuals with the same hearing loss is

40 dB to 50 dB or greater for most hearing loss levels.

Other findings from the Bentler and Cooley (2001) study have clinical importance (multiple regression analysis using almost 2,000 LDLs; subjects ranging in age from 11 to 97 years):

1. LDLs did not vary as a function of the frequency tested (when hearing loss was matched).
2. There were no gender differences.
3. There were no age differences.

As mentioned above and readily observed in Figure 6–7, the variability of LDLs for individuals with the same degree of hearing loss is very large. For example, if we take a common 50 dB hearing loss, we see that LDL

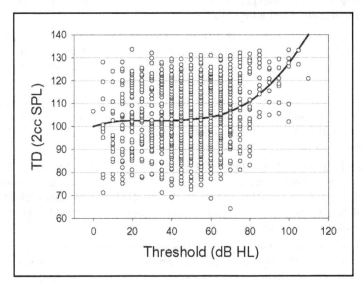

Figure 6–7. Display of LDLs (TDs) referenced to a 2-cc coupler as a function of hearing loss obtained from 710 individual ears. Data points averaged for frequencies 500 Hz to 4000 Hz. *Source:* Adapted from Bentler and Cooley, 2001. From *Speech Mapping and Probe Microphone Measurements* (p. 205), by H. G. Mueller, T. A. Ricketts, and R. Bentler, 2017, San Diego, CA: Plural Publishing. Reprinted with permission.

values ranged from the mid-70s to more than 130 dB—nearly a 60 dB range. Perhaps more important than the range per se, is that there were not just one or two outliers, but a fairly even distribution between the lower and upper values. If we were to use average values to predict the correct MPO setting in this example, the value would be around 102 dB (re: 2-cc coupler; see regression line in Figure 6–7). Bentler and Cooley (2001), however, report that only 32% of measured LDLs fell within ±5 dB of this average. Assuming that we would not want an MPO mistake of greater than 5 dB, this clearly points out the problems that can exist when average values are used.

If you have a patient who states that their hearing aids make loud sounds too loud and that some loud sounds are uncomfortable, our bet is that the hearing aid MPO did not get programmed correctly, possibly because average rather than measured LDLs were used. They need to go back to their audiologist, as this is something that is very fixable.

Conducting the Testing

Although measuring LDLs is usually considered a fairly simple task and can be conducted effectively by a technician, there are two important procedural conditions that, if not followed correctly, will significantly reduce the validity and reliability of the task: the use of loudness anchors and appropriate instructions.

Loudness Anchors

Loudness anchors are used to give the patient a reference for the loudness perceptions that he or she will be experiencing. It indicates

boundaries and intermediate steps, which facilitates the understanding of the task and improves reliability; the patient has words to attach to a perception. The loudness anchors that we recommend, shown in Figure 6–8, are from Robyn Cox (1995) and were used in the development of the Cox Contour Test. The Cox loudness anchors also have been adapted for children, where faces with different expressions accompany the different loudness levels (Figure 6–9). In general, research has shown that reliable LDL values can be obtained with children as young as 5 to 6 years.

Prior to the testing, the patients are familiarized with the loudness anchors, and they are provided the chart to use during testing. They can respond either by stating the loudness category or by simply giving the number.

Loudness Anchors	
#7.	Uncomfortably Loud
#6.	Loud, But Okay
#5.	Comfortable, But Slightly Loud
#4.	Comfortable
#3.	Comfortable, But Slightly Soft
#2.	Soft
#1.	Very Soft

Figure 6–8. Loudness anchors used for LDL testing. Anchors adapted from those used for the Cox Contour Test. *Source*: Adapted from Cox, 1995. From *Speech Mapping and Probe Microphone Measurements* (p. 206), by H. G. Mueller, T. A. Ricketts, and R. Bentler, 2017, San Diego, CA: Plural Publishing. Reprinted with permission.

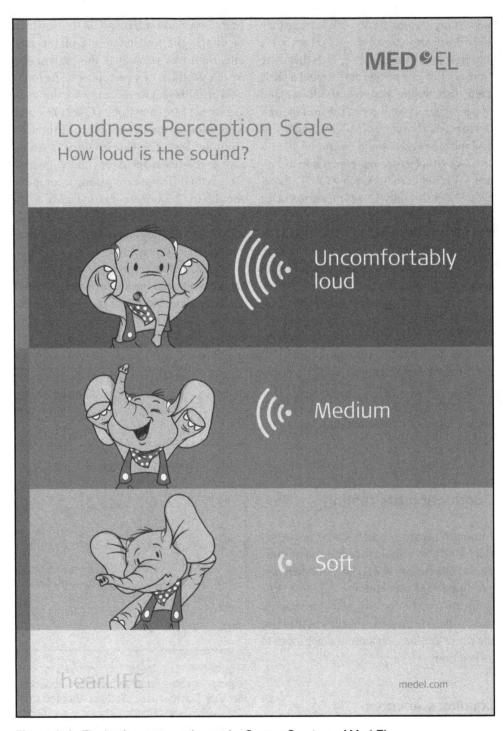

Figure 6–9. The loudness perception scale. *Source*: Courtesy of Med-El.

Instructions

Going hand-in-hand with the anchors are the instructions. The measured LDL can vary by 15 dB to 20 dB simply based on the instructions that are used. Given that we are using the loudness anchors of Cox (1995), it is appropriate to also use the instructions that were developed in association with these anchors. They are provided in Figure 6–10. What we are looking for is when the sound is *first* uncomfortable, not what the patient can tolerate. The difference between *uncomfortable* and *tolerate* can be 10 dB to 20 dB for some patients.

Test Procedures

Typically, LDL testing is conducted in the test booth, as that is where the equipment is located and the patient is already seated and hooked up to earphones for the diagnostic testing. Each ear is tested independently, using pulsed pure tones at two or three key frequencies. An ascending approach is used, usually starting around the patient's MCL (e.g., 60 to 70 dB HL), and then going up in 5 dB steps. The testing for a given run stops when a #7 rating is given. The procedure is repeated for reliability. If the #7 rating of the second run is within 5 dB of the first (it usually is), the two are averaged and the LDL is recorded. This test also gives good information about loudness growth. It not only gives LDL measurement but also the most comfortable level (MCL) reported by patients. This information can be used during fitting as well. It usually takes 5 min to test two to three frequencies for both ears (typically a low frequency like 500 Hz and a high frequency like 3000 Hz)—we think it is time well spent.

Clinical Application

So what does the audiologist do with the measured LDLs? It requires some second

---

LDL Instructions

THE PURPOSE OF THIS TEST IS TO FIND YOUR JUDGMENTS OF THE LOUDNESS OF DIFFERENT SOUNDS.

YOU WILL HEAR SOUNDS THAT INCREASE AND DECREASE IN VOLUME. YOU MUST MAKE A JUDGMENT ABOUT HOW LOUD THE SOUNDS ARE. PRETEND YOU ARE LISTENING TO THE RADIO AT THAT VOLUME. HOW LOUD WOULD IT BE?

AFTER EACH SOUND, TELL ME WHICH OF THESE CATEGORIES BEST DESCRIBES THE LOUDNESS. IT IS OKAY TO REPEAT A LOUDNESS CATEGORY, AND IT IS OKAY TO SKIP A CATEGORY.

KEEP IN MIND THAT AN UNCOMFORTABLY LOUD SOUND IS LOUDER THAN YOU WOULD EVER CHOOSE ON YOUR RADIO NO MATTER WHAT MOOD YOU ARE IN.

Figure 6–10. Instructions that are read to the patient prior to administering LDL measures. *Source*: Adapted from Cox, 1995. From *Speech Mapping and Probe Microphone Measurements* (p. 207), by H. G. Mueller, T. A. Ricketts, and R. Bentler, 2017, San Diego, CA: Plural Publishing. Reprinted with permission.

grade math, but nothing too difficult. A continual disconnect in the fitting of hearing aids is that we conduct testing in HL, manufacturers commonly provide hearing aid software referenced to 2-cc coupler levels in SPL, and we verify hearing aids in ear canal SPL. As a result, we are continually converting between the three references. For our current task, we want to set the software AGCo, which is in 2-cc coupler SPL, but the numbers we have are in HL. Fortunately, there are corrections called *RETSPLs*, an acronym for the Reference Equivalent Threshold in SPL and is pronounced *Rhet-Spull*. All the audiologist needs to do is add these RETSPLs to the HL LDLs, and he or she will have the needed 2-cc coupler values to set the MPO correctly. Recall from Chapter 5 that the MPO sets the stop sign for output, so if this is set correctly, sounds will never be too loud, they'll also never be too squashed, they should always be "just right"—just like the porridge of the Little Bear!

Speech-in-Noise Testing

It is common in best practice guidelines related to the fitting of hearing aids to recommend speech recognition in noise as a routine measure prior to the hearing aid fitting, and we certainly agree. When you encounter patients who are having trouble understanding in background noise, see if speech-in-noise testing has been conducted. There are several reasons why these tests are important, besides the fact that the speech recognition score in quiet is a very poor predictor of a patient's speech-in-noise performance, or the patient's success with hearing aids. Reasons why speech-in-noise testing always should be conducted for hearing aid patients are as follows:

- To address the patient's complaints: It is very likely that problems understanding speech in background noise are the primary reason why the patient is seeking assistance. Conducting this testing conveys to the patient that we understand this, and are interested in learning about his or her problem.
- To select the best technology: The results of these tests can impact your selection of the fitting arrangement (e.g., unilateral vs. bilateral), the hearing aid style, level of technology (entry vs premium) and/or the need for special features such as remote microphones.
- To establish a baseline: The information collected during this testing can be used as a baseline for measuring aided benefit.
- To monitor performance over time: A patient's ability to understand in background noise may become significantly poorer without an associated change in hearing thresholds or speech understanding in quiet.
- To assist with counseling: How does the patient's score compare with individuals with normal hearing, or other individuals with the same degree of hearing loss? Part of the fitting process is to maintain realistic expectations for the patient. The results of speech-in-noise testing will assist in identifying real-world situations where the patient may or may not do well.
- To help a patient make a decision: Many times, a patient may be on the fence regarding the use of hearing aids and maybe has heard that hearing aids do not work. An aided versus unaided speech test during the initial visit provides an example of potential benefit (see example later in this chapter), and often provides that shot in the arm to encourage the patient to move forward.

There are several good speech-in-noise tests available that could be used to accomplish the goals we stated above. Most audiologists select one or two favorites for routine use. When picking a test, there are several factors to consider, some of which might impact the clinical effectiveness of the test.

◼ Words or sentences? Sentences have more face validity, but single words are not impacted by context. There are some tests that are low predictability sentences like the AZ Bio Sentences that has stimuli like: The purple velvet curtains were very expensive OR He crushed a can on his head. However, the co-articulation and sentence structure does make the words more predicable than single words.

◼ Type of background noise? Speech noise is a better masker, but multitalker babble is more realistic. There can also be a varied number of speakers in the background; four speaker babble has been shown to be the most effective as it is both information masking (masks the signal because of overlapping speech sounds) and spectral masking (masks the signal because of overlapping acoustic energy).

◼ Adaptive versus fixed SNR? Fixed is more real world, but floor and ceiling effects can be an issue. Adaptive eliminates the floor and ceiling effect (if scoring is at 50% correct), but resulting SNR might not be realistic. The scoring for adaptive results in an SNR, which is difficult to communicate to the patient.

◼ What intensity for the presentation level? There seems1 to be four choices:
  ◻ Choice #1: Conduct testing at the level at which the norms were collected. This is the most reasonable choice, as it allows for comparison with the norms and should ensure the best interlist reliability.
  ◻ Choice #2: Conduct testing at the level at which the best performance is predicted. This should provide the best indication of true recognition ability and best predict potential performance with amplification. This is usually done at the level at which the word recognition testing, as described in Chapter 2, was completed.
  ◻ Choice #3: Conduct testing at the average real-world levels, which should provide the best prediction

---

DID YOU KNOW: Olive, Twist, or Cherry?

For most speech-in-noise testing, it is common to use a multitalker babble, sometimes referred to as *cocktail party noise*. You probably also have used the phrase *the cocktail party effect*, which if you didn't know, is a scientific term! In the early 1950s, much of the early work in this area was related to the problems faced by air traffic controllers. At that time, controllers received messages from pilots over loudspeakers in the control tower. Hearing the intermixed voices of many pilots over a single loudspeaker made the controller's task very difficult. The effect was first defined in a Journal of Acoustical Society paper in 1953, where it was named the "*cocktail party problem*" by Colin Cherry.

of how the patient performs in the real world. (Note: we say best, not *accurate*—clinical testing is not too good at predicting real-world performance.)

▫ Choice #4: Conduct testing at the specific level that relates to a patient complaint; a patient with a mild hearing loss whose primary complaint is understanding soft speech might be tested at the level of soft speech.

What Test(s) to Use?

Some of the more common speech-in-noise tests are included in the following list:

▪ QuickSIN: Six sentences in each list, with five key words in each sentence. The patient is scored for correctly identifying the key words. Each sentence is recorded at a more difficult SNR, going from +25 dB to 0 dB in 5 dB steps. Test is scored in SNR.

▪ BKB-SIN: Similar to the QuickSIN, but with a much easier vocabulary (first-grade reading level). More commonly used for children, but appropriate for adults.

▪ AZ-Bio: Similar to the BKB-SIN. Sentence tests with low and high predictability sentences. Can independently adjust the speech and the noise. Commonly used as part of a cochlear implant evaluation. Scored in total number of key words correct.

▪ HINT: Ten sentences in each list. Patient must correctly identify all key words in each sentence for the sentence to be scored correctly. Scored in SNR. Administered adaptively using a fixed noise signal. Commonly used in research, but seldom in the clinic.

▪ WIN: An adaptive test using NU#6 monosyllables with multitalker babble. Seven lists of 10 words are presented at 7 different SNR levels (0 dB to 24 dB in 4 dB steps). Scored in SNR loss.

▪ CST: Paragraph on a meaning topic, based on children's reading material, presented at a fixed SNR (e.g., +8 dB). There are 25 key words in each paragraph. It is scored in percent correct.

We just provided a quick review of six different speech-in-noise tests. That's just the beginning. Mueller, Bentler, and Ricketts (2014) review in detail 12 different speech tests that could be used in the prefitting process. For one reason or another, an argument could be made for using any one of these. The most common test used by audiologists in the clinic is the QuickSIN or the WIN. We're not saying these necessarily are *the best*, but they are the most popular; they are the ones you'll most likely encounter, and they meet most of the criteria that we believe are important.

Quick Speech-in-Noise (QuickSIN) Test

The QuickSIN was designed to be short enough for routine clinical use, and provide a reliable way to measure a listener's speech understanding ability in noise. The test certainly is quick, as a single list only requires about a minute to administer after instructions—we recommend using two lists/ear, but we're still looking at less than 5 min for both ears. The presentation level of the speech is fixed, and the level of the multitalker background varies when SNR is adjusted (+25 to 0 dB). The competing signal is somewhat unique, as it is not a true babble as used with some of the other tests commonly used. It is only four talkers, and one of the talkers, a female, sounds very similar to the talker who is presenting the target sentences. You might say that this makes the test "unfair," but this type of background noise is not unlike what many of our hearing aid patients frequently experience in their daily life. The test is easily scored (with minor math applications) using the standard score sheet, copies of which are available online. The clinician simply marks the number of key words correctly repeated for each sentence and then sums these numbers to calculate a total score, shown in Figure 6–11.

The QuickSIN is scored as SNR loss, rather than SRT-50 because the score is adjusted based on average performance for normal hearing individuals. That is, the number of correctly repeated key words is subtracted from 25.5 (SNR loss = 25.5–correct key words). This number reflects the SNR at which a patient correctly repeats approximately 50% of the key words, with the normal hearing correction. For example, take a look at the scoring shown in Figure 6–11, which is fairly typical. Notice that this patient got 5 of 5 words correct for the two easy SNRs (+20 dB and +25 dB), and didn't get any of the 5 words correct for the most difficult SNR (0 dB). In total, he got 19 of the 30 words correct. We then subtract this from 25.5 (to correct for normals, who do not score 100% on this test), and we have an SNR Loss of 6.5 dB. This means that when this patient is in background noise, he needs the noise to be 6.5 dB softer for him to perform the same as someone with normal hearing. In case you see QuickSIN scores in patient records, the following is a general key for interpretation:

- 0 dB SNR to 2 dB SNR Loss Normal
- 3 dB SNR to 7 dB SNR Loss Mild
- 8 dB SNR to 14 dB SNR Loss Moderate
- \>14 dB SNR Loss Severe

The guidelines say that something like a 12 dB SNR loss is "moderate," but we have found that this patient will have considerable trouble in background noise, even with well-fitted hearing aids. Recall that we said back in Chapter 5 that directional technology is effective in improving the SNR—in reverberation, this advantage could be 4 dB. So our patient would still have an 8 dB SNR loss, and this is only where he can understand

List 1   **Score**

1. A <u>white</u> <u>silk</u> <u>jacket</u> goes with <u>any</u> <u>shoes</u>.   S/N 25   _5_
2. The <u>child</u> <u>crawled</u> <u>into</u> the <u>dense</u> <u>grass</u>.   S/N 20   _5_
3. <u>Footprints</u> <u>showed</u> the p̶a̶t̶h̶ he <u>took</u> up the <u>beach</u>.   S/N 15   _4_
4. A v̶e̶n̶t̶ near the <u>edge</u> brought in f̶r̶e̶s̶h̶ <u>air</u>.   S/N 10   _3_
5. It is a <u>band</u> of s̶t̶e̶e̶l̶ t̶h̶r̶e̶e̶ i̶n̶c̶h̶es <u>wide</u>.   S/N 5   _2_
6. The w̶e̶i̶g̶ht of the p̶a̶c̶k̶age was s̶e̶e̶n̶ on the h̶i̶g̶h̶ s̶c̶a̶l̶e̶.   S/N 0   _0_

    25.5 - TOTAL = _**6.5**_ SNR Loss   **TOTAL** _19_

Figure 6–11. Sample scoring of the QuickSIN for one list of six sentences (30 words). Normally two lists would be used for each ear and the SNR-Loss would be averaged. *Source*: From *Fitting and Dispensing Hearing* Aids (2nd ed., p. 176), by B. Taylor and H. G. Mueller, 2017, San Diego, CA: Plural Publishing. Reprinted with permission.

50%. Many restaurants and social gatherings have an SNR more negative than 8 dB, so we'd predict that this patient will still have problems in these settings. A remote mic for his hearing aids would probably solve the problem, if he was willing to use it.

Words in Noise (WIN) Test

Wilson (2003) describes that several factors entered into the development of the WIN test, including: a test that would use traditional word stimuli, that would fit a clinical protocol, that would evaluate recognition performance at multiple SNRs, and that would generate a performance metric that was easy to compute and easy to interpret. The WIN then evolved with the following characteristics (Wilson, 2003):

- The NU#6 monosyllabic materials recorded by a female speaker were selected. This test was already in widespread use in VA clinics and, therefore, familiar to clinicians. This word list also was selected because of its sensitivity to the variety of word-recognition performances in quiet exhibited by individuals with hearing loss. This enables word-recognition data to be obtained in quiet and in the background noise using the same speaker, speaking the same words.

- The justification for selecting multitalker babble as the competing background noise was because based on evidence that multitalker babble is the most common environmental noise encountered by listeners in everyday life. The multitalker babble used with the WIN test was recorded by audiologist Donald Causey and consists of three female and three male speakers talking about various topics.

- The level of the multitalker babble is fixed relative to the varied level of the speech signal. This is designed to mimic the real world, in which background noises are maintained at fairly constant levels for given listening situations. To reduce test variability, the words were time-locked to a unique segment of babble for reduced variability.

- To achieve the goal of clinical time efficiently, the test was designed to use multiple speech presentation levels in which 10 words were presented at each of seven levels (a total of 70 words). Since the original development, this has now been shortened to 35 words.

- Finally, the WIN test design was amenable to quantification in terms of percent correct at each signal-to-babble ratio, of the overall percent correct, and of the 50% correct point of the signal-to-babble function.

The clinical WIN test of today is mostly the same as reviewed by Wilson (2003). It has been shortened to 35 monosyllables, which are presented in seven groups of five with a fixed babble level; the level of the words change in 4-dB steps equating to SNRs ranging from 24 to 0 dB.

To score the WIN, the number of words repeated correctly is counted for each signal-to-babble ratio (five possible for each of seven levels). Some audiologists also plot the number of correct responses on the WIN normative chart. This graphic representation can be helpful for patient counseling. The scores for each level are then added to determine the total correct and the SNR-50 (SNR for 50% correct) is then obtained from the chart on the right-hand side of the score sheet (see Figure 5–11). These thresholds correspond to the descriptors used in the threshold chart on the score sheet (e.g., normal, mild, moderate, severe, or profound), and these terms can be used to describe the patient's performance. As stated, the test is scored in SNRs, and the categories are as follows:

- Normal: ≤6.0 dB.
- Mild: 6.8–10.0 dB.
- Moderate: 10.8–14.8 dB.
- Severe: 15.6–19.6 dB.
- Profound: >20 dB.

Prefitting Self-Assessment Scales

We have all heard the old saying, "You can't judge a book by its cover." A saying that is maybe not as well known, but even more true is, "You can't judge a hearing aid candidate by his audiogram." Patients differ in so many ways that are not displayed in *X*s and *O*s or word recognitions scores. There is an excellent battery of validated preselection self-assessment inventories available. They are easy to administer and score. The results of these scales will shape the fitting process, assist in technology decisions, and become invaluable for developing counseling strategies and a relationship with the patient along the way. The routine use of these scales is not only a good thing to do, it is the right thing to do.

In some ways, these scales are not much more than an extended case history, but they allow the clinician to collect information in an organized manner, and in most cases, the patient's responses can be compared with average data from large samples. The information collected using these inventories can significantly influence prefitting counseling and in some instances alter fitting decisions. In some cases, the scores collected before the fitting serve as a baseline, as they may be compared with results measured after a patient wears hearing aids for a period of time to directly quantify subjective hearing aid benefit, reduction in hearing handicap, or other outcomes of interest.

Here are a few areas where self-assessment prefitting measures might be helpful for the overall hearing aid fitting process:

- They assist in determining if a patient is a candidate for hearing aids. Is the patient's report of communication problems consistent with the audiogram? Do they even report that they have problems?
- They assist in determining if a patient is ready to be helped. If a person denies they have communication problems, will he or she accept the use of hearing aids? Is counseling needed before even attempting to move forward?
- They assist in establishing realistic expectations. A patient is obtaining hearing aids because of problems understanding speech in background noise. His or her expectations show that he or she believes that the use of hearing aids will resolve 100% of these communication problems. It is probably best to readjust the patient's expectations before he or she begins to use hearing aids.
- They assist in establishing a baseline. Many of the same inventories used in the prefitting process also are used as outcome measures following the fitting. Obtaining prefitting unaided data will then be helpful in determining aided benefit.

There have been a large number of inventories that have been introduced over the years. We have selected a subset that we believe are useful, and each of which provides unique information. These tests are all explained in detail in Mueller et al. (2014), complete with guidelines for administration and scoring, and related seminal references. Here is a brief summary:

- Hearing Handicap Inventory for the Elderly/Adult (HHIE/A): Measures the degree of handicap for emotional and social issues related to hearing loss.
- Abbreviated Profile of Hearing Aid Benefit (APHAB): Provides the percent of problems the patient has for three different listening conditions involving speech understanding (in quiet, in background noise, and in reverberation) and problems related to annoyance of environmental sounds (aversiveness scale). (See Appendix E.)
- Expected Consequences of Hearing Aid Ownership (ECHO): Measures the patient's expectations for four different areas: positive effect, service and cost, negative features, and personal image. (See Appendix F.)
- Client Oriented Scale of Improvement (COSI): Requires patients to identify three to five very specific listening goals/communication needs for amplification. This can then be used to measure patients' expectations related to these specific goals (See Figure 6–19 for sample patient use).
- Hearing Aid Selection Profile (HASP): Assesses eight patient factors related to the use of hearing aids— motivation, expectations, appearance, cost, technology, physical needs, communication needs, and lifestyle.
- Characteristics of Amplification Tool (COAT): Determines the patient's communication needs, motivation, expectations, cosmetics, and cost concerns.

- Profile of Aided Loudness (PAL): Assesses the patient's loudness perceptions and satisfaction with these perceptions for 12 different everyday environmental sounds.

Real-Ear Coupler Difference

This prefitting test involves two different pieces of equipment that we have yet to discuss in detail: the 2-cc coupler test box and the real-ear probe-microphone system. As the name indicates, the purpose of this testing is to determine how the output of a hearing aid in a standardized coupler differs from the output of that hearing aid (with all parameters set the same) in the patients ear. We know that with a hearing aid/earmold in place, the residual volume of the ear canal will be less than 2-cc. This is true for even an adult with a large canal. So basic acoustics tells us that the output will then be greater in the ear—the smaller the volume, the greater the output. Boyle's law tells us that if you halve the volume, the output goes up by 6 dB. We tend to agree. You can imagine, that for an infant's ear, the residual volume is much smaller than 2-cc, maybe only a quarter as big, meaning a 12 dB increase in output.

Consider that all the data for hearing aids is expressed in 2-cc coupler lingo. Audiologists therefore need to mentally correct this to the real ear, or measure the hearing aid directly in the real ear. There are average RECD values available for adults, and for children, specified by age for the months 1 through 60. To give you an idea of why this matters, at 2000 Hz, for a 3-month-old, we would predict the RECD to be 17 dB, whereas for a 5-year-old, it would be 10 dB. But this varies considerably from person to person, which it's best to measure it. There are two main uses of the measured RECD:

■ The primary utilization is for infants and toddlers, where probe-microphone verification is not possible. If we know the RECD, then we can fit the hearing aid in the coupler. We'll describe how it works. We put the child's pure-tone thresholds into a prescriptive fitting algorithm (more on that later), and prescriptive fitting targets are generated. We'll say that for this child, the algorithm says that she needs an output of 82 dB at 3000 Hz. We measure her RECD and find that it's 12 dB at 3000 Hz. We now know that if we set the hearing aid to 70 dB in the coupler at 3000 Hz, we'll match our desired target in the real ear. Pretty simple, huh? We would do this for all frequencies of course. Now what about the MPO? Let's say that we don't want the maximum output of the hearing aid in the real-ear to be greater than 120 dB for this patient at 3000 Hz (where the output is at its real-ear max). We then would again test the hearing aid on the coupler, and set the coupler MPO to 108, which would give us our desired real-ear limiting.

■ The second reason for making RECD testing part of the prefitting process applies to adults as well as children. When we do our real-ear verification, we convert our HL thresholds to ear-canal SPL thresholds. We have an example of that back in Figure 6–6. But how is this correction made? First, HL is converted to coupler SPL (our friend the RETSPL from earlier), and then the *average* RECD is added. If we actually measure the individual RECD, the probe-mic equipment will use these values rather than average, and the threshold represented will be more accurate.

Quality Control: 2-cc Coupler Testing

You've maybe heard mention of the "test box," which is a small tabletop device with sound isolation where hearing aids can be tested on a coupler. It really isn't much of a "box" anymore, although as recent as 20 years ago, these enclosures were more like 2' by 2' (or bigger) and really did resemble boxes. Today, the test box often is coupled with the probe-mic equipment in one system. Figure 6–12 shows the complete system on the left, and on the right the test box is opened (pictured closed in the left photo).

All hearing aids must meet certain performance requirements based on an *electro-acoustic analysis*. There are standards from the American National Standards Institute (ANSI) that describe how hearing performance is measured. In general, this involves attaching the hearing aid to a 2-cc metal coupler and using sweep tones and noise signals to test the aid in an isolated sound enclosure. When new products are developed, detailed specifications are established. These specifications (e.g., the gain and output results from the test box evaluation) are used for quality control when each product is manufactured. In other words, the product is not shipped to the audiologist unless it meets the specifications. In some clinics all hearing aids are tested on the coupler when they arrive from the manufacturer to determine if they meet standards. This testing normally would be conducted by a technician. Given that most clinics don't have a technician and audiologists have

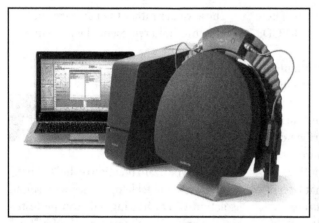

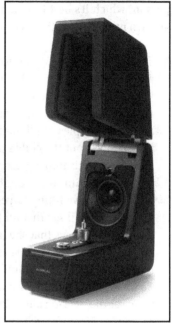

Figure 6–12. A. Typical test equipment for conducting 2-cc coupler and probe-microphone measures. **B.** The 2-cc test box with the cover open. *Source*: Images provided courtesy of Natus Medical Denmark ApS.

better things to do, this quality control testing usually isn't conducted. Rather the test-box check is reserved for when a problem is suspected.

The standard 2-cc coupler may either be an HA1 or HA2 style. With an HA1 coupler, the receiver of the hearing aid is placed into a large opening, and puttylike material is placed around the case of the hearing aid to seal off the opening. An HA2 coupler can be used for attaching to a BTE hearing aid by using an additional snapon earmold tubing attachment and a standard length of tubing. Other couplers are available for more specialized testing. In research settings, audiologists use a manikin known as the Knowles Electronics Manikin for Acoustic Research (affectionately known as the KEMAR—"Kee-Mar"). The KEMAR has a different smaller coupler, believed to be more representative of the ear.

In general, audiologists use 2-cc coupler measures for three reasons:

- To assess the performance of the hearing aid when it arrives from the manufacturer to ensure that it is performing according to specifications.
- To assist with the fitting process, that is, corrections are made to the 2-cc coupler findings to predict performance in the patient's ear. This approach is commonly used with infants and young children in cases where direct probe-microphone verification is not possible (see our previous RECD section).
- To troubleshoot a patient complaint of a faulty hearing aid, or to simply conduct an annual check of the hearing aid's performance.

Hearing Aid Programming

Today, the audiologist clicks on handles or buttons in the computer software to change the hearing aid settings. The hearing aid settings are programmed digitally between the computer and the digital hearing aid circuit using a Bluetooth device—no wires needed! The programmed settings can be saved to the hearing aid's memory and to a patient database in the software and stored on either a local hard drive or network server. With digital hearing aids, it is now possible to make changes on 20 or more different parameters for a single hearing aid. Moreover, the changes are significant, for example, changes in gain of up to 70 dB are achievable.

The computer software for hearing aids is nearly always manufacturer specific, that is, each manufacturer develops and maintains ongoing versions of a software application for fitting its hearing aid products. These software applications may either be standalone or may be programming modules within a larger, more universal computer software platform called *Noah* (not an acronym—named to encourage audiologists to "get in the boat."). Standalone software programs are installed and assessed much like other software programs on a computer. Noah, on the other hand, is a software system that has programming modules from different manufacturers, and a dispenser may see a wide variety of patients fit with different brands of hearing aids; thus, nearly all software programming modules need to be available. The downside to multiple standalone software applications is the difficulty it imposes on maintaining one central patient database, as each stand-alone application has its respective patient database. In contrast, Noah allows for execution of many different manufacturer software modules, and uses only one central patient database. Think of Noah as a file management system. It is nice to have one patient file with all of their hearing aid programming saved, particularly if they have more than one set of hearing aids from more than one manufacturer.

As we mentioned, there are thousands of adjustments possible on today's hearing aids, and for programming efficiency, audiologists usually only fit one or two brands of hearing aids (even within these brands there may be 10 or so different models with different programming features; consider that manufacturers add new products every year, which also involves software updates). It would be impossible (and unnecessary) for an audiologist to be proficient in programming all brands of hearing aids. It is not uncommon, therefore, that if a patient walks into a clinic with Brand X hearing aids that need to be reprogrammed, but the audiologist only fits Brand Y, the audiologist will likely send the patient down the street to a colleague who fits Brand X. Although many audiologists will state they fit "any hearing aid manufacturer" as discussed previously, there are so many things to keep up on with hearing aids it is virtually impossible. Therefore, most audiologists only know two or three hearing aid manufacturers well.

Prescriptive Fitting Methods

In the preceding section, we discussed "programming" of the instruments. A reasonable question might be: "What do we program them to do?" Desired hearing aid gain and output for the patient is first selected using a validated *prescriptive fitting method* (for review, see Mueller, Ricketts, & Bentler, 2017). This is a mathematic model of selecting gain and output based on the patient's hearing loss that has been shown to provide the best outcome. Ear canal gain and output target levels are used as the prescription; the goal of the fitting is to have the optimal frequency-specific gain and output for soft, average, and loud speech inputs. Additionally, the maximum power output

(MPO) of the hearing aid cannot exceed the patient's loudness discomfort levels (LDLs). Although the exact prescriptive targets may not be the *ideal fitting* for all patients, it has been shown that they will optimize the fitting for the *average* patient. Given the large variety of hearing aid settings, it is important to have a good starting point. You have to start someplace.

The following are two fitting methods that are currently used:

- National Acoustic Laboratories' (NAL) NonLinear method v.2 (NAL-NL2). See http://www.nal.gov.au
- Desired Sensation Level method v.5 (DSLv5.0). See http://www.dslio.com

In general, most audiologists use the NAL method with adults and the DSL method with children. However, in Australia, where the NAL-NL2 method was developed, it is also used with children; whereas in Canada, where the DSLv5 was developed, it remains popular for adult hearing aid fittings. In essence, the methods are appropriate for both populations and ongoing comparison work between the two methods continues. The two methods are more similar than they are different.

We do need to mention that each manufacturer tends to have their own proprietary fitting method (called "Phonak-Fit, Oticon-Fit, etc.). While the NAL-NL2 and the DSLv5 have been validated with hundreds, if not thousands, of patients, these proprietary fits have no basic research behind them. Yet, the reps from the companies encourage audiologists to use these algorithms. Why? Because often, the manufacturer's method is designed to make the use of the hearing aid "more pleasing." For example, if a given manufacturer has a crappy feedback reduction system, in their algorithm, they simply reduce gain in the area where they know feedback will occur—no feedback, but no audibility or effective speech recognition either. Would an audiologist ever use these fitting methods rather than the ones validated by research? Unfortunately, it happens.

The Day of the Fitting

As mentioned in the preceding section, hearing aids typically are programmed according to a prescriptive fitting method that is appropriate for the patient's hearing loss. It is important to verify that the prescriptive fitting method produces the appropriate ear canal output when the hearing aids are actually being worn by the patient. In other words, just because prescriptive targets are met on the simulated version shown on the computer fitting screen, does not assure that the SPL values are correct in the individual's ear. In fact, there is considerable evidence that what the manufacturer has displayed in the fitting software as "simulated real-ear output" often deviates by 10 dB or more from the true real-ear output (Mueller et al., 2017). Real-ear verification is essential, and not to do so is considered unethical practice by some, including us. This is the cornerstone of the fitting process.

Probe-Microphone Verification

When this testing is conducted, a thin silicone tube is placed in the ear canal and is attached to a measurement microphone, which measures the aided ear canal levels for externally produced signals such as speech. The goal is to have the tip of the tube about 5 mm from the eardrum. The preferred method is to deliver calibrated real speech at input levels ranging from soft to loud (e.g., 55–75 dB). This procedure is often referred to as "speech mapping." Using this approach, we attempt to place the LTASS at a level that matches the mathematically derived fitting targets that we discussed earlier. The most commonly used signal today is the International Speech Test Signal (ISTS), which we discussed earlier. It was derived to resemble average speech of an international speech spectrum. Unlike pure tones, speech has a large range, with many valleys and peaks. The range of the signal delivered is normally around 30 dB SPL, which is the 30th to 99th percentiles of the speech itself.

When we verify the fitting using probe-microphone measures and real speech, the procedure we use is referred to as the real-ear aided response, or the REAR. Using the REAR to verify the fitting is quite logical, as everything is referenced to ear canal SPL, and we can easily visualize the portion of the speech signal that is audible for individual patients in their own ear. The SPL-O-Gram fitting format, as shown in Figure 6–13, means that louder outputs indeed fall above softer outputs. If you're new to using an SPL-O-Gram, the common "upward sloping" audiogram takes some getting used to because it seems upside down compared to the traditional HL audiogram, but it's well worth the effort.

Shown in Figure 6–13 is a typical fitting screen from the probe-microphone equipment

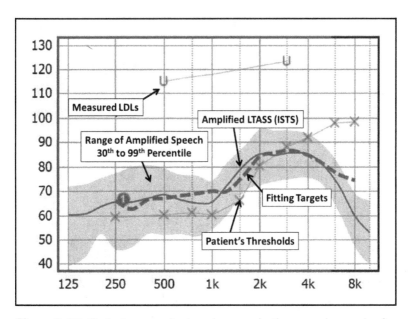

Figure 6–13. Typical screen display when conducting speech mapping for hearing aid verification. Shown is the patient's thresholds and LDLs converted to real-ear SPL, the fitting target, and the measured aided speech spectrum. Display is for 65 dB SPL ISTS input; testing would normally also be conducted for inputs of 55 and 75 dB SPL, with output then adjusted to match corresponding targets. *Source*: From *Speech Mapping and Probe Microphone Measurements* (p. 123), by H. G. Mueller, T. A. Ricketts, and R. Bentler, 2017, San Diego, CA: Plural Publishing. Reprinted with permission.

using the REAR for verification. The example here is for a real speech 65 dB SPL input—the complete verification process would also include a soft and loud input signal (e.g., 55 dB and 75 dB SPL). The HL audiometric thresholds and the patient's LDLs have been converted to ear canal SPL (the equipment does this for us using average correction factors). In this example, we are looking at the NAL-NL2 fitting targets. The shaded area represents the amplitude range of the amplified signal (30th–99th percentiles), with the LTASS as the dark line near the middle. The goal, accomplished very nicely here, is to make the LTASS equal to the prescriptive targets. The amplitude range of the amplified speech signal also provides some insights regarding compression (discussed in Chapter 5); note that the range is smaller for the higher frequencies, where compression is the greatest (e.g., 500 Hz vs. 4000 Hz).

The usual goals of this verification procedure is to be within fitting targets by +/– 3 dB, if possible, at least through 4000 Hz, for soft, average, and loud speech inputs. There are times when the degree of hearing loss might prevent this. There are also times when a perfect fit to target is obtained and the patient says "this isn't acceptable." Compromises do have to be made, and remember the automatic gain increase feature we talked about in Chapter 5. Finally, these fitting targets are a range and are for average. It's okay if the patient's preferred loudness levels deviate a little from average. A big part of the verification process is to talk the patient through the goals and the test results, reminding the patient of the importance of audibility. Many audiologists utilize a large monitor displaying the results to facilitate this, as shown in Figure 6–14. A patient might first

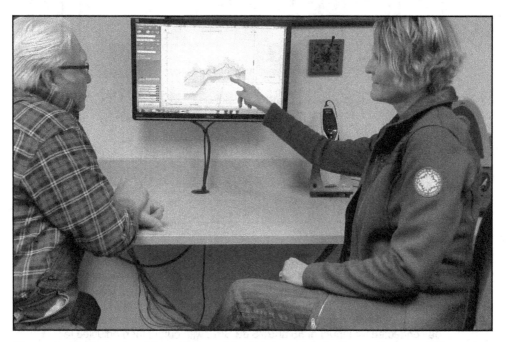

Figure 6–14. Example of how display of speech mapping findings can be used for patient counseling. Small laptop data can be routed to a larger monitor for this purpose. *Source*: From *Speech Mapping and Probe Microphone Measurements* (p. 86), by H. G. Mueller, T. A. Ricketts, and R. Bentler, 2017, San Diego, CA: Plural Publishing. Reprinted with permission.

CLINICAL TIP: Acclimatization and Adjustment

We know two things about new hearing aids users. They often are not fond of the sounds of the hearing aids when they first start using them, and they often like their hearing aids more after a few weeks or months of use (to the extent of being quite rude when a repair is delayed). What happens? It's probably not brain plasticity, but there certainly is some type of adjustment. This adjustment usually involves getting used to hearing sounds that they were not previously hearing. Many people with normal hearing sit and listen to the fan of their computer all day long, and are not bothered at all. If you didn't even know that the fan made noise, and now you can hear it, that could be a big deal and distracting. So, if you encounter someone who is having problems getting used to his or her hearing aids, the following is a slogan we can loan you:

YOU HAVE TO HEAR WHAT YOU DON'T WANT TO HEAR TO KNOW WHAT YOU DON'T WANT TO HEAR!

---

complain that a new hearing aid sounds tinny, but after seeing the amplified speech in his real ear, and realizing all the sounds he will be missing if that output is not above his thresholds, tinny may not sound so bad anymore.

Other Probe-Mic Tests

What we have just gone through is the basic hearing aid fitting process using probe-mic measures. There are many other tests that are conducted with this equipment, and each has its own unique term. There is no reason that you need to know much about these tests, but you very well could see them mentioned in a report related to hearing aid fitting. What follows is a brief description of the different terms (ANSI, 2013).

■ **REUR:** Real-ear unaided response— SPL as a function of frequency, at a specified measurement point in the ear canal, for a specified sound field, with the ear canal unoccluded. Commonly referred to as "ear canal resonance."

■ **REUG:** Real-ear unaided gain— *Difference* in decibels between the SPL as a function of frequency at a specified measurement point in the ear canal and the SPL at the field reference point, for a specified sound field with the ear canal unoccluded. This measurement serves as a baseline for calculating the hearing aid insertion gain.

■ **REOR:** Real-ear occluded response— SPL as a function of frequency, at a specified measurement point in the ear canal, for a specified sound field, with the hearing aid in place and turned *off*. Reveals how the earmold/custom hearing aid is attenuating sound. Used to examine the effect of a vent on the canal resonance, or how "open" an open fitting really is. It is NOT a direct measure of the occlusion effect, although if the REOR is similar to the REUR, there is a high probability that there is no occlusion effect.

- **REOG:** Real-ear occluded gain— *Difference* in decibels, as a function of frequency, between the SPL at a specified measurement point in the ear canal and the SPL at the field reference point, for a specified sound field with the hearing aid in place and turned off.

- **REAR:** Real-ear aided response—SPL as a function of frequency, at a specified measurement point in the ear canal, for a specified sound field, with the hearing aid in place and turned *on*. This is the primary method of hearing aid verification. When we do "speech mapping" we are using the REAR.

- **REAG:** Real-ear aided gain—*Difference* in decibels, as a function of frequency, between the SPL at a specified measurement point in the ear canal and the SPL at the field reference point, for a specified sound field, with the hearing aid in place and turned on. That is, if you use a 60 dB input signal, and the REAR at 3000 Hz is 90 dB SPL, the REAG would be 30 dB. Don't confuse this with the REIG!

- **REIG:** Real-ear insertion gain— Difference in decibels, as a function of frequency, between the REAR and the REUR, or the REAG and the REUG, taken with the measurement point and the same sound field conditions. Used to validate gain-based prescriptive targets. Because gain is always a difference value, and never an absolute value, there is no REIR, just REIG.
  - □ REAG – REUG = REIG
  - □ REAR – REUR = REIG

- **REAR85 or REAR90:** Previously known as the real-ear saturation response (RESR)—SPL as a function of frequency, in the ear canal, with the hearing aid in place, turned on, with the VC adjusted to full-on (or just below

feedback), with an 85 dB or 90 dB input signal (signal of an intensity to cause the hearing aid to reach it's MPO). This measurement is to determine if the maximum output of the hearing aid falls within the desired levels across frequencies based on the patient's LDLs. Also to determine if the maximum output of the hearing aid is at a "safe" level. You can predict the real ear MPO from the coupler OSPL90 if you measure the patient's RECD.

- **RECD:** Real-ear coupler difference— Difference in decibels, as a function of frequency, between the output of the hearing aid in the real ear and in the 2-cc coupler, taken with the same input signal and hearing aid VC setting (see previous discussion).

- **REDD:** Real-ear dial difference— *Difference* in decibels, as a function of frequency, between the output from an earphone (either insert or supra-aural) in the real ear and the audiometer dial setting. The purpose is to convert the patient's HL results (e.g., audiogram, LDL's, etc.) into ear canal SPL values, sometimes referred to as an SPL-O-Gram.

- **RETSPL:** Reference equivalent threshold in SPL. *Difference* in decibels, as a function of frequency, between the output from an earphone (either insert or supra-aural) in the calibration coupler (either 6-cc or 2-cc) and the audiometer dial setting. For example, if the hearing aid dial was set to 60 dB HL at 2000 Hz, and the output in the 2-cc coupler for the insert earphone was 62.5 dB, the RETSPL would be 2.5 dB. The RETSPL is not technically a *real-ear* term, but it is used for some corrections related to real ear measures.

If all that was too much, the following are some shorter, practical versions:

- **REUG:** The natural hearing aid the patient walked in the door with; the amplification his or her pinna and ear canal have been giving him or her all their life.
- **REOG:** What the hearing aid or earmold does to the patient (acoustically) *before* the hearing aid is turned on; how the REUG is altered, and how the coupling is acting like an earplug.
- **REAG:** What the hearing aid gives the patient when turned on—but not accounting for what might have been taken away, or what the patient had before the instrument was inserted.
- **REIG:** What the patient has when he or she walks out of the office (relative to gain at the eardrum) that he or she didn't have when he or she walked in. If the output of the hearing aid (REAR) does not exceed his or her REUR (what he or she walked in with), it's possible that he or she could walk out with less than what he or she came with (and then the audiologist will have to write *him or her* a check—very embarrassing!).
- **REAR85:** This is the maximum output of the hearing aid in the real ear of the patient for the current programmed settings.
- **RECD:** This is the difference between the *output* in the coupler and the *output* in the real ear. How is this patient's ear different from a coupler? It is also used to accurately convert the dB HL of the audiogram to the dB SPL of the hearing aid fitting.
- **RETSPL:** This is the difference between the audiometer dial setting and the output in a coupler.
- **REDD**—This is the difference between the audiometer dial setting and the output in the real ear (HL + RETSPL added to the RECD).

Aided Speech Testing

Because the patient usually enters the hearing aid fitting process due to difficulty understanding speech, particularly speech in background noise, it seems logical that the verification procedure should measure his ability to understand aided speech. Although this seems logical, because of the poor sensitivity of most speech material, it is difficult to use outcomes of speech testing in clinical practice for selecting the best hearing aid frequency response or signal processing strategy—the probemic measures must be used for this. Although this is not useful for selecting the best hearing aid setting or arrangement, it may be useful in demonstrating to the patient the benefits of amplification. The aided speech results, especially when background noise is included, also adds useful information for counseling. We also can't forget that simply using this measure in the fitting process seems to increase patient loyalty to the provider, satisfaction with the fitting process, and ultimately, increased satisfaction with amplification over time (see Mueller et al., 2014).

The general purposes for completing aided speech recognition testing include the following:

- demonstrate that the hearing aids improve audibility leading to improved speech recognition;
- demonstrate that a technology aimed at improving SNR (directional microphones, beamformers, FM

KEY CONCEPT: Aided Sound Field Testing—Just Say "NO"

There was once a time when audiologists would test aided thresholds in the test booth. In fact, there sometimes would be a completion between two products to see what was best. This of course has little value, as there is considerable masking in the real world, and what is 5 dB to 10 dB better in the booth doesn't really matter. Fortunately, with the development and use of probe-microphone measures, aided sound field testing no longer is needed. This is good, because there are many factors that make these results invalid, or at the least, questionable. The American Academy of Audiology Clinical Practice Guidelines on Pediatric Amplification had a fair bit to say on this topic, so we'll review the comments here. They start off by saying: "Measurement of aided sound field thresholds should not be used as a method of hearing aid verification."

That statement pretty much sums it up, but they go on to list some of the reason why:

- Aided testing only samples hearing aid characteristics at widely-spaced intervals (octave/half-octave) and does not indicate the presence of peaks or troughs in the hearing aid response characteristics.
- Test–retest reliability, commonly referred to as +/– 5 dB in the adult population, may be significantly greater in the pediatric patient. Depending on the child's developmental level, interest in the test procedures, and other variables, test reliability may be large

enough to obscure meaningful test information.

- Children are likely to move (both head position and possibly body position) during testing, which may result in significant increase or decrease in the test signal intensity at the ear or hearing aid microphone.
- The input stimulus, depending on its intensity, may interact with the hearing aid signal processing in a manner such as to over- or underestimate the aided response. In children with normal or near-normal hearing in any portion of the frequency spectrum, but in particular the low-frequency region, the noise floor of the test booth may obscure (lessen) the apparent gain provided by the hearing aid in that frequency region.

As reviewed by this committee of experts, anytime you see aided sound field thresholds for a child, view the findings with skepticism. The aided audiogram isn't really needed, as the speech mapping will clearly show what has been made audible. If someone *must* see aided results, it is possible for the audiologist to use the real-ear insertion gain and construct "predicted" aided thresholds. Given all the problems with doing the testing in the sound field, these predicted thresholds are probably more accurate than if an attempt had been made to actually assess thresholds behaviorally. An example of the probe-mic predicted thresholds are shown in Figure 6–15.

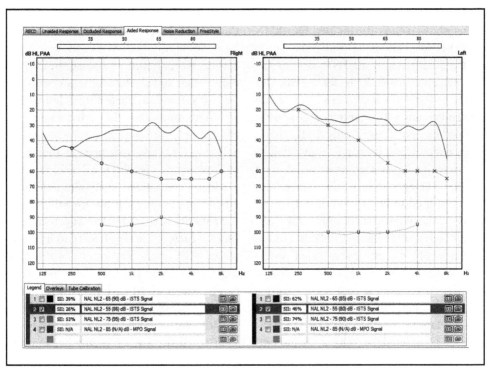

Figure 6–15. Example of using the results of probe-microphone testing to predict aided thresholds based on the earphone unaided thresholds and the aided insertion gain measured. The upper dark line represents the predicted thresholds for each ear. *Source*: From *Essentials of Modern Hearing Aids: Selection, Fitting, and Verification* (p. 684), by T. A. Ricketts, R. Bentler, and H. G. Mueller, 2019, San Diego, CA: Plural Publishing. Reprinted with permission.

systems, remote microphones, etc.) can lead to improved speech recognition in noise; and

- demonstrate the limitations of performance in noise (even with SNR improving technologies) to aid in counseling related to realistic expectations.
- complete a cochlear implant candidacy evaluation.

Illustrative Case Study

Here is a patient that we saw in the clinic recently that makes a good case for aided speech testing. Our patient is a 72-year-old male who is obtaining his first pair of hearing aids. He recognizes that he has problems, but is still somewhat apprehensive about the use of amplification. He has a typical downward sloping hearing loss bilaterally, going from 25 dB to 35 dB in the low frequencies, to 60 dB to 70 dB in the 3000 Hz to 4000 Hz region. Our probe-microphone testing showed that we were able to obtain a good match to NAL-NL2 targets bilaterally through 4000 Hz for soft, medium, and loud inputs. At this point, we decided to conduct some supplementary speech testing as part of the verification process. As mentioned earlier, this will not be used to alter the fitting, but rather to gather useful information that can be used in counseling.

Our prefitting test results from a week earlier showed that his unaided QuickSIN performance (conducted under earphones at 70 dB HL) was 8 dB SNR loss for the right ear, and 9 dB SNR loss for the left. Our testing today in the sound field (conducted aided bilaterally with an input of 65 dB SPL) revealed an SNR Loss of only 4 dB. This is a very encouraging finding. It shows that he is performing better with hearing aids than his best-ear earphone performance, and the input used today is considerably softer (conversational speech). Moreover, for many "noisy" environments, the SNR is around +5 dB to +10 dB, and these aided results suggest that he now should be able to follow a conversation in these settings. So, from a verification standpoint, these findings are more or less a pat on the back for the audiologist who selected the technology and pro-

grammed the hearing aids. But what about the patient? He probably doesn't realize that he is doing any better—he still is missing several words—and of course, he doesn't realize that today's testing was conducted ~20 dB softer than the testing of last week.

To demonstrate the aided benefit to the patient, we conduct a second Quick-SIN measure. We now present the signal at a soft-speech level (50 dB SPL) and test unaided versus aided bilaterally. Additionally, to make things more meaningful for the patient, we score the test as percent correct for each of the six SNRs (two lists = 10 words/SNR level). The results of this testing are shown in Figure 6–16. Once these results are graphed and placed in front of the patient, we can have a meaningful discussion. We would start by first pointing out than when there is very little background

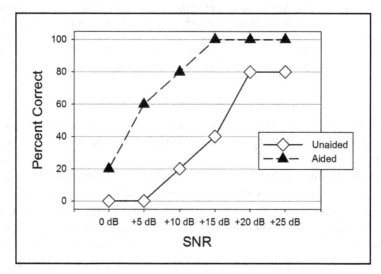

Figure 6–16. Worksheet to show patient scores as a function of the SNR for both the aided and the unaided conditions. This testing was conducted with a soft speech level, so even if the scoring for the Quick-Sin initially was represented as SNR-loss, it is possible to see the percentage correct across the various SNRs using this approach, to show the patient the positive effects of increased audibility. *Source*: From *Speech Mapping and Probe Microphone Measurements* (p. 220), by H. G. Mueller, T. A. Ricketts, and R. Bentler, 2017, San Diego, CA: Plural Publishing. Reprinted with permission.

noise (e.g., SNR +20 and +25), he does okay without hearing aids (he probably already knew that). We then might mention that even with hearing aids, he won't do very well in the very difficult listening situations—the 0 dB SNR condition—but we also need to mention that neither do people with normal hearing! We then focus on the center portion of the chart, the most commonly encountered SNRs in daily activity, where the use of hearing aids improved his understanding by 60%. It's probable that he has already mentioned this to us on his own, as this degree of improvement is very noticeable to the patient during the procedure. The 5 min to 10 min spent conducting this testing and explaining the results to patients can have a lasting impact on their attitude toward the use of hearing aids.

Verification of MPO

Our "day-of-the-fitting" testing is almost over. The final thing in our tool kit is verification that the maximum output (MPO) was set appropriately. Recall that earlier, we measured the patient's LDLs, converted these values to 2-cc coupler, and then set the MPO in the fitting software to match these values. We know we're not going to be too far off, but verification is still needed.

For this testing, we suggest the use of loud obnoxious noises. By obnoxious noises, we mean everyday sounds such as door slam, toilet flushing, baby crying, dog yapping, dishes clattering, and so forth. There are two reasons for using these types of signals. First, some of the noises are composed of relatively narrow bands—this will drive the hearing aid to a higher MPO than a broadband signal such as speech. Secondly, the quality of the signal can impact the LDL; LDLs tend to be lower for noises that are not pleasant to listen to. In the clinic, on the day

of the fitting and verification, we typically want to create a "worst case scenario" so that the patient has no unpleasant surprises when he or she starts using the hearing aids in his or her everyday environment.

The testing is conducted using the same Cox Loudness Anchors we discussed earlier. One by one, several obnoxious noises are presented to the patient at a level of 80 dB SPL to 85 dB SPL, and rated on the Cox scale. Patients should rate the noise to be a #6 on the chart. If the patient rates a given noise as #7 (and this is verified on retest), the output (AGCo kneepoint) of the hearing aids (or at least one hearing aid) needs to be adjusted downward. If the peak of the noise signal is known, only the AGCo for this frequency region is lowered. This process is continued until consistent #6 ratings are obtained. If the patient consistently gives a #5 rating (which rarely happens), then the AGCo kneepoint would be adjusted upward, to increase the dynamic range of amplification (termed headroom).

Hearing Aid Orientation

For most fittings, considerable time and effort needs to be dedicated to the hearing aid orientation, as there are several things to review. This can be a laborious process, but it is critically important. As a speech-language pathologist, it is possible that you will need do this with some of your clients with cognitive decline, as they might not remember what they were told in the audiologist's office. We have organized the orientation phase of the fitting appointment into three general areas:

Hearing Aid Use

- The patient is instructed on the insertion and removal of the devices. Have them attempt to conduct this task in your office in front of you. You will have to show the patient how to hold the hearing aids during the insertion process (conduct this training over something "soft," as the hearing aids will be dropped). You will have to instruct them on adjusting the volume control, the remote, and any additional switches the hearing aids may have. More and more, the pairing to their smartphone is also part of this procedure.

■ Demonstrate to the patient how to use the telephone with their new hearing aids. It's important to create a real-world situation, for example, they answer a ringing telephone. If the hearing aids have wireless streaming, assure that the patient knows how to operate this feature.

■ Instruct the patient on care and maintenance. The patient needs to be shown how to clean the hearing aid. This will involve showing the patient how cerumen is removed from the end of the hearing aid. Part of care and maintenance is also instructing the patient on how to change the battery, or how to place them in the charger, and how to store the instruments when they are not being worn.

CLINICAL TIP: Verification Versus Validation?

If you look up dictionary definitions of verification and validation, you may be hard pressed to discriminate between the two words, which mean essentially the same thing. However, in the world of quality control, there has been a great deal of discussion on the topic, and several industries have provided definitions for these two words that are specific to their work. In most cases, verification is used when discussing if specific goals—often design or manu-facturing goals—were met. In contrast, validation is used to describe whether the end user/target audience obtains what they wanted or needed. Stated simply

■ Verification: Are we building the system right?
■ Validation: Are we building the right system?

Applied to the selection and fitting of hearing aids, hearing aid verification is often used to refer to the process of ensuring that the hearing aid meets specific criteria (are we building the system right?). For example, we verify that we achieve our target prescriptive gain and output, we verify that aided loudness does not exceed threshold of discomfort, or we verify that aided thresholds meet expected levels. In contrast, hearing aid *validation* is the process of ensuring we meet the goals set forth in the communication needs assessment (are we building the right system?). Think of your mom's chocolate chip cookie recipe. You can start by following the recipe perfectly, and measure each ingredient perfectly—that's *verification. Validation* is when you take the first bite after they come out of the oven.

Establish Realistic Expectations

- A new hearing aid user might be on a wearing schedule. A wearing schedule allows the patient to gradually adjust to the new sounds they will be hearing. As a rule of thumb, new hearing aid users should start out wearing their hearing aids at home in a relaxed and quiet situation for a few days before wearing them in more demanding listening situations, like a restaurant. Usually, the average new user needs about a week to begin full-time use. The main point is that they need to go from relatively easy to more difficult listening situations.
- We know that new users often tend to be bothered by louder noises when they start using their hearing aids, even if you have programmed gain for loud sounds correctly. Encourage them to attempt to adjust to these sounds, as over time, the annoyance level will be reduced.
- We know that many new users expect the hearing aids to provide improved speech understanding in all listening environments—including extreme background noise. We recommend that you remind them during this initial orientation that there are certain situations where improvement will be limited.

Offering Reassurance

- There are potential negative emotions surrounding hearing loss and hearing aid use. Many of these emotions are still present after the fitting. It's important to be patient and offer support for each individual, especially during their initial foray with hearing aids.

After the Hearing Aid Fitting

We are now to the point of discussing what occurs after the patient has been fitted with his or her new hearing aids and has left the clinic or office. There will likely be follow-up counseling required, and maybe a little troubleshooting for some problems that were discovered during real-world use. In this section, however, we are going to focus on self-report validation measures. Recall that earlier in this chapter we encouraged the use of some type of formal questionnaire to be completed by the patients that relates to their hearing difficulty and communication needs. Many of these same prefitting tools are used as outcome measures in the validation stage. The results of these outcome measures are useful in and of themselves, and when compared to prefitting test results, they allow us to determine the benefit afforded by the intervention.

An outcome measure allows us to quantify the impact of the management or treatment scheme. They can be useful for answering the following important clinical questions:

- How did the intervention impact the individual?
- Did the management improve the communication abilities of the individual?
- Did our intervention improve the person's overall lifestyle?
- And most important clinically, did we meet our intervention goals that were identified during the hearing needs assessment?

You might ask why do we really need self-report measures of real-world outcomes? Why not just stick with probe-microphone measures and speech perception scores as indicators of success? We can think of at least four reasons why self-report outcomes are a good idea:

■ First, for largely economic reasons, health care is becoming more consumer driven. In this evolving system, the consumer decides what treatment is selected and when it is complete. The major index of quality of service is self-reported outcome and satisfaction. Consumer-driven health care places an added emphasis on the patient's point of view. Therefore, it is critical to measure the real-world benefit and satisfaction of hearing aid use. Because today's patients are, on average, more savvy and better informed than our grandparents, they want to know how much benefit they are receiving in everyday listening situations. Using a self-report of hearing aid outcome allows us to measure and report to patients how they are doing compared to an average.

■ Second, self-report measures of outcome are gaining importance, due in part to the fact that many real-world experiences simply cannot be measured effectively in laboratory conditions. The traditional hearing aid outcome measures (e.g., speech recognition in quiet and in noise) do not capture the true experiences of hearing aid use in everyday listening situations. Consider hearing aids with automatic and adaptive beamforming and directional technology. The effectiveness of features such as these depends heavily on the lifestyle and listening environments of the individual patient. In order to quantify the true impact of hearing loss and its associated treatment on activity limitations, lifestyles, and so on, self-report measures need to be used.

■ Third, even when laboratory conditions are used to simulate real-world listening situations, they do not always resemble the patient's impression of the actual real-life situation. Assessing speech perception in noise with a defensible signal-to-noise ratio is rarely perceived by patients as bearing any resemblance to their own experiences. Self-report outcome measures give us a scientifically defensible way to measure the real-life success of the hearing aid fitting.

■ Finally, if you choose not to use outcome measures, it is likely that your patients will find other ways to report their satisfaction, or lack of satisfaction. There are several Internet sites devoted to rating doctors and other health-care providers, and we suspect that these will become even more commonly used in upcoming years. Increasingly, hospitals and clinics are sending out provider satisfaction surveys following a clinic visit. Figure 6–17 shows an example of an audiologist's rating from the website http://www.healthgrades. com, showing the rating for "likelihood to recommend this audiologist to family and friends." Many prospective patients will likely view these ratings before making an appointment—just like your patients now use TripAdvisor or Yelp to decide where to have dinner. It makes good sense, therefore, for the audiologist to obtain these ratings themselves so that, if there are problems, they can take care of them before they are made public on the Internet.

The following are some practical reasons for using standardized scales as part of the fitting and validation process:

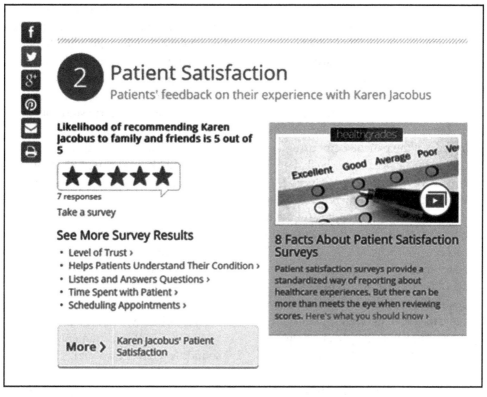

Figure 6–17. Sample rating of patient satisfaction for audiologist from the website http://www .healthgrades.com, following the fitting of hearing aids. Although not a direct measure of satisfaction with amplification, it is unlikely that dissatisfied hearing aid users will recommend a given audiologist to their family and friends. *Source*: From *Speech Mapping and Probe Microphone Measurements* (p. 227), by H. G. Mueller, T. A. Ricketts, and R. Bentler, 2017, San Diego, CA: Plural Publishing. Reprinted with permission.

- Assist in determining the success of the hearing aid fitting by comparing the patient's score to normative data. Example: A patient has a very mild hearing loss; normal hearing through 2000 Hz, dropping down to a 40-dB loss in the 3000 Hz to 6000 Hz range. His unaided scores showed significant handicap and considerable communication problems. Following the fitting of new hearing aids and a reasonable adjustment period, the patient's aided scores suggest fewer communication problems. In fact, the patient's aided scores reveal that he is performing at the 40th percentile of people with normal hearing.

- Assist in determining if prefitting goals are met or if additional intervention is needed. Example: The patient identified "easier to understand my daughter on the phone" as a prefitting goal. After 3 weeks of wearing the hearing aids, the patient indicates continued difficulty and no benefit in this area. Additional hearing assistive technologies including amplified telephones, wireless streaming, and speakerphone solutions are explored.

■ Assist in determining if prefitting goals are met or if additional counseling is needed. Example: The patient established the goal of wearing his or her new hearing aids in more listening environments. Because the inventory can be used to monitor progress, it becomes apparent after three months of use that the patient is not using the hearing aids as he or she had hoped. More counseling regarding the difficulties encountered, as well as ways to achieve more successful use of the hearing aids could be key to future success.

■ Assist in determining need for postfitting adjustment. The patient's postfitting results revealed that he has a low tolerance for loud sounds with his new hearing aids (e.g., he judges sounds to be "uncomfortably loud" that most individuals wearing hearing aids consider "loud but okay"). This was not the case on the prefitting assessment. This information might suggest adjusting the hearing aid MPO settings again, but might also represent a newfound perception of loudness that will be only appreciated after a few weeks of adjustment, and maybe some extra counseling.

Cox (2005) provided an excellent article regarding guidance for using hearing aid outcome measures—including how to grade the overall effectiveness of each measure. Ricketts et al. (2019) review in detail eight different self-assessment scales that easily can be used for real-world validation of the fitting. We have selected three of these to mention here. They are not only our favorites, but are the most commonly used.

■ Client Oriented Scale of Improvement (COSI): Measures early and final abilities for specific communication situations important to the patient; used as a pretest to define goals and to plan management and quantify expectations, and as a posttest to assess the success of the management in meeting the patient's goals. The form starts off as a blank sheet, as the patient nominates situations (usually 3 or 4) where he or she would like to see improvement in communication (see Figure 6–18 for example).

■ Abbreviated Profile of Hearing Aid Benefit (APHAB): Provides "percent of problems" the patient has for three different listening conditions involving speech understanding (in quiet, in background noise, and in reverberation) and problems related to annoyance of environmental sounds (aversiveness scale). There are a total of 24 items, six in each of the four categories. These ratings can be obtained as a prefitting or unaided measure, as an aided measure, or—by looking at the aided to unaided difference score—as a benefit measure. See Appendix E for the APHAB form.

■ International Outcome Inventory for Hearing Aids (IOI-HA): The scale is indeed international, as it is available in 29 different languages (https://icra-audiology.org/Repository/self-report-repository/Survey). It can be downloaded for no charge. This makes it an excellent tool for comparing hearing aid fitting outcomes around the world. The IOI-HA covers a minimal set of seven core outcome items that are sufficiently general to apply to all patients and many different types of investigations carried out in different countries in the world. Each question is designed to relate to a different domain.

DID YOU KNOW: Comfortable with Your COSI?

It has been suggested that the COSI outcome measure has become popular in part because of the positive warm feeling the name suggests—after all, who wouldn't want to be "cozy"? Of interest, however, is that the COSI was developed in Australia, and in Australia, "cossie" (or "cozzie") is a term sometimes used to refer to one's swimsuit—a shortened version of costume, as in "swimming costume." So if you say, "Let's take a look at your 'COSI'" to your Australian patient, it might take on a somewhat different meaning!

The domains assessed are as follows:

- Benefit from hearing aids
- Daily use
- Satisfaction with amplification
- Impact of using hearing aids on significant others
- Residual activity limitation
- Residual participation restriction
- Impact on quality of life

Client Oriented Scale of Improvement (COSI)

The COSI is one of the most frequently used self-assessment tools utilized in the prefitting stage of auditory habilitation, and is the most commonly used postfitting outcome measure. In fact, as a pretest and posttest, this tool has both efficiency and specificity (to the individual)! One issue related to most all standardized self-assessment scales is that the items must be relevant for the hear-

ing aid user. This is the main strength of the COSI. Since it's the outcome measure you'll most likely encounter, we'll go into its use in a little more detail.

The COSI items usually are nominated on the day of the fitting. It's also possible to measure the patient's expectations for these nominated items, something we recommend, as it might lead to meaningful counseling if expectations are not realistic. In Figure 6–18 we show the five items selected by this patient, and to the left of each item is the importance rating given to that item. We have modified the original COSI form, so now the ratings that you see to the right of each item are the patient's *expected outcomes*, rather than actual degree of change. This form was completed on the day of the fitting.

Notice that understanding grandchildren, was the last item this patient thought of, yet after some thought and discussion with his wife, it was given #1 priority. Conversely, the first thing he mentioned was understanding at his favorite watering hole (an event that had just happened the night before), yet this ultimately was given #5 priority, as upon reflection, he realized he only visits the Ryder bar a couple times a month—a very small percentage of his total communication needs. Bingo, however, is every Friday night in the school gym! Note that overall, his expectations are fairly high, maybe a little unrealistic. We tell him this, but assure him we will give it our best shot.

Regardless of whether expectations were initially assessed, when the patient returns for his or her postfitting visit, the previously completed COSI form is then brought out for the patient's ratings. It is common that the patient doesn't remember all of the exact items he or she selected (and may have new items based on recent listening experiences). It is easy to cross out listening tasks that are no longer meaningful, add new ones, or simply have the patient rate

NAL

CLIENT ORIENTED SCALE OF IMPROVEMENT

National Acoustic Laboratories
A division of Australian Hearing

Name: Kirby Mueller   Category.   New   X
Audiologist: Return
Date: 1. Needs Established
         2. Outcome Assessed

Aided Expectations

Final Ability (with hearing aid)
Person can hear
10%   25%   50%   75%   95%

SPECIFIC NEEDS

Indicate Order of Significance

	Specific Needs	Worse	No Difference	Slightly Better	Better	Much Better	CATEGORY	Hardly Ever	Occasionally	Half the Time	Most of Time	Almost Always
#5	Hearing friends while shooting pool in Ryder Bar.					✓						
#4	Understanding numbers called during Bingo.				✓							
#2	Understanding wife when she is in another room.				✓							
#3	Not have to turn the TV up so loud.				✓							
#1	Understanding soft voices of grandchildren when they visit.				✓							

Figure 6–18. The prefitting COSI for a patient. The patient selected five areas for improvement, rated them in priority, and then rated his expectations following the fitting of hearing aids. *Source:* From *Speech Mapping and Probe Microphone Measurements* (p. 232), by H. G. Mueller, T. A. Ricketts, and R. Bentler, 2017, San Diego, CA: Plural Publishing. Reprinted with permission.

NAL
CLIENT ORIENTED SCALE OF IMPROVEMENT

National **Acoustic** Laboratories
A division of Australian Hearing

Name: **Kirby Mueller**
Category. New X Return ___
Audiologist:
Date: 1. Needs Established ___
2. Outcome Assessed ___

SPECIFIC NEEDS

Indicate Order of Significance

Order	Specific Need	Degree of Change	CATEGORY	Final Ability (with hearing aid) Person can hear
		Worse / No Difference / Slightly Better / Better / Much Better		Hardly Ever 10% / Occasionally 25% / Half the Time 50% / Most of Time 75% / Almost Always 95%
#5	Hearing friends while shooting pool in Ryder Bar.	Slightly Better (X)		Half the Time (X)
#4	Understanding numbers called during Bingo.	Much Better (X)		Almost Always (X)
#2	Understanding wife when she is in another room.	Slightly Better (X)		Occasionally (X)
#3	Not have to turn the TV up so loud.	Much Better (X)		Almost Always (X)
#1	Understanding soft voices of grandchildren when they visit.	Much Better (X)		Most of Time (X)

Figure 6–19. The postfitting COSI for a patient. Prior to the fitting, the patient selected five areas for improvement and rated them in priority. Shown here are the patient ratings of benefit obtained with the hearing aids for each communication situation. *Source: From Speech Mapping and Probe Microphone Measurements* (p. 234), by H. G. Mueller, T. A. Ricketts, and R. Bentler, 2017, San Diego, CA: Plural Publishing. Reprinted with permission.

191

only the situations that are consistently on the list.

Benefit on the COSI can be assessed in two different ways: degree of change (improvement provided by the hearing aids) and final hearing ability with hearing aids (an absolute measure of communication ability). It is typical to see a similar pattern for these two different ratings, but sometimes, a difference is noted. For example, a patient with a fairly severe hearing loss who works in a demanding listening situation might rate his degree of change as "much better," but have only a final hearing ability of 50%. We suggest having the patient rate both categories because doing so may bring up key issues that need to be addressed.

Pool-Playing Grandfather

Our patient is back in our office after using his hearing aids for 3 weeks. The first thing he said when he walked in the door was "these things are great"—that's the news we want to hear, but we still move forward and sit down with him to complete the COSI. We don't show him the sheet he completed earlier regarding his expectations—we'll bring that out later. His completed COSI is shown in Figure 6–19.

The good news—he reports doing "much better" in 3 of the 5 categories. He notes some improvement with hearing his wife from a different room, but we are falling below his expectations for this category (see Figure 6–18). It may be that given his degree of hearing loss and the difficulty of this listening situation, this might be as good as it gets. We already have soft sounds programmed to NAL-NL2 fitting targets, but we could try increasing them a few dB. Overall, we would consider this a successful fitting,

and indeed, we met or exceeded expectations for most of the nominated categories. Moreover, the use of the COSI in this manner facilitates postfitting counseling. The form for the COSI can be downloaded from https://www.nal.gov.au/wp-content/uploads/sites/2/2016/11/COSI-Question naire.pdf.

In Closing A to Z

We promised that we'd do "hearing aid fitting A to Z" in this chapter, and we think we came pretty close. Obviously, understanding the speech signal is a critical goal for determining candidacy and amplification strategies. We then did some speech-in-noise testing, loudness assessment, and RECDs. Prefitting self-assessment inventories are also important, assist with the fitting, and offer opportunities to measure benefit. Selecting a validated prescriptive method is one of the keys to the overall process, assuming that the goals of the prescription are verified with probe-mic measures. Ensuring that soft sounds are audible and that speech has been amplified to optimize benefit, is the cornerstone of the overall process—there is no alternative to using real-ear verification. And finally, we need to use outcome measures to validate that all of our hard work on the day of the fitting paid off. Hopefully, we have both benefit and satisfaction—our self-assessment scales will tell us this. Of course, there still may be some post fitting counseling, and maybe some aural rehabilitation—which we'll talk about in Chapter 10. But we did make it close to Z—certainly at least to W, which isn't bad for one chapter!

7 Implantable Amplification Devices

As we have discussed in previous chapters, there is a wide array of amplification technologies available, and these solutions provide significant benefit for the majority of individuals with hearing loss. There are some cases, however, when the traditional treatment is less than satisfactory. The most common of these cases is when the hearing loss is so severe that conventional hearing aid technology does not provide adequate gain and output. This often is treated with a cochlear implant. Another example might be a medical condition of the middle ear, when an implantable device will be more effective. Other devices are designed more for cosmetic purposes, or unique patient conditions.

Several different types of implanted devices are currently available, and it is probable that you will work with patients, both children and adults, using some type of implantable device. While you don't have to be an expert in this area, you will want to understand the basic parts and function of the device so that you can ensure function. Further, it's possible that you may assist with determining candidacy for the devices, referring for testing, or providing initial counseling for an interested patient.

Cochlear Implants

The most common implantable device that you will encounter is the cochlear implant.

Cochlear implants have been considered by many to be the most significant technological advancement for the treatment of significant hearing impairment. Prior to cochlear implants, the only available technology for people with significant hearing loss was superpowered hearing aids, along with visual communication (speech reading or sign language) or tactile devices. By nature

> **DID YOU KNOW: Electrodes and Blades of Grass**
>
> As mentioned elsewhere, one of the pioneers of the world of cochlear implants is Dr. Graeme Clark, who developed the multiple electrode device. Clark's first multichannel cochlear implant operation was conducted at the Royal Victorian Eye and Ear Hospital in Melbourne, Australia, in 1978. It's reported that while developing the procedure, Clark had difficulty identifying a way to place the electrode bundle in the cochlea without causing any damage. His breakthrough came during a walk on the beach, by using a seashell which had the same spiral shape as the human cochlea and grass blades to represent the electrodes. The blades of grass were flexible at the tip and gradually increased in stiffness.

of the candidacy selection procedure, people who use cochlear implants receive minimal benefit from traditional amplification, and, for these individuals, a cochlear implant often is life changing.

The purpose of a cochlear implant is to change acoustic information to electrical impulses presented to the auditory nerve that can be perceived as sound for those people with a sensorineural hearing loss. Cochlear implants have been around for decades, but have more recently been available to the general public.

The name "cochlear implant" is a little misleading, as it somewhat suggests that the goal of the procedure is to stimulate the damaged cochlea. This is not the case. The implant bypasses the impaired cochlea and directly stimulates the auditory nerve. The surgically implanted internal component consists of a receiver placed under the skin in the temporal bone area and an electrode array inserted into the cochlea. The external components consist of a microphone, sound processor, transmitter, and power supply. A diagram is shown in Figure 7–1.

For the cochlear implant to function appropriately

- The microphone receives the acoustic sound and sends the input to the sound processor.
- The sound processor digitally analyzes the sounds and processes the signal as programmed (mapped) by the audiologist.

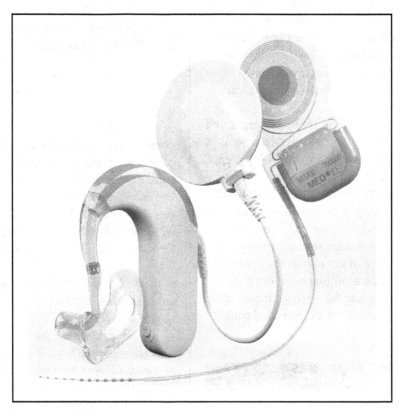

Figure 7–1. The internal and external components of a cochlear implant. *Source*: Image courtesy of Med-El.

■ The signal is then transmitted across the skin to the internal component. A magnet holds the external component near the internal component for appropriate radio signal transmission and to ensure that the two sides stay aligned.

■ The internal radio signal receiver picks up the signal and transmits the signal down the electrode array to the appropriate electrode. The electrodes are tonoatopically organized like the cochlea in which it is inserted.

■ The electrodes produce an electrical pulse thus stimulating the corresponding portion of the auditory nerve.

This basic function of a cochlear implant is similar across all manufacturers of cochlear implants; however, there are significant differences in electrode array, external and internal components, processing, software, and assistive devices between the three different manufacturers currently approved in the United States.

There are three general types of cochlear implants that currently are available on the market in the United States. While we described their general function earlier, their physical look differs (see examples in Figures 7–2 and 7–3):

■ Ear-worn devices consist of a behind-the-ear processor and a coil that attaches to the head. The microphones are on the ear-level device.

■ There also is a head-worn device that is only one piece that is solely attached to the head with nothing behind the ear. In this design, the microphones, processor, and magnet are all in the same unit that attaches on the outside of the head.

■ The third type is a body-worn device. This device has a head-level coil like the ear-worn device, but the processor is attached to the patient's shirt or is worn in a harness. This device is commonly used in children or as a waterproof device made for swimming. In the body-worn system, the microphone is located on the headpiece.

There also are "hybrid" devices that are available that include a cochlear implant component and a hearing aid component (Figure 7–4). These devices specifically are designed for patients who have aidable residual hearing ability in the low frequencies, but have limited/no hearing in the high frequencies. In these cases, the two components of the device—hearing aid and cochlear implant—work in conjunction to provide the patient a complete auditory signal through electrical stimulation of the high frequencies and acoustical stimulation for the low frequencies.

**THINGS TO REMEMBER:
A Little History About
Cochlear Implants**

Electrical stimulation of the auditory system was first reported in 1959. This first stimulation included placing active lead on a segment of the auditory nerve, and using an induction coil, stimulation was provided to the nerve. Although speech perception was not reported, the recipient did report that they were more aware of sounds. A cochlear implant race ensued between William House in the United States and Graeme Clark in Australia. House performed the first single-channel cochlear implant surgery in 1961 and the first implant in a child was performed in the early 1980s. Clark developed the first multichannel cochlear implant and implanted an adult in 1978 and a child in 1985.

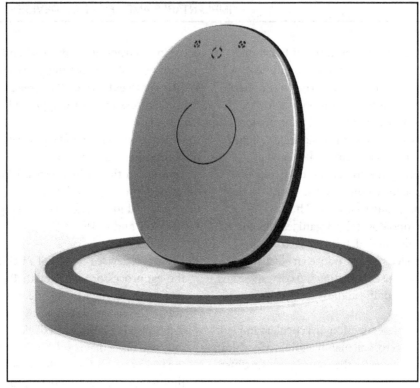

A

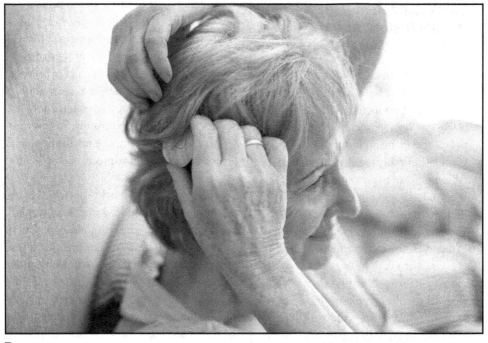

B

Figure 7–2. A–B. A head-worn device that is only one piece that is solely attached to the head, with nothing behind the ear. In this design, the microphones, processor, and magnet are all in the same unit that attaches on the outside of the head. *Source*: Images courtesy of Med-El.

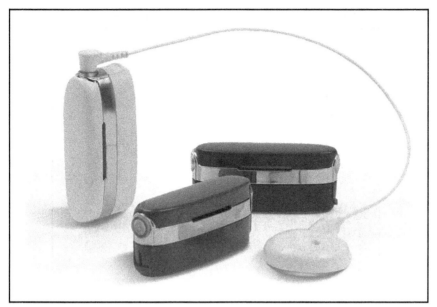

A

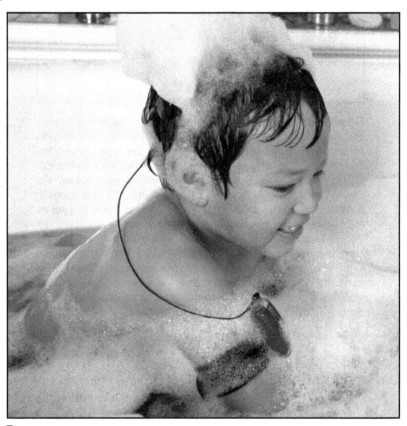

B

Figure 7–3. A–B. A body-worn device. This device has a head-level coil like the ear-worn device, but the processor is attached to the patient's shirt or is worn in a harness. In the body-worn system, the microphone is located on the headpiece. *Source*: Photos provided courtesy of Advanced Bionics, LLC © 2019.

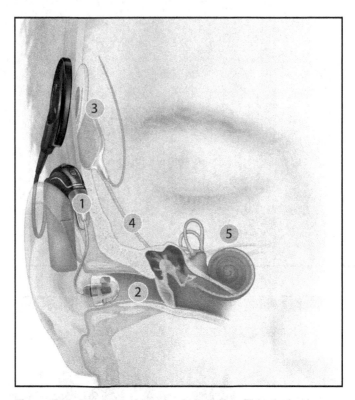

Figure 7–4. Hybrid cochlear implant device. This device has an electronic cochlear implant component and an acoustic hearing component. The person typically receives the high frequencies from the implant and the low frequencies from the hearing aid. (1) Microphone on the processor picks up the sounds they are missing and converts them into digital signal. (2) The acoustic component amplifies the sounds that the person hears and sends them through the ear canal in the normal pathway of hearing. (3) The missing sound information is sent through the coil to the implant under the skin. (4) The implant sends the electrical signal to the electrode that is implanted into the cochlea. (5) The hearing nerve fibers in the cochlear combine the acoustic signal and the electrical signal and sends it to the brain to be heard as sound. *Source*: Courtesy of Cochlear Americas.

Cochlear Implant Candidacy

Cochlear implants are a surgically implanted device and, therefore, in the United States, are classified as an FDA Class III medical device. The FDA oversees the selling, distribution, marketing, and labeling of medical devices, and are most strict about Class III devices.

The currently approved cochlear implant devices can be found on the FDA website (FDA, 2019). This also means that there are strict guidelines on who qualifies to receive the device. Early clinical trials only approved those patients who demonstrated no benefit (0% correct on open-set speech tests bilaterally) from traditional amplification. Current qualification for cochlear implants are generally based on open-set speech reception scores obtained by an audiologist with the patient using a best-fit amplification device. This tends to move the criteria away from audiometric thresholds and toward function with appropriately fit hearing aids. While the FDA sets the minimum criteria, many clinics and insurance agencies set more stringent criteria.

Most clinics define qualification as word recognition scores with less than 50% accuracy in the ear to be implanted and less than 60% accuracy in the nonimplanted ear in the best aided condition. Insurances may dictate more strict criteria, or on the other hand, allow for more relaxed qualifications. The criteria are also changing as cochlear implants become more prominent in persons with unilateral hearing losses; people who have hearing loss in just one ear with normal hearing ability in the opposite ear. It is important for audiologists who complete the testing for cochlear implants to remain informed about the changing guidelines, as advances are made in the device coding strategies, internal and external component technology, as well as changes in surgical techniques. If you are referring a patient who you think might be a candidate, it is important, therefore, for the patient to see an audiologist who routinely works in this area.

In the early days, patient qualifications for a cochlear implant were based solely on bilateral audiometric thresholds, but as mentioned earlier, now qualification is based on performance for the best aided condition. Best aided condition includes appropriately fit hearing aids, as we previously described in Chapter 6. Current qualifications are based on a variety of factors and are listed in Table 7–1 for children and 7–2 for adults.

Table 7–1. Cochlear Implant Candidacy for Children

	Qualification
Age	12 months of age or older
Audiometric	Significant sensorineural hearing loss that would limit educational success
Device Use	Little or no benefit as demonstrated by lack of sufficient progress (e.g., 3 months' progress in 3 months' time) on development of auditory, speech, and language skills; suggested a 3 to 6-month trial with appropriately fit devices
Medical	No medical or radiological contraindications to surgery
Support	Sufficient educational support and motivated self/family with appropriate expectations
Testing	Younger children where open-set speech testing is not possible, decision for cochlear implant is often made based on developmental progress, audiometric thresholds, and caregiver reports
	Older children: <50% accuracy in the ear to be implanted and <60% on the nonimplanted ear using the Pediatric Minimum Speech Test Battery (PMSTB), unless different criteria are dictated by insurance

Table 7–2. Cochlear Implant Candidacy for Adults

	Qualification
Age	No age restriction
Audiometric	Significant sensorineural hearing loss that impacts daily communication ability
Device Use	Little or no benefit after 3 to 6 month trial with appropriately fit devices
Medical	No medical or radiological contraindications to surgery
Support	Motivated patient with appropriately set expectations
Testing	<50% accuracy on open-set sentence recognition testing using the hearing aid alone in the ear to be implanted and <60% on the nonimplanted ear using the Minimum Speech Test Battery (MSTB), unless different criteria are dictated by insurance

While these are the general guidelines, these can be changed if there are extenuating circumstances such as likelihood of cochlear ossification due to bacterial meningitis. Best practices for cochlear implants are available through professional organizations such as the American Academy of Audiology Cochlear Implants Best Practices Guideline (https://www.audiology.org/publications /guidelines-and-standards).

CASE STUDY: Candidate for Hybrid Cochlear Implant

As we mentioned and as the name suggests, the "hybrid" cochlear implant includes the low-frequency benefits of traditional amplification, coupled with high frequency audibility delivered electrically. The ideal candidate has an aidable hearing loss in the low to mid frequencies, and a profound loss in the higher speech frequencies. The general audiogram that determines candidacy is shown in Figure 7–5. Observe that if someone had this degree of hearing loss, it would be very difficult to make speech audible with traditional amplification (except maybe loud speech). Also recall from Chapter 2, that the frequencies of 2000 Hz to 4000 Hz contribute substantially to speech understanding. A second issue to consider is that this patient most likely has "cochlear dead regions." What we mean by this is that in the regions where the loss is severe, there may be very few functional hair cells in the cochlear. This means that even if we did make speech signals audible in this region, it would not contribute to speech understanding. In fact, in some cases, it results in significant distortions and speech understanding goes down, not up, when audibility is present. This again, would lead the cochlear implant team to consider a hybrid implant if the patient was interested. The recommendation, of course, would also depend on the hearing status of the other ear.

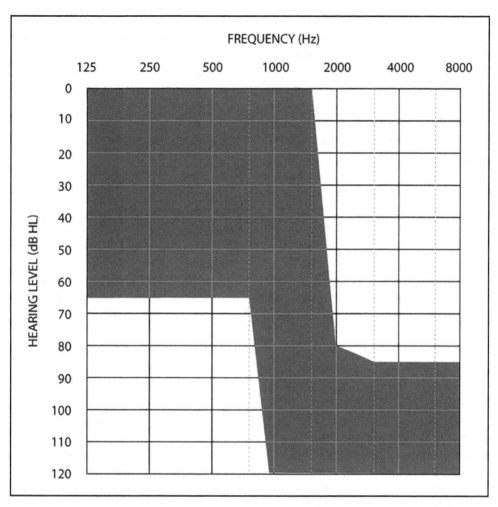

Figure 7–5. Audiogram for candidacy for a hybrid cochlear implant. *Source*: Courtesy of Cochlear Americas.

Preoperative testing is used to determine if the patient is medically and audiologically suited for a cochlear implant. Such information also can be compared to postimplant results to determine the adequacy of the implant and current programming as well as patient progress through rehabilitation. The determination of cochlear implant is typically made by a group of individuals including an audiologist and a surgeon. However, particularly in pediatric cases, a speech-pathologist, deaf educator, and psychologist may be involved. Opinions of other profes-

sionals may also be taken into account. Testing completed prior to implantation is briefly described in the sections that follow.

Medical Evaluation

A medical evaluation must be completed prior to implantation. This evaluation includes a complete physical exam and obtaining a complete medical history. The patient's overall health is assessed to determine if they are healthy enough for surgery and the cause of the hearing loss may be investigated. Cochlear imaging (CT or MRI) will be completed to evaluate and visualize the mastoid and inner ear structures for implantation. The scans are used to identify anatomical anomalies and may be used to help determine ear and method of implantation. Knowledge of the anatomy may also help the team determine the surgical technique and may influence the implant selection. Cochlear malformations rarely preclude patients from obtaining a cochlear implant, and in fact are the least common reason that would preclude patients from obtaining them (Jackler, 2015). The results of the medical evaluation will allow clinicians to assess the medical, physical, structural, and functional ability of the auditory system. Through thorough preoperative medical testing, the clinician is able to better counsel patients about the surgery and physical limitations and allow clinicians to set better expectations for postsurgical outcomes.

Audiologic Evaluation

As discussed in Chapter 2, the audiometric test battery should include a comprehensive behavioral and objective test of a patient's auditory ability. A complete case history is obtained to assess the patient's motivation for seeking a cochlear implant, hearing device history and use, prenatal and perinatal medical concerns, current medical com-

---

CLINICAL TIP: Are Two Better Than One?

In the early days, only one ear was implanted, even when a profound hearing loss existed bilaterally. We know, however, that with hearing aids, performance with bilateral fittings exceeds that with unilateral ones. Is the same true for cochlear implants? The answer appears to be yes! Starting around 2000, we started to see bilateral cochlear implantation occurring. There are significant benefits of bilateral hearing! Hearing with two ears helps hearing in noise. The auditory system is able to combine and compare the information coming to each ear and filter out what we are trying to hear from what we are trying to ignore. Also, hearing with two ears allows the person to localize or tell where sounds are coming from. The ability to tell where the sounds are coming from has significant safety implications such as localizing a car when crossing the street. There have also been significant reports of improved ease of listening and decreased frustration in social settings for people who receive bilateral cochlear implants. Currently, it is more common to see bilateral implants in children than it is in adults. Current data suggests that 36% of surgeries are bilateral cochlear implants with 70% of those being in children. Most commonly, these children have been between 3 and 10 years of age. Seventy-two percent of all bilateral cochlear implant surgeries were completed sequentially (70% of children and 76% of adults). Children less than 3 years of age are the only group where simultaneous implantation occurs more frequently than sequential (58% simultaneous).

plications, as well as educational and cognitive level. Individuals with significant medical or cognitive problems are not precluded from receiving a cochlear implant, but special consideration should be given and expectations should be discussed. Testing includes a full audiometric test battery including air conduction, bone conduction, and speech in quiet ability. Additionally, auditory speech perception testing is completed using appropriately fit amplification (American Academy of Audiology Pediatric Amplification Protocol, 2013) as was described in Chapter 6. Although we discouraged aided speech testing in Chapter 6, testing using hearing aids must be done to satisfy the FDA regulations that govern cochlear implantation. Testing is completed using developmentally and linguistically appropriate materials that are sensitive enough to measure differences in technologies and performance over time.

Specific recommendations for adults are provided in the manual of the Minimum Speech Test Battery (MSTB) and for children in the Pediatric Minimum Speech Test Battery (PMSTB; Uhler et al., 2017). Given that you might see the results of these different tests in reports, we have included a brief review of the tests that are part of the battery.

Adult Minimum Speech Test Battery

- AZ-Bio: Open-set, not-predicable sentence list. For example: (1) Her nails are unnaturally thick; (2) You must live in a gingerbread house; (3) Only the ants' coiled carcasses remained after the extermination. The testing may be completed in quiet or in noise.
- CNC word list: Open-set, not-predicable word list. For example: (1) Say the jar again; (2) Say the boil again; (3) Say the tough again.

- BKB-SIN: Open-set, not-predictable sentence list. These tend to be easier than the AZ-Bio. For example: (1) The clown had a funny face; (2) Children like strawberries; (3) She cut with her knife. These can be completed in quiet or in noise.

Pediatric Minimum Speech Test Battery

This battery has a hierarchy based on the child's age and cognitive level. The hierarchy is listed below in order of ease from easiest to most difficult.

- Speech discrimination: Used typically with infants using visual reinforcement. For example: "Bababa" said through a speaker or insert on the left side and when the child turns their head a video is played to reinforce the behavior.
- Early speech perception test (ESP): A multipart test that was created for children who are hard of hearing. It includes a pattern perception (hop, hop, hop vs. ahhhhhhh); spondees (icecream, baseball); and monosyllables (bat, baby).
- Lexical neighborhood test (LNT): Single-syllable words that are lexically appropriate for children.
- CNC word list: Open-set, not-predicable word list. For example: (1) Say the jar again; (2) Say the boil again; (3) Say the tough again.
- BKB-SIN: Open-set, not-predictable sentence list. These tend to be easier than the AZ-Bio. For example: (1) The clown had a funny face; (2) Children like strawberries; (3) She cut with her knife. These can be completed in quiet or in noise.
- Pediatric AZ-Bio: Open-set, not-predicable sentence list. For example:

(1) Her nails are unnaturally thick;

(2) You must live in a gingerbread house;

(3) Only the ants' coiled carcasses remained after the extermination. These can be completed in quiet or in noise.

Aided speech perception testing is completed in each ear independently to assist with the determination of ear for implantation; additionally, testing is completed in the binaural condition. Additional objective testing may be completed such as optoacoustic emissions, immittance, and auditory brain stem response (see Chapter 2 for review of these tests). Given that the implant may have an impact on the vestibular system, some clinics also perform a vestibular assessment; this information may also be used to assist in ear selection and to identify those patients who may be more susceptible to vestibular issues postimplantation.

Speech and Language Evaluation

A speech and language evaluation may be useful in the adult population, but is critical for pediatric patients. This evaluation is performed by a licensed speech-language pathologist and will be used to determine the patient's current level of speech and language function. Repeat assessments can be used to determine candidacy for pediatric patients as candidacy for children can be based on auditory, speech, and language competency. Children with hearing loss need to not just show progress of skills, but also demonstrate that these skills are in line with their normal hearing peers in the rate at which the skills are obtained. Further, an educational evaluation may be used to assist with the determination of language proficiency. The assessment may include current performance as well as assessing their future needs for educational support. The assessments conducted by the speech pathologist and edu-

cation team are essential for the pediatric patient to ensure that the child receives the care they need for success with their implant.

Psychological and/or Social Work Evaluation

Given that hearing loss is associated with depression, social isolation, dementia, reduced social engagement, and poor health-related quality of life, an evaluation by a social worker or psychologist may be warranted. The psychologist or social worker may be able to reveal any mitigating circumstances that would impact the outcomes of the person receiving the implant. They may also be able to determine motivation for seeking the implant and help set outcome expectations of the person and their family. Assessments can include social, emotional, educational, vocational, and adaptive abilities of the family and the person with hearing loss. Further, for older adults and others with cognitive impairment, a cognitive assessment may be warranted. The information gleaned from a cognitive evaluation or screener may help the team in their plan for rehabilitation and assist in setting appropriate expectations.

As you are seeing patients, it's important to take note of those who might need a cochlear implant; that is, someone who has a significant hearing loss and is not receiving adequate benefit from traditional amplification. In the adult population, this means that they are struggling to understand daily communication and have a difficult time communicating without visual cues, such as on the phone. This lack of hearing ability may have a significant impact on their health, safety, and social life. In the pediatric population, criteria also dictate the lack of success with traditional amplification. However, given that children are developing speech and language, you will want to also attend to their progress in speech, language, and auditory ability. It is not just making progress in their skills, but adequate and proportional progress. This is often described as three months' progress in three months' time.

Initial Appointments

The initial appointments after surgery are nerve-wracking for patients and family at best. After surgery, the patient returns to the programming center for initial activation. The amount of time between surgery and activation varies depending on center; some wait days while other recommend several weeks. The time between surgery and activation allows for healing and decrease of the swelling around the surgical site. The actual activation procedure will vary depending on the patient's age and cognitive level as well as the device that was implanted.

In all implant activations, the external device is connected to the head and the magnet strength is determined. The magnet needs to be strong enough to ensure that the device stays in place, but does not cause skin breakdown. The implant is then activated and programmed through a computer interface. There are several objective and subjective measures that can be completed to ensure that the device is providing the best sound to the patient. At the initial activation, patients who have previously had normal hearing may report that things sound different than they expected. While online videos may make one think that this appointment always has a happy response, it is more common for little ones to cry given that they are not used to hearing. The device is not hurting them, but they may be dismayed at the new access to sounds. Programming of the device, also called mapping, is done by an audiologist in a systematic method. Depending on the type of device, the audiologist will measure com-

fort levels and/or thresholds of the device in the attempt to provide sound across a variety of pitches and a range of loudness. Various programming techniques are used to refine the programming.

By the end of the appointment, patients, parents, and caregivers have been instructed on the basic care and function of the device and given instructions to return in a week or so. Patients will return often in the first few months for refinement of their programming and for further instruction on the device. The greatest gains in perception and function occur within the first few months; however, perceptual changes and improvements have been demonstrated even several years after implantation.

The number of times a patient returns to their implant center for continued programming can vary greatly and depends on many factors. Patients often return on 6-month intervals for cleaning and checking of the device and to ensure function. Audiometric testing can also be completed to ensure that the device is providing appropriate stimulation. Often, the same measures that were completed at pretesting/candidacy testing will be completed for comparison of function. This testing enables the clinician to compare pre- versus postoperative outcomes, but also is able to identify if any speech cues are being misperceived by the patient. This information will also be used to determine rehabilitation plans and future speech-language needs.

Cochlear Implant Companies

Unlike hearing aids, where you might find 20 to 30 different manufacturers or brands, there are currently only three different cochlear implant companies whose product is available in the United States. We have included some blurbs from their websites, so there may be some marketing hype included, but it does give you an idea of who the players are:

- Advanced Bionics Corporation: Advanced Bionics is a global leader in developing the cochlear implant systems. Acquired by Sonova Holding AG and working with Phonak since 2009, AB develops cutting-edge cochlear implant technology that restores hearing to those with severe-to-profound hearing loss. With operations in more than 50 countries and a track record for developing high-performing, state-of-the-art products, AB's talented group of technologists

and professionals are driven to succeed, work with integrity, and stay firmly committed to quality while delivering unmatched customer service. Their headquarters is in Los Angeles, California. (Sonova, 2019)

- Cochlear Americas: Since launching the world's first cochlear implant system more than 30 years ago, Cochlear Limited has brought the miracle of sound with its entire product portfolio to more than 450,000 hearing-impaired individuals across the globe. They work with more than 2,000 of the top hearing professionals around the world and have more than 100 active research

POINTS TO PONDER: Cochlear Implants and the Deaf Culture

There is a long history of disagreement over spoken versus visual language, and between those who see deafness as a medical condition and those who see it as an identity. Cochlear implants often are at the center of this discussion. Deaf (with a capital D) refers to the culture, while deaf (with a lowercase d) refers to hearing ability. Those who are Deaf does not necessarily refer to the status of hearing, but being part of the culture. Deaf often use some form of sign language as their primary means of communication. Historically, those who had minimal hearing ability and did not receive benefit from a hearing aid used sign language as their primary means of communication. Therefore, if someone is implanted and can effectively use auditory cues and

spoken language, one could understand the concerns of those in the Deaf community. Some people who are Deaf feel that a cochlear implant would be overwriting their culture, while some with a cochlear implant report that they can use a cochlear implant and still be part of the Deaf culture. Current trends suggest that the majority of persons who are born with hearing loss are born to normal-hearing parents. Therefore, it is not unexpected that the majority of these parents choose to pursue cochlear implants for their children. It is important to note that those who are implanted early are more successful with an implant and, should the child choose to not use the implant in the future, if the external piece is not worn, they do not hear.

partners in 20 different countries to continuously innovate and provide breakthroughs to those with hearing loss. The result is the most chosen cochlear implant system in the world. Cochlear's promise: "Hear now. And always," reflects their philosophy of a lifetime commitment to those individuals who choose our products. Their U.S. headquarters are in Denver, CO; their company is based out of Sydney, Australia. (Cochlear, 2019)

▪ MED-EL: MED-EL is a global technology company in the field of hearing loss. They develop and manufacture implantable hearing systems. These include cochlear implants, middle ear implants, bone conduction hearing implants, electric acoustic stimulation hearing implant systems, and auditory brain stem implants. The company is headquartered in Innsbruck, Austria and was founded in 1990. The U.S. headquarters is located in Durham, North Carolina. (Med-El, 2019)

Middle Ear Implants

In 1935, Alvar Wilska placed iron fillings on a patient's eardrum and then elicited electromagnetic sound from a headphone; the patient reported hearing. The iron fillings caused the tympanic membrane to move, which in turn caused vibration to the cochlea. At that time, Dr. Wilska reported it as a middle ear transmission device. After that discovery, little was done in the area of middle ear implants until the 1980s. Middle ear implants offer several advantages; of partic-

ular interest is the cosmetic advantage given the completely invisible implanted design. Further, some patients report that they can obtain a better sound quality due to reduction of feedback and little or no occlusion because of where the device is situated in the ear. Given that hearing aid technology continues to change, with better feedback control and more open fitting, these reported benefits might not be as great today as when the basic research was conducted.

There are currently two available types of middle ear implants: partially implanted and fully implanted. The primary difference is whether the device requires a microphone outside of the ear. In the partially implanted device, there is a portion of the device that is attached to the middle ear bones (ossicles) while the microphone sits behind the ear in a BTE-style device. This device picks up the sound and transmits the signal to a surgically implanted transducer that moves the ossicles in a manner and force consistent with hearing loss. The audiologist programs the device to meet the audiometric needs of the patient. The advantage of this style is that the microphone device has its own battery that can easily be changed. Further, this external microphone can be upgraded and may take advantage of many of the features of modern hearing aids. Conversely, it is visible and sits outside of the ear like a hearing aid and this may be unsuitable for some patients.

The other type of middle ear implant is a fully implantable device. This device does not have an external microphone. The entire device including the microphone is implanted into the middle ear. These devices have the advantage of 24/7 hearing ability. Further, patients with this kind of device are able to participate in water sports without the concern of ruining the device. Conversely, the battery is implanted internally and must be changed after several years; this may require a second surgery.

Candidacy

Although it is a middle ear implant, current recommendations are only those with a sensorineural hearing loss qualify for the surgery. Technically, anyone with a sensorineural hearing loss could benefit from the implant, but only those who perceive a communication difficulty would likely go forward with the surgical process. The target population of the middle ear implant are those with a moderate to severe sensorineural hearing loss whose hearing loss impacts their daily life. Those with more significant hearing loss are not typically recommended a middle ear implant as a cochlear implant would likely be of more benefit given damage to the cochlea. The middle ear implant is best recommended for those who require amplification, but likely do not qualify for a cochlear implant.

Given the need for self-report, the middle ear implant is only recommended for those who have the cognitive ability to report sound quality. The current recommendations are that the middle ear implant is only for adults. Further, the person needs to have normal middle ear function given that the ossicles are required to drive the sound to the cochlea. See Table 7–3 for the criteria.

Initial Appointments

Similar to cochlear implant activation, the appointment of the initial activation is often filled with anxiety for the patient and family. The device is activated and the patient can immediately "hear." Currently, there is not a way to verify that the device is providing adequate amplification to ensure audibility; therefore, testing is completed to determine if the device is working appropriately.

In situ measurements are first completed to determine audiometric thresholds with the device activated. By "in situ" we mean that an audiogram is completed using the device. Sounds are presented through the implant and thresholds are recorded. The

Table 7–3. Candidacy Criteria for Middle Ear Implants	
	Qualification
Age	Adult with cognitive ability necessary for accurate self-report
Audiometric	Significant sensorineural hearing loss that impacts daily communication ability; likely in the moderate range
Device Use	Likely will have had some previous amplification history, but not required
Medical	No medical or radiological contraindications to surgery; normal middle ear status
Support	Motivated patient with appropriately set expectations
Testing	Typical audiometric testing

patient is asked to report sound quality and programming is completed accordingly. After these measurements are completed, audiologists often then complete functional gain testing. This is completed by putting the patient in a sound-treated booth and measuring thresholds and speech reception. Given the location of the implant, the testing may be completed through sound field or via headphones/inserts. As described in Chapter 6, this testing is conducted unaided and then again aided (device activated). The difference between the two is termed "functional gain." It should be noted that functional gain testing is not completed as part of typical hearing aid fitting protocols given its poor test–retest reliability; however, in the context of middle ear implants, it is one of the few ways to ensure that the device is functioning, as ear canal probe-microphone measures are not possible. In some cases, the audiologist would only do the "aided" sound field, which does not provide gain per se, but offers an insight regarding audibility of soft speech in the real world.

Counseling to set appropriate expectations is also important for patients with a middle ear implant. It is imperative that the person with the middle ear implant be able to tell the audiologist any changes or differences in hearing ability with the device. No matter how you are providing the sound, a person with a sensorineural hearing loss has a damaged cochlea. Unlike a cochlear implant, middle ear implant surgery has not changed the function of the cochlea. A person with sensorineural hearing loss still has significant distortion of speech and speech perception may still be impaired; like with any implant, ensuring appropriate expectations of the patient and family are critical to success with the device. We believe that all patients considering a middle ear implant first have an extended trial with traditional

amplification, so that they are making a well-informed decision.

Bone Conduction Devices

Taking the bone transduction information described in Chapter 2, the transmission of sound through bone conduction has been studied since the 1500s. The first reports of hearing through the bones can be found in anatomical reports of Vesalius, Fallopius, and Eustachius' physiological studies of the mid- to late 1500s. In 1550, Cardano reported a method of hearing through one's teeth by holding a rod or a spear next to the teeth; however, the discovery has also been attributed to Ingrassia and his mentor Vesalius, the discoverer of the stapes. In the mid-1600s, Cablei and Vulwer were the first to use bone conduction technology to treat hearing loss. A rod was placed between the teeth of the speaker and the teeth of the listener with hearing loss to transmit sounds. These discoveries and inventions were used as a foundation for modern hearing testing and modern bone conduction hearing devices.

The current type of bone conduction device was first implanted in 1977 by Anders Tjellstrom in Sweden. Similar to the process utilized today, a 4-mm screw was inserted into the bone behind the ear and a device was attached to transmit the sound via bone conduction. This screw integrated into the bone via osseointegration. Osseointegration is when the bone tissue actually integrates with titanium, creating direct contact between the living bone and the implant— making them a single unit.

Originally called bone anchored hearing aids or by the acronym BAHA, the trend has moved away from calling bone conduction devices this for several reasons. First, the

DID YOU KNOW: SoundBites and Molar Mic

As you might have noticed in our introduction to this section, we mentioned some of the work in this area from centuries ago, where scientists dabbled with using the teeth to transfer sound to the cochlea. Why not have a hearing aid fitted to the teeth you might ask? A somewhat bizarre idea, but—guess what—such a hearing aid existed as recently as 5 years ago. The name of the product was "SoundBite," and yes, there were a few of them sold (advertised for single-sided deafness patients). The company abruptly filed for bankruptcy in January 2015, and we are not aware of anyone picking up the product—much to the dismay of the people owning this device who need repairs. An interesting offshoot, however, from Sonitus, the manufacturer of the defunct SoundBite, is a new product that has been dubbed "Molar Mic" in research trials. According to Sonitus, Molar Mic creates a unique wireless audio interface by embedding both a tiny microphone for talking and a speaker transducer for hearing in a compact, custom-fit mouthpiece that snaps comfortably around a user's back teeth. This allows the user to both talk and hear without external devices attached to the head. Its unique application is for military and rescue operations when communication is difficult.

use of the term "hearing aid" makes insurance billing complicated. Second, the Baha is a registered trademark name for the bone conduction device by one specific manufacturer of the device. That is, the once acronym has turned into a name of a product. Third, a bone conduction device does not have to be anchored to the ear, it could be just be placed on the mastoid for transmission.

Current bone conduction devices consist of a microphone, processor, and transmitter that uses force for transmission. The microphone picks up the acoustic sound, the processor makes changes to the digitized signal, and the sound is transmitted through the mastoid bone through force. The force transmission vibrates the mastoid bone and therefore the basilar membrane inside both cochlea in a method similar to the stapes movement in traditional hearing. As we discussed in Chapter 2, there is little energy lost between ears when the mastoid/skull is set into vibration. Meaning, if the signal is generated on the right mastoid, the vibrations at the left cochlea will be nearly as great as those of the right cochlea. An example of a bone conduction device is shown in Figure 7–6.

In the early days of implantable bone conduction hearing aids, the target patient was one with a significant middle ear condition, but with relatively normal hearing via bone conduction. In some cases, these patients also had draining or infected ears, which further contraindicated the use of traditional hearing aids. The implantable bone conduction device was a reasonable solution. For people with a conductive hearing loss either due to chronic ear disease, middle ear disease, or external ear canal problems, the bone conduction device bypasses the disorder portion of the ear and directly stimulates the normal hearing cochlea.

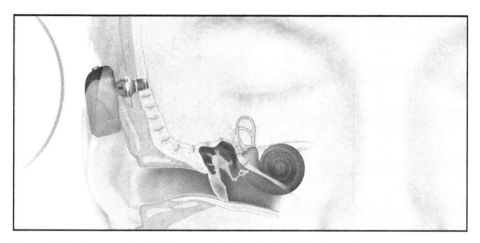

Figure 7–6. An example of a bone conduction device. This device is connected to a titanium screw on the head or a headband worn by the patient. *Source*: Courtesy of Cochlear Americas.

Today, these bone conduction hearing devices also are often recommended for people with unilateral hearing loss (only hearing loss on one side). For this hearing loss population, it is recommended that they are implanted on the "dead" side and the sound is transmitted to the normal hearing ear via the bone vibration. Given that the sound is being transmitted to the good ear, the person will still not be able to localize the sounds, but they will be able to more or less receive sounds equally from both sides in their good ear. Now, this should sound very similar to CROS amplification using small BTE hearing aids or even smaller custom products, which we discussed in Chapter 4 It is. The results for the patient would be similar, although probably better for the traditional hearing aids, as they tend to have more features. So, you have the choice of wearing a couple small hearing aids, or having something implanted into the side of your head. Unfortunately, in some centers, patients with unilateral deafness never are given a trial with traditional CROS before undergoing surgery for a bone conduction device.

There are three primary types of bone conduction devices available on the market:

- Headband devices use pressure to hold the bone transducer via a headband. The devices are clipped to the headband and the sound is transmitted via pressure. It is important that the device be tight enough to transmit the sound appropriately. This is most commonly used for trials and with children.
- Similar to the original device implanted in 1977, a second option is a titanium post placed into the mastoid bone behind the cochlea. The external processor is then attached to the post for transmission to the cochlea. See Figure 7–7 for an example of a titanium post that would be placed in the mastoid bone.
- Finally, a newer method has recently been approved by the FDA using magnetic transmission. Similar to a cochlear implant, a magnet is placed under the skin in the mastoid bone. The force is transmitted across the skin

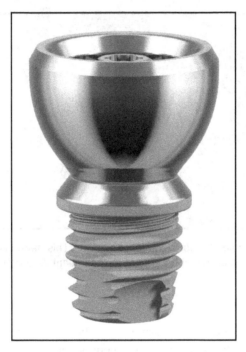

Figure 7–7. One type of titanium post placed into the mastoid bone by a surgeon. This will then be connected to an external device. The external device will vibrate this post to transfer sound to the cochlea. *Source*: Courtesy of Cochlear Americas.

KEY CONCEPT: Bone Conducted Sound Is for Fun Too!

As we mentioned, sending sound to the cochlea via bone conduction can be quite efficient. Bone conduction devices can be used as headphones even for normal hearing individuals. People report loving being able to hear their music and the word around them—they can even use them while swimming. Some early athletes who enjoy running at 4:30 in the morning (looking at Lindsey's father) have daughters who worry about them running in the dark when car traffic cannot see them. Bone conduction headphones may allow the runner to hear their music but also hear any surrounding sounds—like car horns. Some of you older readers might remember the Bone Fone. This device, introduced in 1979, was a wearable radio that draped around the user's neck like a scarf, and as the name indicates, transferred sound via bone conduction. It weighed about a pound, and the "scarf" was made of Lycra. The Bone Fone did not survive too many years, but the device represented an evolutionary step from handheld electronics to wearable hands-free technology for listening to music.

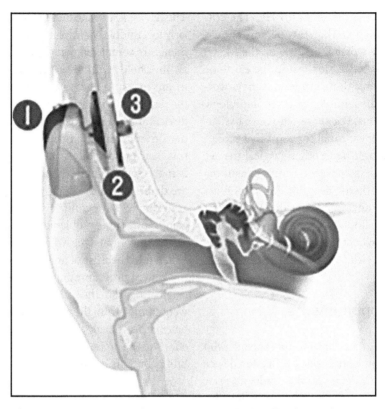

Figure 7–8. A magnetic bone conduction device. The internal component is placed by a surgeon. The external microphone and processor is attached to the internal component via magnetic force across the skin. *Source*: Courtesy of Cochlear Americas.

between the external processor and the internal osseointegrated magnet for transmission via bone conduction to the cochlea. See Figure 7–8 for an example.

Candidacy

The U.S. FDA regulations state that implanted bone conduction devices are for adults and children over the age of 5. The age restriction for children is due to maturity of bone and growth of the head and middle ear. Prior to age 5, children may use the bone conduction device on a band. Devices are approved for

persons with conductive or mixed hearing loss with air conduction thresholds greater than 45 dB HL and those with a difference between air conduction and bone conduction thresholds of 30 dB HL. Studies have suggested that those with at least this degree of difference will benefit more from a bone conduction device than a traditional hearing aid (Mylanus, van der Pow, & Cremers, 1998). Additionally, as we mentioned, patients with a profound unilateral sensorineural hearing loss with normal hearing in the opposite ear, also known as single-sided deafness, are candidates for the device. However, the better hearing ear should have thresholds better than 20 dB HL. The criteria also suggest that the person should have a score worse than 60% on the MSTB CNC word recognition test in the ear to be implanted, but these guidelines may be overridden by the audiologist given audiologic considerations. For those who have ossicular disease or ear canal concerns that cannot be corrected through other surgical means, nerve disorders such as an acoustic neuroma that makes them ineligible for a cochlear implant, or other infections, the audiometric thresholds should be considered, but the percent correct of the implanted ear may be overlooked. Criteria are listed in Table 7–4.

Initial Appointments

Unlike with other implants, most people who receive an implanted bone conduction device have worn the device on the headband prior to implantation, so they have a better idea as to what to expect from the initial sound quality. The device is attached to the post or magnet. The magnet strength is adjusted to ensure that the device stays in place, but is not too tight, as that may cause skin breakdown.

The device is activated and programed similarly to a middle ear implant. In situ measurements are completed to determine audiometric thresholds with the device attached. This means than an audiogram is completed using the device. Sounds are presented through the device and thresholds are recorded. If the person was implanted because of a conductive hearing loss, all the device needs to do is make sounds louder; once the thresholds are determined, the device is programmed accordingly. Some clinics also complete aided gain testing (note problematic issues we have already mentioned regarding this procedure). When fitted because of unilateral hearing loss, the goal of programming is to make sounds originating from the bad side sound as if they were coming from the front of the user (eliminate the head shadow effect). There have been efforts to use probe-mic measures to verify the fitting, but this is rarely done.

Implants Beyond Activation

Like fitting traditional hearing aids, the job isn't finished on the day the product is fit. In

Table 7–4. Candidacy Criteria for Bone Conduction Devices	
	Qualification
Age	Soft band: any age; implanted device: over the age of 5
Audiometric	Single-sided deafness or conductive/mixed hearing loss where traditional aids or surgery will not correct
Device Use	Likely will have had some previous amplification history, but not required
Medical	No medical or radiological contraindications to surgery if receiving surgical implantation
Support	Motivated patient with appropriately set expectations
Testing	Typical audiometric testing; >60% correct on implanted ear unless other medical concerns dictate implantation

some cases, it's just starting. It's possible that you also will see some implant patients who are struggling for one reason or another. We present here some common issues to consider.

Ensuring Implant Function

Like any medical/mechanical device, problems sometimes occur. The audiologist is responsible to ensure that the device is functioning to the best level for the patient through appropriate and best practices programming. They will see the patient on a regular basis, however, the devices may have problems in the interim between appointments.

What the Audiologist Does

Given that many people with an implant have minimal hearing ability without the device, a rapid response is necessary when a device is not functioning. For those with cochlear implants or bone conduction devices, it is possible for the patient to contact the manufacturer of the device and they will send a replacement device. The audiologist provides the programming (mapping) to the manufacturer and a device is mailed to the patient. The turnaround for providing the devices is quite rapid and the manufacturer will require the patient to return their nonfunctional device. For those with middle ear implants, any disruption in function requires an appointment with the audiologist and testing to determine the cause of problem.

Day to Day

Day-to-day function should be verified by the patient or the caregiver. The patient should verify that all sounds have been heard. If necessary, all cochlear implant devices allow for headphones to be plugged into the device to ensure that the micro-

phones are functioning. It should be noted, that listening to the device through headphones only ensures that the microphones are working and not that the sound is being transmitted appropriately. There are devices on the market that can be used to ensure that the internal device is receiving a signal, but this does not inform the user as to the full function of the implant. For bone conduction devices, a device may be connected to a bone conductor, like a bite block, and the caregiver or teacher may listen to the device to ensure function. There is not currently a mechanism for an external person to listen to a middle ear implanted device. Batteries in a cochlear implant and bone conduction device should be changed or charged on a regular/daily basis.

It should be noted the importance of ensuring function of the device in the pediatric patient prior to the educational school day or prior to any therapy. One quick method to check this is to determine if the patient is able to accurately report sounds. We recommend using the Ling 6 (ahh, ooh, eee, sh, s, m; see Figure 8–23). They should be presented without visual cues. These sounds are used because they represent the entire English speech spectrum. The lack of function can lead to reduced speech production or speech-language skills over time. Further, any lack of hearing ability may impact the educational performance in children as well as negate any speech-language therapy services that are being provided. By quickly checking the device at the beginning of the school day and/or therapy sessions, clinicians and educators can ensure that the child is receiving access to the auditory information provided.

Outcomes

The goal of postsurgical rehabilitation for patients with an implant is to maximize their oral communication ability if this is the mode of communication desired by the patient/family. If the desired primary communication is not oral, different rehabilitation strategies can be adopted. There are different rehabilitation strategies that can/should be implemented depending on the device; these will be discussed in other parts of this book, particularly in Chapter 10.

Outcomes assessments can help provide documentation of benefit derived from use of an implant, help identify problems, as well as determine the need for any additional referrals. Therefore, outcomes assessments should be performed at regular intervals. These assessments may be performed by an audiologist, however, there are many instances where assessments by speech-language pathologists may be of great benefit to the individual with hearing loss.

Overview of Current Speech Perception and Language Outcomes

Outcomes for people with implants vary based on several factors. These factors include but are not limited to:

- Length of time with hearing loss
- Use of system that allowed for stimulation of auditory pathway prior to implantation
- Cause of hearing loss
- Age at which hearing loss occurred
- Numerous implantation factors
- Status of the cochlea
- Amount of residual hearing
- Additional disabilities/diagnoses
- Family/personal motivation
- Appropriateness of programming/mapping
- Consistency of follow-up appointments

- Socioeconomic factors
- Education of the patient and/or parents

In children, there are several factors that may significantly influence the outcomes and speech perception ability of children with cochlear implants.

- Age at implantation: In studies of children aged 3 to 5 years of age (Ching et al., 2013), those who were implanted earlier did significantly better; specifically, those who were implanted prior to 12 months do significantly better than those who are delayed being implanted. Further, they reported that a delay in implantation of 6 to 12 months resulted in a half standard deviation decrease in language ability.
- Communication mode: This is specifically the communication mode used by the caregivers. Those whose family communicated through auditory listening and spoken language have better outcomes than those whose family uses sign language.
- Education ability of the mother: Yes, mom matters! Those children who had higher maternal education reported better language outcomes.
- Other disabilities: Those children for whom hearing loss is their only disability demonstrated better outcomes than those who had additional disabilities in addition to hearing loss. Children with neurocognitive had poorer language outcomes than children with other disabilities.
- Normal anatomy: Those with abnormal temporal bones had poorer outcomes than those with normal temporal

bone anatomy. Further, those with normal neural anatomy will have better outcomes than those who have abnormal anatomy.

In adults, speech performance obtained by postlingually deafened adults far exceeds adults who are implanted prelingually. For those prelingually deafened adults who decide to pursue cochlear implant, additional rehabilitation will need to be pursued so they can best utilize the information that they are receiving. For children, a variety of factors will impact outcomes of implanted devices; however, family and education support and time investment are the best predictors of outcomes. Further discussion on habilitation and rehabilitation will be investigated in upcoming chapters.

In Closing

It was not that long ago that implantable devices were considered "experimental" or for special cases only. Today, it's not uncommon to see someone wearing an implantable device at the grocery store or the neighborhood restaurant. This of course is partly due to the advancement of the technology, which then in turn has expanded candidacy. While working as a speech-language pathologist, you won't be directly involved in the fitting of these devices; yet, it's very probable that you will have patients wearing them, both children and adults. We hope that we have provided you with some background that will be useful when working with these patients.

8 Hearing Assistive Technologies and Classroom Considerations

Individuals with hearing loss experience a greater difficulty understanding speech in the presence of competing noise; this difficulty is exacerbated for children when compared to adults. In addition, because of the more randomness of their lifestyle, children with hearing loss may experience the signal of interest originating from one meter or more away, and not always in the direction that they are facing. In order to optimize listening situations, hearing assistive technologies will be of great use.

Hearing assistive technologies are devices that can help individuals with hearing loss function better in day-to-day situations, especially for communication and environmental awareness. They can also be used with individuals who have normal hearing sensitivity, who might have auditory processing difficulties, language deficits, learning disabilities, or attention deficits. An individual who has hearing loss can use these devices with or without cochlear implants or hearing aids. Hearing assistive technologies are beneficial when completing therapy sessions with young children and adults as these systems will allow the signal of interest to be more direct and effective.

Things That Impact Speech Perception

There are several things that can significantly impact speech and would necessitate the need for a form of assistive technology. Some of these factors may be overcome with hearing aids and cochlear implants while others need assistive technology; for most of these, any detriment to speech will be compounded by noise and therefore assistive technologies will need to be used to improve speech understanding.

- Audibility
- Availability of visual cues
- Talker specific characteristics
- Reverberation
- Signal-to-noise ratio
- Distance

Audibility

Arguably, the most important thing for understanding speech is to ensure that the signal is audible. In Chapter 6, we discussed the importance of hearing aid verification. One of the key components of probe-microphone real-ear testing is to ensure that audibility has been optimized. Once the device is verified, and audibility is confirmed, it is assumed that the person will be able to hear soft sounds adequately. However, these tests are conducted in quiet. Once noise is introduced into the environment, audibility will decrease. Noise decreases understanding by masking audible speech cues. A person may then need to rely on assistive technology to improve their audibility for the speaker in the presence of background noise. Moreover, in cases where the hearing loss is more severe, it might not be possible to restore audibility for soft sounds effectively using only the hearing aids.

Availability of Visual Cues

Many studies have been conducted to determine the effectiveness of directional microphones and other hearing aid features. In the laboratory, these features have been shown to be somewhat effective; however, in field studies, these features have significantly reduced benefit. Why is this? One real-world factor is visual cues. Specifically, in most noisy situations where hearing aid features can be activated to improve intelligibility, visual cues are most always available. By utilizing visual cues, the level of a listener's speech recognition performance can increase substantially. Now, imagine you have a child in a noisy lunchroom. The child is sitting across the table from the person they are speaking with. They will get much more information from the visual cues of the speaker than their hearing aid can give them. In fact, the impact of visual cues is not additive but multiplicative. If only 40% of the cues are audible and 20% of the cues

are visual, a person may understand upwards of 90% of the signal. Several researchers have attempted to quantify the impact of visual cues in conjunction with hearing aid features. They found that hearing aid features increased the person's ability by about 10%, while the use of auditory-visual cues increased the perception by more than 20%. As an SLP, ensuring that the student has access to the visual cues by preferential seating and good self-advocacy may improve a student's overall performance.

Lighting may also have an impact on availability of visual cues and the performance of speechreading. In clinical practice, several practical suggestions to facilitate speech performance are based on findings from Erber (1974). For example, the listener and talker may be made aware of the need for appropriate lighting conditions and to arrange for high contrast between the intensity of light on the face of the talker against low background light levels. More recently, similar considerations regarding contrast luminance at the talker's face have been addressed. Another consideration for the listener is that moving from one area to another in which there is a large increase or decrease in light intensity may require short intervals for some visual adaption to occur; however, after adapting, the level of lighting does not appear to be a critical factor given that there is now enough light to see the talker's face. The optimum separation between the speaker and listener is approximately five feet. The synergistic characteristics of background noise or the competition of other people talking coupled with reverberation will obviously degrade the quality of the signal; this will further affect speech reading performance, requiring the listener to rely on visual cues to a greater extent than auditory cues. As an SLP, you may suggest that a teacher not turn off the lights when they are speaking. They may not be aware of the importance of visual cues and the additive affect it has. Your knowledge of spoken communication can influence all children, but even more so those with hearing loss in their ability to use visual cues to enhance auditory perception.

Talker-Specific Characteristics

Numerous reports on talker variability appear in the literature on auditory language processing. One source of variability in auditory speech perception occurs for iterations produced by the same speaker and is associated with a magnitude of 10% of test–retest reliability in speech intelligibility. Talk-specific characteristics, such as physical details about a talker's face and observable patterns of articulation, have also been shown to affect memory for spoken words. There are some suggestions that appearance of facial features (e.g., prominence of lip vermillion, lip thickness, facial hair) may influence the ability to understand the speaker. Additional sources of variance within and across talkers include differences in regional accents or social variation that affect speech sound production and coarticulation, as well as differences in anatomical structures. Consequently, some speakers are easier to understand than others. There is also some evidence that female talkers may produce more visual speech gestures than males, but this gender difference may not generalize to audiovisual speechreading conditions.

Several investigators have used paradigms to elicit different speaking styles to address the impact of speech rate on intelligibility. The majority of the speech tests used in audiology are recorded and "read" speech. Read speech is significantly slower, has less coarticulation, and pauses at word boundaries. This makes the speech more intelligible. As the rate of speech increases, the understandability decreases. On the other hand, when in conversation, speech is often much faster, coarticulated, and less intelligible particularly for those with hearing loss. Figure 8–1 demonstrates this trend. This figure is from a study by Van Engen, Chandrasekaran, and Smiljanic (2012) that compared clear speech to conversational speech. The panels on the left are conversational speech, while the ones on the right are clear speech; the top panel is a meaningful sentence, while the bottom is not. They reported that the clear sentences had higher mean F0s and larger F0 ranges. In the meaningful sentences, furthermore, clear speech was characterized by significantly greater energy in the 1 kHz to 3 kHz range. They also reported a significantly better understanding of the clear speech than the conversational particularly for the sentence that was not meaningful as the participants could not use contextual cues to determine the meaning. "Clear speech" has widespread clinical relevance; however, there is disagreement in the literature as to how to best elicit a clear-speech-speaking style. Clear speech is preferred, but likely conversational speech is used in daily conversation and teaching settings. As an SLP, you may need to assist teachers and other communication partners about the importance of slowed speech. As speech rate increases and speech cues become less prominent, the need for assistive technology may increase.

Reverberation

Another aspect of classroom acoustics that needs to be considered is reverberation. Reverberation is the interpretation of the persistence of sound after it is produced. This occurs because the sound is being reflected off of surfaces in the room, which causes

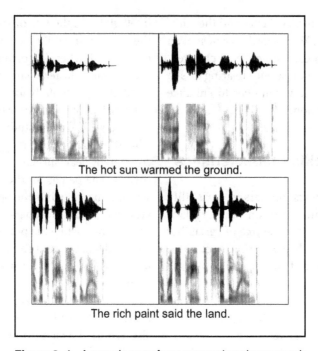

The hot sun warmed the ground.

The rich paint said the land.

Figure 8–1. A sample waveform comparing clear speech (left panel) with conversational speech (right panel) in a contextual sentence (top panel) and noncontextual sentence (bottom panel). *Source*: From "Effects of speech clarity on recognition memory for spoken sentences," by K. J. Van Engen, B. Chandrasekaran, and R. Smiljanic, 2012, *PloS one*, *7*(9), e43753.

temporal smearing of the speech waveform (Figure 8–2). As a result, reverberation tends to produce a prolongation of the spectral energy of vowel phonemes, which reduces consonant recognition. This can have a significant effect on speech recognition because as you know, a vast majority of acoustic information important for speech recognition is provided by consonants. Reverberation is more prevalent in rooms that have hard ceilings without acoustical tiles, ceilings taller than 10 feet, hard flooring, or lack of sound absorbing materials. The effect is a little different from noise, however, because this masking is occurring because echoes from early portions of speech act to mask later portions (overlap masking) or echoes from a speech segment act to mask the same speech segment (speech self-masking). In consequence, shorter reverberation times or early reflection mainly fill in the gaps in speech. Filling in the gaps makes speech more unintelligible. This has the most impact at about six feet from the speaker (Figure 8–3). As an SLP, the impact of reverberation is important for you to know because all children are impacted by reverberation, but particularly those with hearing loss. Hearing aids can actually compound the issues of reverberation due to signal processing and changes in the signal due to hearing aids. So as the SLP, if you have a child with hearing loss, you may suggest that they sit

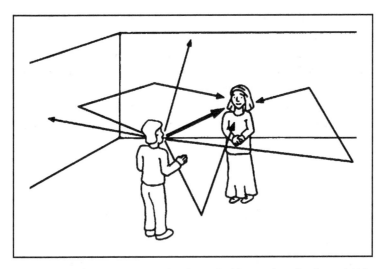

Figure 8–2. A presentation of a direct (bold arrow) and reflected (thin arrows) sound pathways, produced by a talker (illustrated by Wilder Boule). *Source*: From *Essentials of Modern Hearing Aids: Selection, Fitting, and Verification* (p. 92), by T. A. Ricketts, R. Bentler, and H. G. Mueller, 2019, San Diego, CA: Plural Publishing. Reprinted with permission.

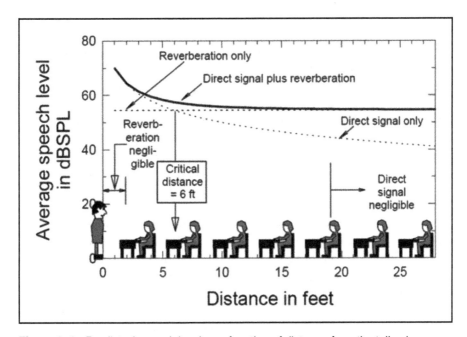

Figure 8–3. Predicted speech level as a function of distance from the talker in a room 3 feet x 20 feet x 9 feet with a reverberation time of 500 ms. *Source*: From *Essentials of Modern Hearing Aids: Selection, Fitting, and Verification* (p. 92), T. A. Ricketts, R. Bentler, and H. G. Mueller, 2019, San Diego, CA: Plural Publishing. Reprinted with permission.

in a specific seat so as to be less impacted by reverberation. You may assist the audiologist in justifying the purchase and encouraging use of a remote microphone system (discussed later on in this chapter) to decrease the impact of reverberation on speech perception in the classroom.

Signal-to-Noise Ratio

These systems provide better access to communication in difficult listening environments as they provide an enhanced signal-to-noise ratio. The signal-to-noise ratio is the relationship between noise and the

---

KEY CONCEPT: Some Points on Reverberation

For the most part, we have been talking about speech signals delivered in ideal surroundings. We know, however, that our hearing aid patients will be out in reverberant conditions. In fact, it often is the poor understanding of speech in these difficult conditions that prompts the patient to obtain hearing aids. How does reverberation impact the speech signal?

■ One of the most common measures of a room's effect on sound propagation is reverberation time. Commonly, reverberation time is defined as the time required for a signal to decrease in level by 60 dB after its offset (ANSI S1.1-1994).

■ Reverberation occurs because sound generated from any source inside a room will be reflected (bounced) off room surfaces. Due to these reflections, there will be multiple angles of arrival for sound energy other than the angle of origin. That is, there will be a direct sound pathway (D) and several reflected sound pathways (R), which in combination are referred to as the reflective or reverberant sound field (see Figure 8–2).

■ There are usually many more reflected sound pathways than shown here, and some sound pathways may never reach the listener before they decay away (become so low level they are not heard).

■ As the distance from the sound source increases, the level of the direct sound will decrease. According to the inverse square law, every doubling of distance will halve the intensity. In contrast, the reverberant sound level remains approximately constant (although this changes with proximity to reflective surfaces—for e.g., the reverberant level might go up near a wall). In consequence, as a sound source and a listener are separated in space, there is an increase in the reverberant to direct sound ratio. The distance at which the level of the direct signal is equal to that of the reverberant signal is referred to as the critical distance (Egan, 1988; Peutz, 1971). An example demonstrating direct sound, reverberant sound, and a combination of the two as a function of distance is shown in Figure 8–3.

primary signal, such as the speaker's voice. Noise is considered to be anything that conflicts with the auditory signal an individual is trying to attend to. Noise could be many different environmental sounds such as refrigerator noise, an air conditioning unit, background speakers, or wind. The quieter and farther away the noise is from the intended signal, the more audible that intended auditory signal will be. Noise tends to mask the weaker consonant phonemes at a significantly higher rate than more intense vowel phonemes. Individuals of all ages benefit from an improved signal-to-noise ratio; however, children need a much higher (better) signal-to-noise ratio when compared to adults due to decreased neurological maturity and lack of communication experience. As the SLP, you may be more aware of the impact of noise on a child's performance. You may be able to suggest individual learning or recommend that the student see an audiologist to determine if they could use a remote microphone. Recall that in Chapter 6 we discussed speech tests that are scored in SNR. For example, if a child has a test such as the BKB-SIN (similar to the QuickSIN, but more appropriate for children), and his or her score is an SNR = 16 dB, this sends a strong message regarding potential success (or lack of it) in the classroom. This score means that the primary speech signal needed to be 16 dB above the background noise for the child to understand 50% of the words. Most classrooms do not have an SNR this favorable, and we easily can predict that this child will have problems.

Distance

Hearing assistive technologies can also help overcome difficulties caused by distance. The farther away someone is from a sound source, the more difficulty that person will have when trying to understand what is being said. This occurs because there is a loss of high frequency consonant information. In addition, distance decreases the amplitude level of speech. In theory, direct sound pressure decreases by 6 dB for every doubling of distance from the sound source. This is known as the inverse square law. For example, in theory, if the teacher's voice is 65 dB SPL for the student sitting in the front row (5 feet from the teacher), it will be 59 dB SPL for the student 5 feet farther back, and only 53 dB SPL for the student in the back, 15 feet from the teacher.

Due to the fact that there is decreasing sound intensity with distance and that some frequencies will be absorbed more than others by absorptive elements in the room (i.e., acoustical tiles, people, etc.), the reflected sound that reaches the listener will have a different acoustic signature in the intensity, frequency, and temporal domains. Hearing assistive technologies are extremely beneficial in overcoming these difficulties whether an individual has normal hearing sensitivity or hearing loss. Although speech-language pathologists are not able to prescribe the use of these devices, it is critical that you understand how they function as some of your clients may utilize these them.

Remote Microphones

The more basic approach of placing the microphone and sound source in close proximity is by far the most effective, if the goal is enhancement of signal-to-noise ratio for a single talker. We will generally refer to these technologies as "remote microphones" since the microphone is placed a distance away from the hearing aid wearer. A hardwire remote microphone was used by listeners with hearing impairment more than a century ago, but less cumbersome wireless techniques have been used for many decades. These microphones allow for better speech understanding over a greater distance, as they are much less susceptible to interference from reverberation and other background noise between the speaker and the listener. Both digital and analog wireless microphones, including "FM systems," have been shown to significantly improve signal-to-noise ratio by as much as 16 dB to 20 dB in noisy environments; however, several studies over the last few decades have demonstrated that the magnitude of signal-to-noise ratio advantage greatly depends on the specific configuration (e.g., mix ratio, use of fixed vs. dynamic microphone gain, directivity of the microphone, etc.) and may be as little as 4 dB to 5 dB for some situations.

When wireless microphones are used without activation of the hearing aid microphones, the signal-to-noise ratio at the ear is determined primarily by the signal-to-noise ratio at the location of the remote microphone. In other words, signal-to-noise ratio is optimized by placing the remote microphone in close proximity to the talker's mouth and/or using microphone array technologies to improve directivity. In contrast, when both the wireless microphone and the hearing aid microphones are activated at the same time (as is typical), signal-to-noise ratio is determined by the highest level of the speech (e.g., location of the remote microphone) and the highest level of noise, which can be either at the location of the remote microphone or the HA microphone (e.g., Norrix, Camarota, Harris, & Dean, 2016). As a result, benefit from a wireless microphone when the listener is surrounded by noise will be greatly reduced by activating the hearing aid microphones, even if the signal-to-noise ratio at the remote microphone is very good. Because of these trade-offs, the optimal configuration for a remote microphone is a balance for each individual patient between:

- The amount of difficulty communicating in noise—how much help do they need?
- The need, desire, and ability to monitor sounds other than the primary talker (which might differ from time to time, location to location).

The function of a remote microphone is similar to the function of a hearing aid. The microphone picks up the speaker's voice and then converts acoustical energy to electrical energy, which is converted to a digital signal. The digital signal is then transmitted to the hearing assistive device or personal receiver. The purpose of the device is to improve signal-to-noise ratio and also decrease the acoustic distance between the speaker and the receiver. In Figures 8–4 and 8–5, you can see that without the remote microphone, the signal becomes weaker as we move further away from the speaker. With a remote microphone system, the signal stays a consistent strength despite increased distance.

As mentioned previously, remote microphone systems can improve the signal-to-noise ratio by up to 20 dB; however, most systems are set so that the listener also hears through the microphones of their hearing device along with the transmission of the remote microphone system. The audiologist can set the ratio of remote microphone transmission signal to microphone signal. These can be equal, meaning that the sounds from the microphone are amplified to the same degree as the remote microphone signal; they may also give an advantage to the remote microphone system, meaning that the signal from the remote microphone is louder than the signal coming from the microphones. Depending on the age of the child and cognitive ability, remote microphones

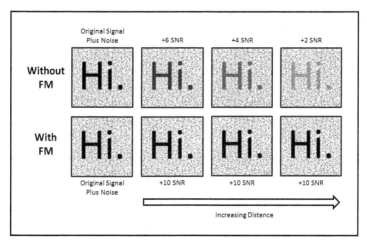

Figure 8–4. How FM systems provide improved signal-to-noise ratio. In each box is a gray shaded area to present background noise. The word 'Hi" represents the speech signal of interest. In the top panel from left to right, you can see the effect of increasing distance on the clarity of the word "Hi." The bottom panel would be an example of the use of the remote microphone system. Despite increasing distance, the signal does not decrease in boldness. *Source*: From *Hearing Assistive and Access Technology* (p. 100), by S. R. Atcherson, C. A. Franklin, and L. Smith-Olinde, 2015, San Diego, CA: Plural Publishing. Reprinted with permission.

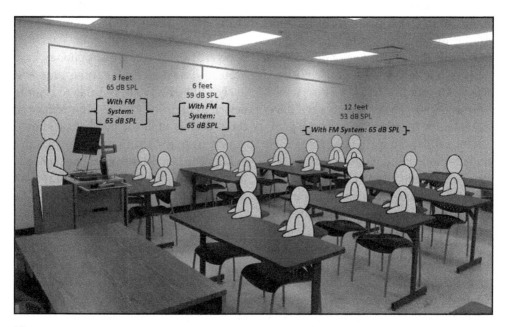

Figure 8–5. The loss of sound energy as a function of distance without a remote microphone system. With a remote microphone system, the speech signal is maintained at a constant level (65 dB in this case) such that the students in the back row can have the same access as the students in the front row. *Source*: From *Hearing Assistive and Access Technology* (p. 101), by S. R. Atcherson, C. A. Franklin, and L. Smith-Olinde, 2015, San Diego, CA: Plural Publishing. Reprinted with permission.

> ### DID YOU KNOW: The Vagabond from the 1950s
>
> While today, we rely on wireless microphones for our hearing-impaired patients, but not surprisingly, this technology initially was introduced for the entertainment industry. The first practical wireless microphone for performers was the Shure Vagabond 88, which was introduced in the 1950's. Interestingly, it was powered by two hearing aid batteries. It could transmit within a performance circle of approximately 700 square feet. It operated in the 2 MHz FM band, weighed one pound, and was 1.4 inches in diameter and 12 inches in length. It had five subminiature vacuum tubes and worked for 25 to 30 hours on its batteries. According to promotional material, the name Vagabond was chosen because "it is a microphone that makes the entertainer foot-loose and fancy-free."

can be set to allow for different ratios, this will be discussed further in Chapter 9.

There are, however, a few disadvantages of remote microphones. One of the most obvious disadvantages is that they require an external device that must be worn by a talker. While this is not a problem in and of itself for some hearing aid wearers, most express concerns about cosmetics and drawing unwanted attention to their hearing loss. Another disadvantage related to the use of the remote microphone is that benefits are typically limited to conversing with a single talker of interest. Remote microphones may not be optimal when listening to multiple talkers or when "overhearing" other conversations is the listening goal. As we described, combining the input from the remote microphone placed near the speaker of interest with the input from an "environmental microphone" placed near the listener (e.g., activating the hearing aid microphones) has long been advocated to overcome this problem. However, data have shown that this combination provides an improvement in signal-to-noise ratio that is far smaller, resulting in limited benefit in noise from this configuration (Lewis, Crandell, Valente, & Horn, 2004). Multichannel remote microphones allowing for automatic switching between two or more microphones have been in development for some time and likely will be routinely available to hearing device wearers very soon. However, even these devices limit the number of sources of interest to less than perhaps four to five talkers. Further, the listener cannot enhance the signal-to-noise for secondary sources of interest with a simple head turn.

There are numerous methods of transmitting the signal from the digital microphone to the listener. In most cases, the remote microphone is worn by the speaker and is transmitted to the listener's ears through their hearing aids, cochlear implant, or individual ear-level receivers. Some devices are able to directly transmit the signal to the hearing device, while others must use a receiver. We can divide the types of remote microphones into two categories: FM systems and proprietary wireless devices. With both of these, an antennae must be present within the hearing device to receive the signal from the remote microphone. This is commonly called a receiver.

Receivers

A receiver is an electronic device that receives signals wirelessly from a microphone transmitter. In some cases, like proprietary wireless devices (discussed later in the chapter), the receivers are built into the hearing aid or cochlear implant. This is because the remote microphone is made by the same manufacturer as the hearing technology. On the other hand, most schools prefer to use universal remote microphones. This is because they are able to use them between students once the student leaves the school or school district. In this case, a receiver needs to be added to the device so that the signal from the remote microphone may be received. There are several available receivers in current hearing aid and cochlear implant technology. We will discuss each of these individually.

- Integrated antennae in the hearing device
- Integrated into the hearing device
- Universal receiver
  - Connected by an audio boot/shoe that slips on and off the device
  - Connected by a port on the device
  - Connected via company-specific intermediary device
- Connected via device that converts the energy into electromagnetism so that the telecoil of the aid can pick up the signal

Integrated Antennae

As the name suggests, this receiver is integrated into the hearing device. In this case, the manufacturer has built in the receiver antenna and no additional equipment is needed. Given that the transmitters and transmitter signal are proprietary, integrated antennae are typically only available from hearing devices made by the same manufacturer as the remote microphone. In this scenario, when the hearing device is received from the manufacturer and programmed by the audiologist, the device is already able to receive the remote microphone signal. There are two possible methods of remote microphones, which we will discuss in depth later on in this chapter: proprietary wireless technology and frequency modulation transmission. In this case, if the signal is not being received by the device, the entire device must be sent in for repair.

Integrated Into the Hearing Device

With this receiver, it is typically a replacement of the battery door or other part of the hearing device that includes the antennae for reception. In this case, a receiver is added to the device after the device is purchased by the audiologist (Figure 8–6). The battery door is changed out for a longer one that includes the receiver. If the receiver is not working, the receiver can be removed and sent in for repair separately from the hearing device. In this case, if there is only one receiver, the person will only hear it in the ear where the receiver is placed. This is a significant disadvantage as, in nearly all cases, speech understanding is enhanced when it is delivered bilaterally. These are advantageous, however, because they stay

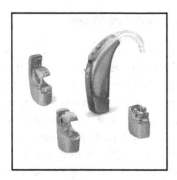

Figure 8–6. Example of integrated receiver. *Source*: Image © Sonova AG. Reproduced here with permission. All rights reserved.

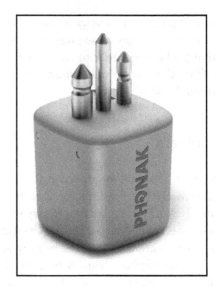

on the device permanently and the fewer times you have to take the device on and off, the less likelihood of damage.

Figure 8–7. Example of universal receiver. *Source*: Image © Sonova AG. Reproduced here with permission. All rights reserved.

Universal Receiver

A universal receiver (Figure 8–7) is typically preferred by schools because it can be transferred between students. This type of receiver is universal and can be paired with many devices. When you have a person with a hearing aid or cochlear implant, check with the audiologist to see what kind of connection is needed to make the universal receiver work. Keep in mind that if the channel of transmission is changed on the remote microphone, that the channel also needs to be changed on the receiver. For some receivers, they use Bluetooth technology and the receiver will need to be paired with the transmitter. There are several means by which the universal receiver can be connected to a hearing device.

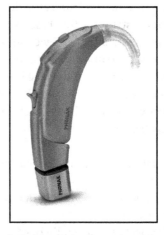

Figure 8–8. Example of a universal receiver, audioshoe, and then these both fit on a hearing aid. *Source*: Image © Sonova AG. Reproduced here with permission. All rights reserved.

Connected by an Audio Shoe/Boot That Slips On and Off of the Device. This shoe or boot slips over the bottom of the hearing device (Figure 8–8). This method of connection is sometimes preferred by schools as it could be used between students. The disadvantage of this is that, in most cases, the boot has to be removed every day which causes wear and tear. Additionally, it is only on one device and the person will only hear the signal through the ear in which it is attached.

Connected Via a Port on the Device. In some cases, there can be a port on the device that allows for the universal receiver to be attached directly to the device. In this case, as it is only attached to one ear and, thus, only one ear will be receiving the information. The advantage of this system is that it uses a universal receiver and connects directly into the hearing device. This means that there are fewer connections and, in theory, would result in less problems.

Connected Via a Company Specific Intermediary. There are several reasons that someone may choose to use a company-specific intermediary device to connect the receiver. One is that there might not be a method for the device to integrate or connect the universal receiver. The advantage is that there is one intermediary and it can go to two devices. In the case where someone uses bimodal technology, a hearing aid in one ear and a cochlear implant in another, this may be one method that both devices can receive the signal. In this case, the universal receiver is attached to the intermediary. The universal receiver receives the transmission from the remote microphone and transmits to the proprietary intermediary that converts the signal to one that can be received by the hearing devices directly (Figure 8–9). This intermediary's signal is proprietary and will only transmit to the specific devices made by the same manufacturer. The disadvantage of this type of device is that it can only be used by people with that device; on the other hand, many people with hearing devices have these intermediaries as they also can be used to connect to other devices like cellular phones.

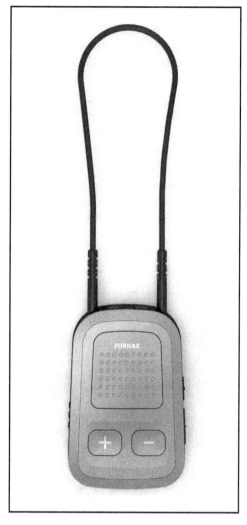

Figure 8–9. Example of a company-specific intermediary with a universal receiver plugged into the bottom. *Source*: Image © Sonova AG. Reproduced here with permission. All rights reserved.

Connected Via Electromagnet Device

This is a last resort for some people to be able to receive remote microphone transmission. In this case, a proprietary device is used to receive the signal from the remote microphone. The device then converts the signal into an electromagnetic signal to be picked up by the telecoil of the hearing device. The device may be worn around the neck, also called an induction neckloop (Figure 8–10, device labeled "E"), or it may fit behind the ear next to the hearing device, also called an induction silhouette (Figure 8–10, device labeled "D"). The reason that this is the last resort is that electromagnetic transmission has significant disadvantages when using it for remote microphones. The original intention of electromagnetic transmission is the telephone. Because of the frequency range of the telephone (300 to 3300 Hz), the electromagnetic transmission cuts off the high frequencies and these are not transmitted. Additionally, there is a lot of low-frequency noise in the transmission of electromagnetic signals. Finally, the person may report that they also pick up other magnetic noise from fluorescent lights in the classroom. Because of these disadvantages, many audiologists use this as a last resort to receive transmission from remote microphones. However, in some cases, this is the only available means of using a remote microphone.

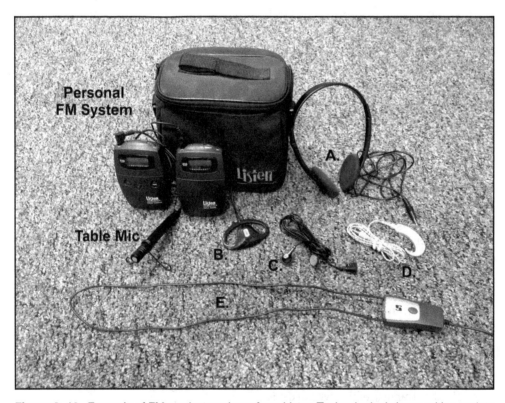

Figure 8–10. Example of FM product package from Listen Technologies' shown with a variety of coupling options. Coupling options are labeled A–E as the following: headphones, earphones, earbuds, induction silhouette (ear hook), and induction neckloop. Photo Credit: Samuel R. Atcherson, Ph.D. *Source*: From *Hearing Assistive and Access Technology* (p. 103), by S. R. Atcherson, C. A. Franklin, and L. Smith-Olinde, 2015, San Diego, CA: Plural Publishing. Reprinted with permission.

> **CLINICAL TIP: Do All Hearing Devices Connect to Remote Microphones?**
>
> Unfortunately, not all devices can connect to remote microphone technology. Particularly when fitting children, most audiologists pay attention to what devices are fit so the child has the opportunity to use remote microphones in school. The disadvantage is that for some devices, this makes the device slightly larger to allow for the connection ability or the antennae to be integrated. So, no, not all hearing devices can use a remote microphone. In some cases, a person may have to purchase new devices that can work with a remote microphone. In the pediatric population, if listed on the IEP, the school must provide the remote microphone system. But, they are not required to provide the hearing aids, and in most cases they do not.

Ear-Level Receivers

For individuals without hearing aids or implantable devices, a pair of headphones, earbuds, or ear-level devices will provide acoustic coupling and the user should be able to adjust the remote microphone volume to optimize listening. (See Figure 8–10, devices labeled "A," "B," and "C.") Ear-level receivers are appropriate for people with normal hearing who do not need hearing aids but struggle in noise and, therefore, would benefit from remote microphone technology (Figure 8–11). These devices are generally used for people with auditory processing disorder or those who have other learning disabilities like ADD or ADHD. In these cases, the ear remains open and the person can hear the sounds that are around them, but they hear the person who is wearing the remote microphone better even though they are at an increased distance.

It may not apparent, but it is important for you to understand the different coupling options with remote microphones. This is because as an SLP, you may be responsible to troubleshoot such devices. Having an under-

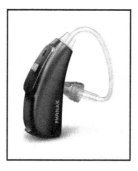

Figure 8–11. Example of an FM receiver that is not a device that also amplifies sound. *Source*: Image © Sonova AG. Reproduced here with permission. All rights reserved.

standing of how the remote microphone connects to the hearing device will help you with troubleshooting and instructing the person wearing the microphone on the use of the device.

Frequency-Modulated (FM) Systems

Although there are many forms of hearing assistive technologies, one of the most utilized is a frequency-modulated system, or FM system. Over the last 40 to 50 years, FM systems have made the most dramatic change. FM systems have commonly been used in the educational system for children with hearing loss. The teacher wears a microphone transmitter, and the student wears one of the previously discussed receivers. In the past, FM systems were also called *auditory trainers* when the student wore a single unit that served as both an FM system and hearing aid. Today, some of the most advanced FM systems are used not just in the classroom, but also in daily life. A person may use them in large lectures, at church, or at family gatherings. People report that any time that they are in noise and they need a better signal-to-noise ratio, they find themselves using an FM system.

An FM system utilizes electromagnetic radiation frequency bands for transmission of audio signals. The transmission of audio frequencies is modulated by a carrier frequency between the two spectral frequency regions discussed in the following text. When the modulation is occurring, the wavelengths become shorter and longer in length as the audio signal frequency changes. The intensity of the audio signal is represented by the deviation of the center frequency (Figure 8–12 proves a comparison of frequency modulation versus amplitude modulation). As the center frequency of the carrier deviates up and down, the audio signal intensity (soft or loud) is represented. The transmitter combines the carrier and audio frequencies, while the receiver dissembles them (Figure 8–13). This is very similar to how a FM radio station functions in your car.

Some systems, although they are called FM system, do not use traditional means of FM transmission. Some use a low energy (LE) Bluetooth-like signal instead. Traditional Bluetooth would not work in current hearing device technology due to the size of the antenna. In a Bluetooth LE device, the devices are paired with the receiver and use frequency jumping across a limited range of frequencies (40 channels spaced 2 MHz apart as opposed to 79 channels on the 2.4 GHz ISM radio band). However, the paired jumping allows for the devices to only transmit between each other and is rather secure. In Bluetooth LE pairing, a process referred to as "discovery

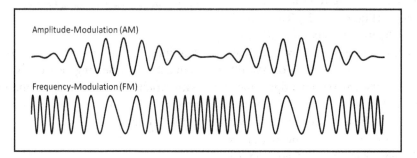

Figure 8–12. Comparison of amplitude modulation and frequency modulation (FM). While both signals have changes in pattern, the FM changes in frequency but not amplitude. Note that the intensity (loudness) of the FM signal is conveyed by moving the carrier frequency up and down. *Source:* From *Hearing Assistive and Access Technology* (p. 97), by S. R. Atcherson, C. A. Franklin, and L. Smith-Olinde, 2015, San Diego, CA: Plural Publishing. Reprinted with permission.

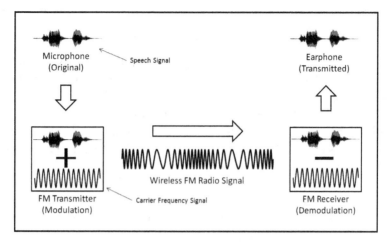

Figure 8–13. How the FM system works. The original signal is picked up by the microphone and sent to the transmitter to be combined with the carrier signal. Once modulated, the transmitter sends the signal wirelessly by radio to the receiver. The receiver will then demodulate the signal and send it to the hearing device. *Source*: From *Hearing Assistive and Access Technology* (p. 98), by S. R. Atcherson, C. A. Franklin, and L. Smith-Olinde, 2015, San Diego, CA: Plural Publishing. Reprinted with permission.

DID YOU KNOW: *Regulation of Carrier Frequencies*

The Federal Communications Commission (FCC) regulates the spectral frequency regions that are allocated for use as carrier frequencies for hearing assistive technologies. The two frequency regions are 72 MHz to 76 MHz and 216 MHz to 217 MHz. The only difference between a FM system and a FM radio station are the frequency regions allocated for their use. The reason the FCC regulates this is that your car stereo cannot overlap with the hearing devices. Initially, only 72 MHz to 76 MHz band was allocated for HAT use. This frequency range was divided into 10 wideband and 40 narrowband channels. However, the separation of those channels was increased further to minimize cross-channel interferences. Hearing assistive devices should take priority and should not pick up any radio transmission. If you have a person report that they can hear the radio, then you might want to send them back to the audiologist—the device might need to be sent in for repair.

---

and handshake," the two devices are then "paired" and can communicate exchanging information like audio signals.

FM systems are extremely adaptable and can be used in various situations. These systems have numerous benefits as speech can be transmitted over long distances and against background noise, improving the signal-to-noise ratio. An FM system consists of two components: transmitting microphone and

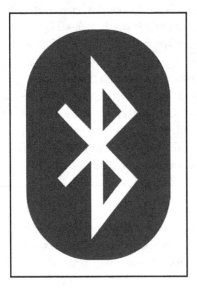

Figure 8–14. Bluetooth logo.

a receiver. The microphone is placed a few inches away from the source, such as a teacher's mouth (Chisolm et al., 2007). The transmitter or microphone could also be placed next to the sound source of interest, such as a television or on a podium. The listener utilizes a receiver that transmits the signal to the listener's hearing aid. As a result, FM systems provide individuals with an improved signal-to-noise ratio, making the acoustic signal louder than the noise.

Over the years, FM systems have changed drastically from having large microphones to small devices that are simple to use. Some FM systems are able to be worn around the speaker's neck or clipped to a shirt as long as the microphone is roughly six inches away

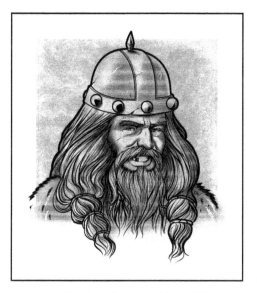

Figure 8–15. An artist's rendition of King Bla-tand. *Source*: Illustration courtesy of Timothy Lim, AuD. From *Hearing Assistive and Access Technology* (p. 150), by S. R. Atcherson, C. A. Franklin, and L. Smith-Olinde, 2015, San Diego, CA: Plural Publishing. Reprinted with permission.

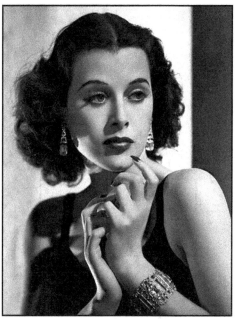

Figure 8–16. Actress/inventor Hedy Lamarr. *Source*: Image courtesy of Wikimedia Commons.

CLINICAL TIP: Two Kids in One School on the Same Frequency

It is possible that you have two children both using FM systems in one school. Depending on the device you are using, it is possible that the children could be on the same frequency. If you have children who are nearby, it is possible that these children will hear both teachers. In this case, you will need to make sure that the students are on different channels. Talk with your educational audiologist on how to adjust the frequencies to avoid any crossover.

---

from the speaker's mouth (Figure 8–17 provides some examples of FM system transmitters). The range of distance that the FM system can transmit varies upon the type of equipment being utilized. In most cases, the small FM transmitter is worn by the speaker and sent to the specific listener.

There are two primary types of FM systems currently on the market: a more traditional FM system and an adaptive FM system. Traditional FM systems use a system that picks up the signal and transmits it to the receiver. It assumes that the noise never changes and that the signal is always in a specific range. For example, if a +10 dB SNR is desired, this means that you would want the speaker to be 10 dB louder than the background noise. The hearing aid alone would

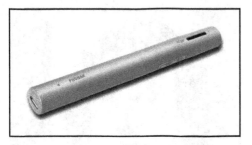

A

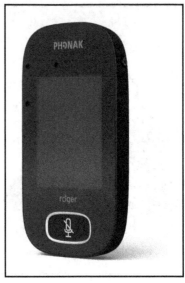

B

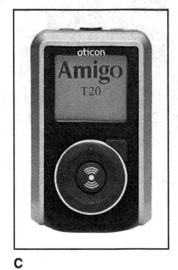

C

Figure 8–17. Examples of FM transmitters. *Source*: **A** and **B** © Sonova AG. Reproduced here with permission. All rights reserved. **C**. Photo courtesy of Oticon A/S.

provide a signal ranging from 60 dB to 70 dB (typical conversational speech level), whereas the speech from the FM microphone would between 70 dB and 80 dB. Such SNR advantages are useful to counteract the effects of distance and noise. However, using a fixed +10 dB SNR advantage in FM systems assumes that the noise will never change and that the SNR setting should never change. This "fixed" +10 dB signal-to-noise ratio approach is a limitation of traditional FM systems.

Recently, dynamic or adaptive FM systems have been developed to overcome the challenges of fixed, traditional FM systems. Dynamic or adaptive FM systems use sophisticated algorithms to enhance speech in varying noise levels and change direction. This is similar to features of hearing aids that were discussed in Chapter 4 In most hearing devices (hearing aids and implantable devices), dynamic/adaptive FM has been shown to be far superior to the traditional FM system, especially when noise levels increase (Thibodeau, 2014; Wolfe et al., 2009). Figure 8–18 demonstrates how dynamic/adaptive FM systems compare to the traditional FM system with both hearing aids and cochlear implants.

FM systems can be utilized in various listening situations. The following are examples of how these systems can be used:

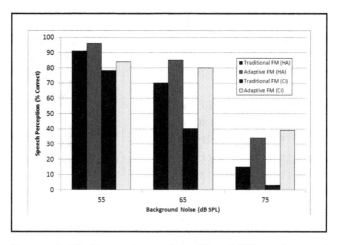

Figure 8–18. Comparison of traditional FM system and dynamic/adaptive FM system in hearing aid and cochlear implant on speech perception as a function of increased background noise levels. *Source*: From *Hearing Assistive and Access Technology* (p. 107), by S. R. Atcherson, C. A. Franklin, and L. Smith-Olinde, 2015, San Diego, CA: Plural Publishing. Reprinted with permission.

CLINICAL TIP: BEWARE of FM Transmission Through Walls

The microphone of an FM System can transmit the auditory signal to the listener through walls. If the person wearing the microphone needs to have a private conversation, or maybe use the restroom, the microphone either needs to be muted or turned off, otherwise the listener will be able to hear what is happening!

- The use of an FM system would allow a student who sits in the back of a classroom to hear the signal just as well as a student who sits in the very front of a classroom.
- An FM system would be beneficial in a cafeteria due to the large space having a lot of reverberation, which would make the signal more difficult to understand.
- If an individual is in a therapy session, the FM system could be used so the listener is better able to hear what the speech-language pathologist, or other professional, is saying.
- A parent or spouse could wear the microphone for the FM system in the car.
- The microphone could be placed in the middle of a large conference room table to have a better signal-to-noise ratio for all the individuals in the meeting.
- In a large area such as an auditorium, the FM system could be connected to an existing public address, or PA, system.

Another way to address problems in large areas would be through the use of a FM sound field system, which will be further discussed in this chapter.

FM systems have both advantages and disadvantages. Most FM systems are easy to set up. They have purposes for both personal and public use. They provide better access to sound and can be used in numerous listening environments. Personal FM systems are portable and simple to install. If the hearing device and the FM system become unpaired, you as the speech-language pathologist can easily repair the devices instead of the child having to go back to the audiologist. They are not susceptible to electromagnetic interference. However, it is possible that there may be some potential interference of radio frequencies by other non-FM systems.

Compatibility issues may arise as some personal hearing aids may not be compatible with public FM receivers or transmitters. FM systems have relatively high-power consumption, which may result in users having to charge the FM system often and charge or replace batteries in their hearing devices. Some personal FM systems have relatively high unit cost. If the system is not an open fit, there may be concerns for localization abilities. There will be a learning curve for use and maintenance. Nevertheless, the advantages of FM systems compensate for the disadvantages.

Proprietary Wireless Devices

Some hearing device companies have developed a remote microphone that will only work with their hearing devices (Figure 8–19 provides examples). This means that a speaker can wear a small microphone and, using proprietary wireless signals, the device transmits the signal to the listener's

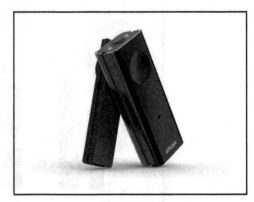

A

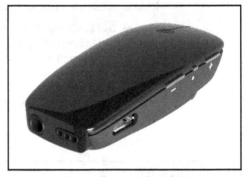

B

Figure 8–19. Examples of proprietary remote microphones. *Source*: **A.** Photo courtesy of Oticon A/S. **B.** Courtesy of Resound.

personal amplification devices. This is used as opposed to an FM system or other general transmission devices. The advantage of this is that they tend to be much less expensive than traditional FM systems. On the other hand, their low cost also means that their ability to process the signal is also less. Most are not the advanced technologies that were discussed in the FM section. They are not able to independently improve the signal. They are able, however, to overcome the problem of distance and signal-to-noise by decreasing the distance between the speaker's voice and the listener's ears at a much reduced cost compared to a traditional FM system. Some companies use near field communication systems to receive the signal, while others are able to directly receive the signal within the hearing device.

Induction Loop

Another type of hearing assistive technology is an induction loop system. An induction loop is a method of wireless transmission of a signal to a hearing aid, cochlear implant, headset, or other assistive device via a loop or wire around a room, building, vehicle, or other selected area. In the United States, induction systems are one of the least used hearing assistive technologies as other systems are more well known and allow for better signal-to-noise ratios. However, induction and loop systems are extremely cost-effective. In order to better understand how an induction or loop system works, we need to discuss the various components of these systems.

The hearing aid telecoil, or t-coil, is a main component of an induction system. A telecoil is composed of a small metal rod encircled by a thin copper wire. Due to how small t-coils can be, they are often built into hearing aids and other implantable devices. In an induction system, the t-coil acts as a receiver. T-coils detect changes in a magnetic field. If a magnetic field is detected and changes within that field occur over time, an alternating electric current is generated in the coil, which is known as induction, hence the name for an induction system. When the telecoil picks up the magnetic signal from an electronic sound source, the signal is amplified and converted from an electric to acoustic signal.

Although every hearing aid and implantable device is different, many can be made with a telecoil. If a device has a telecoil, the telecoil must be activated in order for it to be used. Some hearing aids have automatic telecoils that activate when a strong magnetic signal is placed next to the hearing aid. Most automatic telecoils are manufactured for use with a telephone. If the magnetic signal is weak, a small magnet with an adhesive on one side can be added to the telephone to help activate the automatic telecoil. However, automatic telecoils may not be the most effective for induction hearing loop products. As a result, telecoils will likely need to be manually activated in order to use them with a variety of induction loop hearing products. When an individual has access to a personal telecoil in their hearing aid or implantable device and an induction system, the user can wirelessly pick up sound without the use of additional devices. This will result with an improved signal-to-noise ratio.

Induction technology can be used in a variety of listening environments. Individuals who want to use these systems must have a strong enough t-coil in their hearing aids to do so. The following are just a few examples of where this technology could be used:

- A classroom
- A place of worship
- In an auditorium
- At a sporting event
- On a bus
- In an airport

The magnetic signal can be transmitted to the telecoil in a variety of ways. A small wearable device can be placed next to the hearing device or a wire-based loop can be used for a larger area. If a loop is being used in a large listening area, a sign should be posted so users are aware that a loop system or some other type of hearing assistive technology is available at their disposal. An example of this sign can be seen in Figure 8–20.

Depending on the purpose, location, or skill of the installer, the induction loop system may be able to be installed by the consumer. These systems can range anywhere from $100 to $300 for small areas, or $1,000

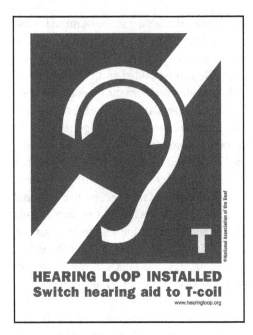

HEARING LOOP INSTALLED
Switch hearing aid to T-coil
www.hearingloop.org

©National Association of the Deaf

Figure 8–20. Hearing loop/telecoil sign. *Source*: HearingLoop.org, with permission of the National Association of the Deaf.

to $150,000 for larger areas. Residential kits can be installed quite easily in rooms within a home, such as a living room or bedroom. The wire loop should be secured to the wall or floor to minimize trips and falls. In addition, it is beneficial to have the wire loop located above or below head level as this maximizes the magnetic signal. It should be noted that individuals on floors above or below the loop may be able to listen to what is being transmitted within the loop with their own telecoils. If it is not possible to loop an entire room, an individual can use a short-range loop or personal loop. In this situation, the personal loop may be placed under a chair or seat cushion. The wires are then connected to an audio loop amplifier, which is then connected to whatever the user wants to hear, such as the television. This type of system would likely only benefit one individual because of its short range. In larger areas, a trained professional will likely need to install

the wire loop because of potential electromagnetic interference. In addition, several loops may need to be added within the various rooms of the larger building. As a result, it is important that a professional install the system to help ensure different loop systems are separated and there is minimal energy "spilled" into adjacent rooms.

Induction technology can be advantageous for a variety of reasons. This technology has low power consumption. Induction loop systems are cost effective and easy to maintain. They can be utilized by all individuals who have telecoils in their hearing devices. However, not every hearing device has a telecoil in it. In addition, it is possible that electromagnetic interference may occur through other electromagnetic sources. Poor sound quality may be an issue if a user is not close enough to the loop wire.

Infrared (IR) Systems

Infrared, or IR, systems are an additional type of hearing assistive technology. These types of systems are most commonly used with television and large meeting spaces, such as a theatre or auditorium. IR systems are based on light waves carrying a signal from one or more transmitters to several types of small, specified receivers.

With IR systems, a transmitter LED and a receiver diode are needed. The receivers can work with earphones, headsets, hearing aids, or cochlear implants. If hearing aids or cochlear implants are being used, a neck loop can be used to send the IR signal to the telecoil inside the amplification device. A direct audio input patch cord can be hardwired to the pocket-sized receiver for cochlear implants. It should be noted that the type of connection to the amplification device and receiver will depend upon the manufacturer of the hearing device and that

---

KEY CONCEPT: T-coil Awareness

As we discussed in Chapter 4, a large portion of the hearing aids dispensed in the U.S. today are the mini-BTE style. In most cases, the goal is to keep the product small, which means that there is not room for an effective t-coil. Many consumer groups are concerned that patients are buying these products without ever knowing that a slightly larger product could be equipped with a t-coil. That is, it is possible that when audiologists are presenting the array of features available in modern hearing aids, the t-coil isn't mentioned, or at least, isn't full advantages of having a t-coil are not explained. Recently, New York State changed the continuing education requirements for dispensing audiologists and hearing instruments dispensers to include one hour of instruction on t-coil and other assistive listening devices, and added a requirement that consumers must be informed regarding the availability of t-coils. Five other states: Arizona, Florida, Rhode Island, Utah, and Delaware have adopted similar laws. The New York law also requires that a sign notifying consumers of this requirements be posted in each office. It is to read: "State law requires hearing care professionals to inform consumers of the benefits of telecoil technology, looped environments, and assistive listening devices."

DID YOU KNOW: Television Remotes Use IR Lights

IR technology is utilized in remote controls for televisions (TV), cable boxes and other related equipment. The remote control has a small LED bulb on the front, which must be aimed at the TV. By pressing a button on the remote, a specific flashing light pulse pattern is sent to the TV and, as a result, the TV will complete the command given. However, this is why a TV remote will only work when it is directly pointed at the TV, and why there must be a line-of-sight without a barrier. If you want to keep your cable box behind a closed cabinet door, you'll want a remote that uses FM signals.

---

not all connection types are compatible with all amplification devices. If a hearing aid or cochlear implant is not being used, a mono or stereo set of earphones can be plugged directly into the receiver.

IR technology works very well indoors in well-lit and darkened rooms; however, sunlight can interfere with transmission. In addition, there cannot be any objects block-ing the transmitter LED and receiver diode. As a result, this type of system may not be best suited for a classroom. If a listener were to be in a much larger room, such as a theatre or auditorium, an IR system could be utilized. The transmitter would be plugged into the sound source (i.e., existing sound system) and the signal is carried within the transmitted light beam to the IR receivers worn by the individuals in the audience. When compared to FM systems and other wireless assistive technologies, IR systems are much less widely used in these settings.

Other Devices

There are few other devices that can send signals to hearing aids and cochlear implants depending on the manufacturer, device, technology level, and so forth. The FCC regulates the function of phones to ensure that they are usable by patients with hearing loss. Even though these laws have been around for a long time, the FCC has only recently brought the accessibility laws up to date with more current technology.

Phones

As discussed in Chapter 5, in addition to direct streaming, there are two primary ways that the signal goes from a phone into a person's hearing devices: acoustic telephone and induction (telecoil). Whether one chooses the acoustic coupling or the induction coupling method to communicate using the phone, it will be important to consider how compatible these methods are with the desired phone. Some of the information on compatibility may be found publicly on an Internet search, and other pieces may require assistance from the phone provider or audiologist. The FCC requires that hearing aid compatible phone providers indicate a quality measure of how much emission is produced by the phone.

M-rating will be important for those who choose acoustic (microphone) transmission while T-rating will be important for those who plan to use the induction coupling method via telecoil. The ratings are M1 to M4 and T1 to T4. An M4 or T4 rating will have the least interference and will be the most compatible with hearing device use. Either way, a person using a phone will want to hold the phone closer to the hearing device. This is not intuitive to most people who are used to holding the phone next to their ear; they will need to hold it higher, next to the microphone of the device behind the ear if their device sits behind their ear.

In the United States, many states may have a state-funded telecommunications equipment distribution program (TEDP) that provides free or low-cost telecommunication devices to qualified residents with disabilities. Although their equipment and process vary from state to state, in general, there is an application process that requires certification of disability by a qualified professional and, possibly, certification of financial need. You are encouraged to look at the TEDP website (http://www.tedpa.org) to determine what you can help your patients receive. In most cases, the person will still be responsible for the monthly bill associated with the device use.

Cell Phones

As our society becomes more mobile and spread out, many people report that they communicate with friends and family via telephone more than in person. Therefore, other than the purchase of hearing devices, the most important decision may be what mobile device to purchase. If available, the person may want to experiment with the acoustic phone (microphone) option as compared with the induction coupling (telecoil) option. For mobile phone purchase, there are two websites available to prescreen for hearing aid compatibility: http://www.phonescoop.com and http://www.accesswireless

.org. Both of these websites help you search or narrow your search for phones by searching for specific features (e.g., phone compatibility or touchscreen).

Landlines

Hardwired phones remain commonplace in some homes and offices. There are a few hardwired amplified phones designed for people with hearing loss. Additionally, many states have assistance programs to provide phones for people with communication impairments. You may be able to recommend these devices to people. Some of these phones have large digital displays, large buttons, a powerful handset, and more than one control for volume and tone. Additionally, these devices may be able to be used for live captioning.

Digital Enhanced Cordless Telecommunications

The microwave technology known as digital enhanced cordless telecommunication (DECT) uses another frequency designation for wireless communication. DECT uses the 1.9 GHz and is less susceptible to interference than other technologies. Presently, the most common use of DECT technology appears to be in cordless phones and baby monitors. Using a base station, the signal is routed to each device within a distance of about 600 meters, large enough to cover a sizable building. A hearing device wearer may be able to listen bilaterally through DECT, rather than just though one ear (Figure 8–21). While present application is limited to certain manufacturers, DECT technology is improving. In a similar manner as Bluetooth, improved energy consumption in Bluetooth-enabled devices

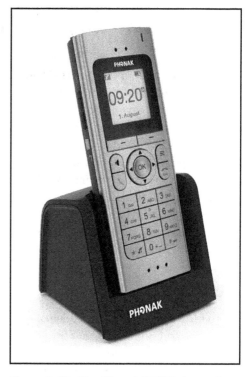

Figure 8–21. The Phonak DECT phone allows the hearing device user to hear phone conversations through both devices. *Source*: Image © Sonova AG. Reproduced here with permission. All rights reserved.

with Bluetooth LE, a low-energy version of DECT (DECT ULE) is also available. These types of technologies will likely be used in other platforms in the future.

Streaming Devices

There are some Bluetooth devices designed to receive a signal but with no intent or capacity to return a signal. When this one-way transmission occurs, it is called streaming. Streaming requires the second device to receive a signal, but does not require that the device be able to transmit a signal. We stream when listening to music from our

---

KEY CONCEPT: Hearing Device Apps

Many hearing aids can be connected to phones, tablets, and computers. These provide significant advantages to listening directly to these devices but also pose challenges in the educational setting. As we discussed in Chapter 4, it's common today to use smartphone apps to adjust hearing aids during use. And of course, who better to do this than a teenager, who typically knows more about the operation of smartphone apps than 90% of adults. Imagine the 14-year-old with a moderate hearing loss wearing bilateral hearing aids who is working in a large room on a science project with several other students. He will want his hearing aids on omnidirectional—equal amplification from all directions—as in this situation, he will not be attending to a talker from a specific location. His next class is history, set up in a traditional classroom manner with the teacher lecturing from the front. He now will want a narrow-directional focus to the front, which not only is reducing any extraneous noise (like the students whispering to each other in the back), but adds additional gain to the focal point (wherever the student is looking—hopefully at the teacher). So all this student has to do is pull out his smartphone and use the adjustment we reviewed in Chapter 5 (see Figure 5–10). However, this poses significant difficulties in educational settings for several points. Many schools ban the use of cell phones in the classroom; yet, for these students, the only way to change the settings on the hearing aids are via the app on the phone. Additionally, they are able to stream from the device. So what about during testing? They could be connected to another student feeding them the answers, or maybe they are listening to a prerecorded lecture. These kinds of features in hearing aids are important for the function of the aid and for the person to be able to best hear, but do pose some considerations for use in the classroom. As the SLP, you will likely be more knowledgeable than many teachers about the ability of hearing aids and what they should be aware of when it comes to equal access, but appropriate use.

---

smartphone or a smart device. We stream audio directions from our GPS systems. In both of these signals, there is no return signal, only one-way signal allowing us to listen to music or driving directions. With hearing aids, the streaming device is often placed in a pocket or worn around the neck. The streaming device transmits to the hearing aids from another device, such as a mobile phone. Because of the reduced energy consumption of Bluetooth LE, the hearing aids have the capacity to interact with external devices without a streaming device. The hearing aids can send information both ways to mobile phones if connected via Bluetooth. That being said, some hearing aid manufacturers only allow for one-way transmissions. While potentially intimidating, the technology is quite user friendly. As an SLP, you may be a resource for pairing and unpairing devices such as mobile phones or computers. In the classroom or during therapy, if the computer or tablet is Bluetooth enabled and the hearing aids are able to so, you can pair the devices for direct connection. In this case, the student would be able to hear directly from the device, improving their ability to understand what is being said. As noted in the Key Concept, however, this should be done with caution.

Sound Field Equalization Systems

Sound field equalization systems are beneficial because the amplified sound can acoustically fill the entire room instead of the signal only being transmitted to one individual. These systems are similar to a PA system. Typically, the speaker utilizes a microphone and transmits the signal to a receiver or amplifier. The amplified sound is distributed to all listeners through loudspeakers. A sound field system can use either FM or IR technology. If the sound field system is using FM technology, the speaker's voice is sent via radio waves to the receiver connected to the loudspeaker. If the sound field system is using IR technology, the speaker's voice is sent via light waves to the receiver connected to the loudspeaker.

This type of system is extremely beneficial in classrooms. All students, whether they have normal hearing sensitivity or hearing loss, benefit from sound field systems because the amplified sound creates an improved signal-to-noise ratio. However, it is important to note that FM systems are still able to provide a more advantageous signal-to-noise ratio than sound field systems. Children with hearing loss often use high levels of energy in classroom instruction as they attempt to learn, making this type of system helpful in decreasing listening effort. Furthermore, the teacher is able to wear the transmitting microphone and freely move around the classroom while lecturing because the system is wireless. This allows the children to attend to the instruction they are receiving and have increased opportunities to learn more efficiently as they are no longer straining to understand what is being spoken. These systems can also be beneficial when children are developing literacy skills as there were fewer at-risk readers in classrooms that regularly used sound field systems. Utilizing a sound field system facilitates improved vocal hygiene of the speaker due to the reduce strain on vocal folds secondary to the increased loudness necessary to provide adequate volume for listeners.

These systems can be integrated into classroom activities as well. Children can use them when presenting information in class. The teacher could use it while lecturing or making an announcement. It could be used to amplify the volume of a video by placing the microphone next to the audio source (Figure 8–22). Not only can these systems be used in the general classroom, they can also be used for specialized subjects such as art, music, physical education, or a foreign language class.

Another type of sound field equalization system that can be more directed at certain individuals is a targeted sound field equalization system. The target system has a single speaker that can be directed toward a single listener. In a classroom setting, the speaker could sit on that student's desk. This type of system could be beneficial in therapy sessions as well. The speech-language pathologist could wear the microphone and have the speaker directed toward the client. This would allow the client to have better access to the clinician's voice.

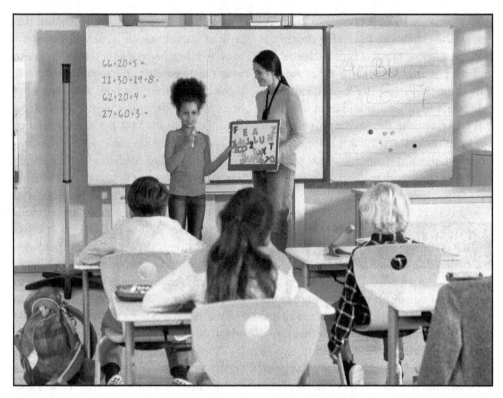

Figure 8–22. Example of sound field system with a teacher wearing the microphone around her neck with a loudspeaker at the front of the classroom providing all students with amplified sound and an improved signal-to-noise ratio. *Source*: Image © Sonova AG. Reproduced here with permission. All rights reserved.

Like other types of hearing assistive technologies, sound field equalization systems have their advantages and disadvantages. One major advantage is that these systems benefit all listeners in the room. They can benefit children whose primary hearing devices are not functioning appropriately. This type of system does not stigmatize certain listeners. Teachers and speakers often report less vocal strain. These systems are not susceptible to electromagnetic interference. Both the listener and speaker can move freely throughout the room while a sound field system is in use. One disadvantage of this type of system is that it may not provide exemplary benefits while in noisy or reverberant environments. In addition, certain rooms may not have the correct arrangement and/or number of loud speakers. Unless it is a personal sound field equalization system, it may not be portable.

Classroom Considerations

The following are recommendations you as a speech-language pathologist can implement to help children with hearing loss in the classroom. These adaptations are beneficial as they will assist children in overcoming the difficulties they may encounter as a result of their hearing loss. Although these recommendations are geared toward the classroom, it is important to note these recommendations and considerations can also be utilized with adults. The following considerations were adapted from an Iowa Area Education Agency document compiled by Tom Mitchell (Davis, 1977; Gildston, n.d.; Luckner, 2002):

- Advocacy. You should help the child to take ownership of his or her hearing loss. By doing so, the child will become his or her own advocate. The child needs to notify the teacher when he or she is having difficulty following directions or does not understand what is being said. You should help the child to develop effective strategies to use to repair communication breakdowns.
- Eye Contact. The child should try to obtain and maintain eye contact with peers, teachers, and other professionals. In the same sense, the teacher should ensure the child is attending to the teacher when an important topic is about to be discussed. Important information should not be given when the student does not have visual access to the teacher's face.
- Attention. You or the teacher should get the student's attention before speaking as the student may need to prepare himself or herself in order to listen to you. Use the individual's name or tap him or her gently on the arm before speaking. The individual will only be able to hear one source at a time.
- Precise Speech. The teacher should remember to speak clearly and enunciate each word. Speech should not be exaggerated or too loud. The speaker should also talk at a slower pace, but not too slow. This will give the individual time to process what he or she is actually hearing. In addition, the teacher needs to keep his or her mouth empty (no eating or chewing gum) when lecturing.
- Repeat or Rephrase. If a student does not understand what was discussed, it should be repeated or rephrased to ensure the student understood the concept. This is especially important during classroom discussions as the student with hearing loss may have difficulty hearing his or her peers around the room. The teacher should try to restate what the other students have said.
- Preferential Seating. The student should sit as close to the sound source as possible with his or her better ear closest to the speaker and in a position where the student can see the speaker's face. This will allow the student to be closer to the auditory source. The student should be seated as far away from noise sources as possible, such as the hallway or fans.
- Visual or Written Aids. Verbal instruction should be supplemented with visual or written aids. This will help to clarify difficult concepts.
- Comprehension Checks. You or the teacher should periodically perform a comprehension check with the student. This will help to ensure that the student understood.

In Closing

Hearing assistive technologies provide many benefits to all users. They allow for improved access to communication, ease of listening, better signal-to-noise ratios, and so much more. These technologies can be used in a variety of listening situations including classrooms, places of worship, amphitheaters, meetings, or at the dinner table. The type of assistive technology one utilizes will depend upon their hearing aid or cochlear implant. In addition, it is important that sound field equalization systems be beneficial to all that use them. This includes the speaker, individuals with normal hearing sensitivity, and individuals with hearing loss as the amplified sound is distributed throughout the room the system is being utilized in. In this chapter, our focus mostly has been on school-age children. But many of the options we have presented also apply to adults. This is technology that they could use in the home, or for group social events. Assisted living facilities could benefit greatly from many of the options we reviewed.

As a speech-language pathologist, you may have to advocate for the use of these systems for your patients. If these assistive technologies are being utilized within therapy sessions, listening checks using the Ling-6 Sound Test should be performed to ensure proper function of the devices. Figure 8–23 is a useful graphic for using the Ling-6 test. Charts like this are available from

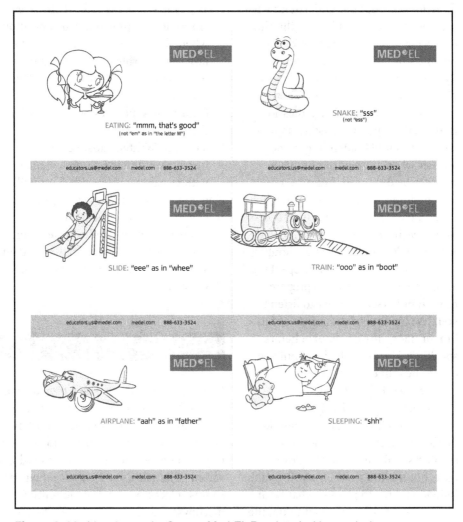

Figure 8–23. Ling-6 sounds. *Source*: Med-El. Reprinted with permission.

several sources, including cochlear implant companies. In addition, teachers should perform daily listening checks of the hearing assistive technologies to ensure that they are functioning appropriately. This can also be done using the Ling-6 Sound Test. More information regarding the Ling-6 Sound Test can be found in Chapter 7. If an individual has access to one of these technologies, the use of that system should be advocated for as they can have a tremendous positive impact on communication.

The classroom considerations discussed above can also have a positive impact on learning and communication. The strategies that you use, the teachers use, and the student use can be very effective in ensuring the listener has access to appropriate communication. The use of these recommendations can also help students become advocates for themselves, which will allow them to take responsibility of their hearing loss. The more a child is able to express what he or she is understanding, the better outcomes that child will have. As a speech-language pathologist, you will be an integral part of this child's development of communication.

9 Hearing Loss, Hearing Aids, and Children

To this point, we have talked in general about hearing loss, hearing aids, and other amplification strategies. Much of it has been focused toward the adult patient. In this chapter, we'd like to focus on children, ranging from infants and toddlers to teenagers. Hearing loss may have a significant impact on the education and vocational pursuits of a child. Children who receive intervention early and often are more likely to succeed in traditional educational environments and have access to a wider array of vocational options. You as the SLP may be the one that identifies the child with hearing loss. You may also be the one who follows the child through their education into adulthood. You may help them learn how to be responsible for their devices, how to advocate for themselves, and make them aware of their rights and responsibilities as an individual with hearing loss. For the school-aged child with hearing loss, it is often the SLP that helps them navigate their educational world with their hearing loss.

Hearing Development

The outer, middle, and inner ears develop at different times in embryologic development, however, all form within the first trimester of fetal growth. By understanding fetal development related to hearing and hearing loss, the SLP may better be aware of the effects of concerns during prenatal development.

Outer ear development

- Week 5 to 20: formation of the external ear (pinnae)
- Week 6 to 22: external auditory canal
  - Portions continue to ossify until 7 years of age
- Week 7 to 23: tympanic membrane
- Week 24: sebaceous glands form to create cerumen (earwax)
- Throughout childhood (until 9 years of age): growth of external ear and external canal develops and grows

Middle ear development

- Typically follows head formation
- Week 3 to 23: formation of the Eustachian tube
- Week 4 to 31: middle ear cavity
- Week: 5 to 30: formation of the ossicles
- Week: 36 to birth: middle ear remains fluid filled
- Birth: middle ear becomes air filled and functional

Inner ear development

- Week 2 to 3: early inner ear structures
- Week 4 to 5: Cochlea and vestibular system form
- Week 6 to 9: cochlear nerve fibers develop
- Week 7 to 8: vestibular semicircular canals from

- Week 12 to 16: lymphatic sacs form within cochlea and fill with polarized fluid (perilymph and endolymph)
- Week 16 to 24: ossification of the inner ear structures

The development of the structures of the ear are important for you to know because if this development is disrupted or an external toxin is introduced (e.g., alcohol), the effects will be seen within these specific structures. Abnormalities can impact hearing ability as well as speech and language development.

Abnormalities

Human pregnancy and development are generally robust processes and, in dealing with abnormalities, this can sometimes be forgotten. All abnormalities of human development can be grouped into three main categories: genetic, environmental, and undetermined (unknown). The complex origins of all parts of the hearing system and the long time-course of development expose this system to a large number of different factors. As the speech-language pathologist, knowing the underlying cause of hearing loss may help you with your course of treatment and recommendations regarding speech, language, auditory, educational, and social recommendations. We provided an extensive table of syndromes and disorders at the end of Chapter 3, but will do a brief review here.

Genetic

In human development, the majority of major genetic abnormalities are thought to be lost in the first 2 weeks of development. Online Mendelian Inheritance in Man (OMIM; http://omim.org) is a searchable database of human genomes and contains explanations and recommendations. Genetic abnormalities may be grouped into:

- Chromosomal aneuploidies (abnormal number of chromosomes)
  - For example, Down syndrome, trisomy 13
- Translocation of chromosomal segments
- Single gene mutations
  - Autosomal
  - X-linked
  - Recessive (carrier)

If a parent chooses, they may have a genetic panel completed to attempt to determine the cause of hearing loss. According to the OMIM, there are more than 900 different chromosomal abnormalities related to hearing and more than 400 clinical diagnoses. Many of these genetic disorders that affect hearing are also part of multisystem genetic syndromes.

Environmental

There are many different environmental factors that affect hearing ability; they are sometimes described as teratogens. Some may be directly due to maternal behavior (e.g., alcohol use, drug use, diet, or smoking) or a pre-existing maternal condition (e.g., diabetes). While others may be due to factors that cannot be controlled by the mother (e.g., infection, contaminants like lead, or radiation).

Abnormality Recognition for SLPs

There are many factors that you could be aware of which may lead you to recommend further testing or recognize as occurring in conjunction with hearing loss. These can be broken down into several factors and may have a varied impact on hearing ability (Figures 9–1 through 9–3).

- External ear
  - Low or uneven ears—indicate developmental abnormality of head development
  - Thickened lobes—consistent with middle ear bone malformations
  - Small ears with absent cartilage—consistent with incus and stapes issues
  - Ear and ear canal anomalies
    - Anotia—absence of ear
    - Atresia—missing most of the ear
    - Microtia—small ear
    - Missing ear canal
  - Facial microtia; for example: Treacher Collins syndrome
  - Preauricular tags and pits—consistent with inner ear concerns
- Middle ear
  - Down syndrome
  - Little person
- Inner ear
  - Tags and pits
  - Variety of syndromes
  - Maternal infections like rubella or toxoplasmosis
  - Maternal cytomegalovirus

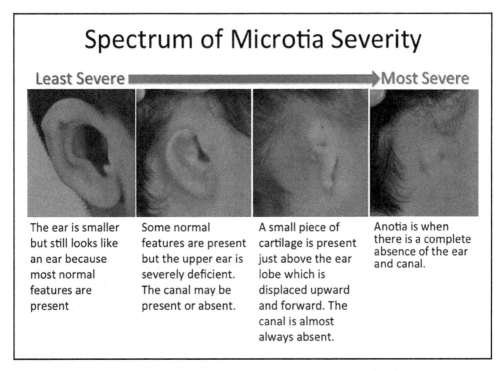

Figure 9–1. Examples of anotia, atresia, and microcia. These are deformities of the external ear, which can have a significant impact on function and could be a sign of other auditory malformations. *Source*: Centers for Disease Control and Prevention (https://www.cdc.gov).

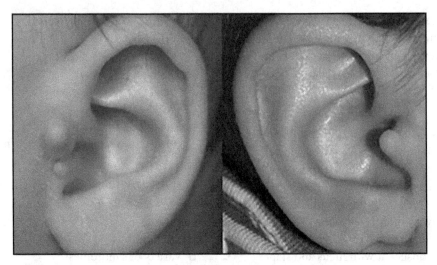

Figure 9–2. Example of preauricular tags. These can be a sign of other auditory malformations. *Source*: National Institutes of Health (https://www.nih.gov).

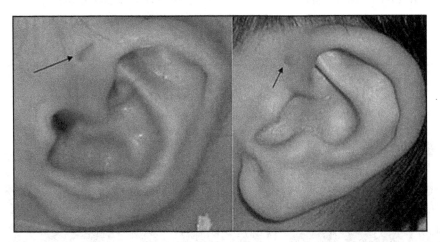

Figure 9–3. Example of preauricular pits. These can be a sign of other auditory malformations. *Source*: National Institutes of Health (https://www.nih.gov).

For many of these conditions, the visual representation may be the only sign of hearing impairment. For some, hearing loss may be part of a sequalae of abnormities. It is important for you to recognize visual signs of abnormalities so they may refer for further testing. However, for most with hearing loss, there may not be a visual representation of hearing concern.

Hearing Loss Identified in Childhood

For the best outcomes, children with hearing loss should be identified early and treatment should be initiated. Current guidelines from the Joint Commission on Infant Hearing (JCIH) suggest that children

---

CLINICAL TIP: Tags and Pits

Also known as an accessory tragus or a branchial cleft remnant, ear tags are benign growths that consist of skin and sometimes cartilage. Ear tags are usually located in front of the ear or on the cheek. The external ear forms early in development before a baby is born when six raised soft tissue swellings (hillocks) fuse together. Additional appendages comprised of skin, fat, or cartilage may form in front of the ear. These are called preauricular tags. Ear tags can occur by themselves, or may occur in association with genetic syndromes such as Goldenhar syndrome, hemifacial microsomia, and first and second branchial arch syndrome. When you are conducting a hearing screening, make sure to look around the ear when placing the earphones. You may be the first to notice a tag or a pit right in front of the ear. You should refer these children for follow-up testing even if they pass the screening.

KEY CONCEPT: A Little About Down Syndrome

According to the Centers for Disease Control and Prevention, approximately one in every 700 babies in the United States is born with Down syndrome, making Down syndrome the most common chromosomal condition. About 6,000 babies with Down syndrome are born in the United States each year. About 90% of those kids with Down syndrome will also have hearing impairment. It has historically been of concern that those with Down syndrome are more disposed to having conductive hearing loss due to facial abnormalities; however, evidence also suggests that they may also be more disposed to having sensorineural hearing loss (Blaser et al., 2006). As with all children, when you are treating children with Down syndrome, it is suggested that you ensure that they can hear prior to any treatment. However, with a child with Down syndrome, you may consider doing a hearing screening more often to account for any transient conductive hearing losses.

For the record, what you see us use here is "Down" syndrome. The name comes from English physician John Langdon Down, who in 1862, helped to differentiate the condition from mental disability. You may have also seen it written as Downs, Downs', or the more logical, Down's. The reason given for dropping the apostrophe is that it indicates ownership or possession, and although it is named for Dr. Down, he didn't have the pathology. Of course, we violate that arbitrary rule all the time—Charles Bell didn't have facial palsy and Carl Wernicke didn't have aphasia. But anyway, the National Down Syndrome Society uses "Down" so it's good enough for us!

born with hearing loss should have confirmed hearing loss by 3 months of age and appropriate treatment by 6 months of age. Further, intervention for habilitation should begin within 1 month of diagnosis; in many cases, this is speech and language intervention by a Birth to 3 SLP. The final chapter in this book focuses on the habilitation/rehabilitation for people with hearing loss.

Hearing loss in children is identified, typically, in one of three manners:

- newborn hearing screening
- school screening
- by an adult that identifies a concern

There are many methods for determining what screening procedures should be used. Hearing screening is an important part of any health screening. The screening identifies a concern that may have a significant impact on the child in their future endeavors.

Newborn Hearing Screening

We discussed hearing screenings in Chapter 2, but given the focus of this chapter, we thought it prudent to cover it again in a more focused manner. The main focus of newborn hearing screening and early hearing detection and intervention (EDHI) programs are to identify those who potentially have hearing loss at birth. As with any screening, it must be viewed in relation to the overall rationale and context. EHDI programs include a newborn hearing screening followed by an audiologic diagnostic evaluation conducted by an audiologist. Those who do not pass the screening are referred to an audiologist for a comprehensive evaluation. Figure 9–4 depicts the progress of identification of hearing loss in newborns.

So what is newborn hearing screening and on whom is it conducted? The goal would be that all children born in the United States have their hearing screened at birth. Newborn hearing screening is typically

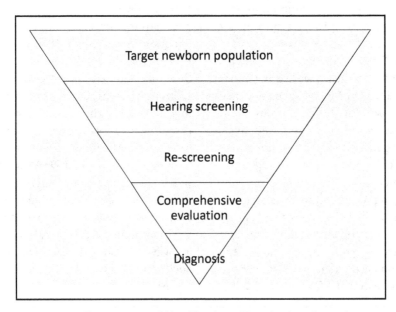

Figure 9–4. The progress of identification of hearing loss in newborns.

> ### CLINICAL TIP: Using the Right Terminology
>
> The importance of communicating results of the hearing screening to both families and physicians is often underestimated. Proper communication of results to parents ensures that they have a positive experience with the newborn hearing screening program, while proper communication of results to physicians helps to ensure that families who are referred from the hearing screening receive appropriate follow-up care. The word *fail* should not be used to describe a child not passing a screening. Instead, consider using *refer* or *no clear response.* The change in terminology has been moved to these terms because it reduced parental anxiety and, despite the outcomes, further testing is needed—therefore the child did not *fail.*

conducted using otoacoustic emissions (OAE) and/or auditory brain stem response (ABR). These tests, while not perfect, typically refer 1% to 2% of those newborns screened; so there will be a proportion of those screened who do not have hearing loss, but will have additional testing. Current data suggest that nearly 4 million babies are born per year with about 98% of those newborns getting a hearing screening. Of those, about 1.7% were referred for follow-up testing. Of those who were sent on for further testing, approximately 68% were diagnosed with hearing loss; an incidence rate of 1.7 children per 1,000 screened.

As with any screening, the impact of false positives should be of concern. A study by Clemens et al. (2000) suggested that the impact of false positives is small. Mothers were surveyed about their responses to the newborn hearing screening even though their children eventually passed. Results of the survey were reassuring with regard to lasting emotional effects of false-positive tests. Only 9% of mothers said they "treated their child differently" before outpatient rescreening, and only 14% reported any lasting anxiety after their child passed the outpatient repeat screen. Of all of the factors they investigated, no single factor was identified as having the most impact on lasting anxiety, but the factors that may play some part include: more educated mothers, a misunderstanding of the meaning of the screening results, and a false-positive during secondary screening. Overall, most parents reported strong support of newborn hearing screening programs.

After Referral on Newborn Hearing Screening

Based on outcomes of the screening, children will be referred for additional follow-up testing. The results of that test will determine if the child will need diagnostic testing. The current JCIH guidelines suggest that the child receive initial rescreening within 1 month of testing, diagnostic testing by 3 months of age, and intervention by 6 months of age. This is commonly called the 1, 3, 6 JCIH guideline. The flow of testing is depicted in Figure 9–5. After newborn hearing screening, the next time that many children will have their hearing screened, unless concerns arise, is in elementary school; therefore, follow-up for those newborns who do not pass the screening is essential. If you have a child who you see as part of Birth to 3 services who did not

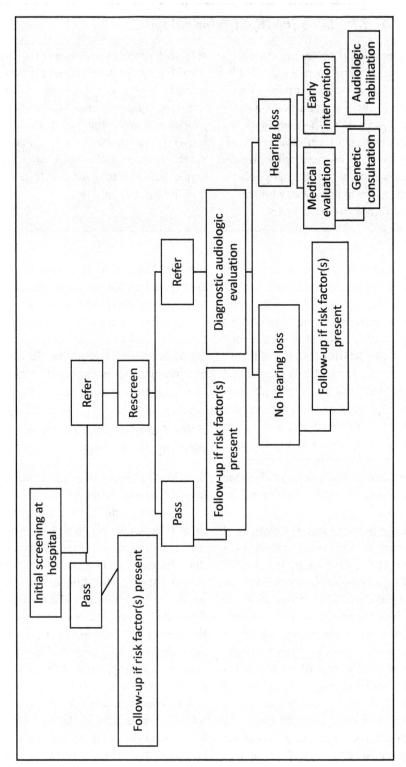

Figure 9–5. Flow of testing for the newborn hearing screening and follow-up. Courtesy of Jessica Messersmith.

> ### CLINICAL TIP: Language Exposure Is Critical
>
> As reported previously, some parents did report treating their child differently after they did not pass the newborn hearing screening. While these children ultimately did end up passing, there is evidence to suggest that those children who are diagnosed with hearing loss do not have as much exposure to spoken language. Research suggests that the parents of children with hearing loss do not talk to their children as much as children who have normal hearing. Normal-hearing children will be exposed to approximately 30 million words by the time they reach kindergarten. However, for those with hearing loss, they may be less exposed to language during their formative years. We know that the first three years are the most critical time for language development. During this time, the brain is most plastic and open. The child's brain develops 80% to 85% during the first 3 years. As children get a little older, the neural con-nections in the parts of the brain that have not been used often will atrophy. If we don't stimulate the brain early, we don't get a do-over. Research strongly indicates that reaching that potential depends on parents and caregivers talking to the children and their overall exposure to language. So if parents of children who have hearing loss talk to them less, those children would be exposed to less language. The language ability of those children have been shown to have significantly fewer word exposures than children with normal hearing ability. This results in a smaller vocabulary, lower reading ability, and overall slower educational progress. As an SLP, you can have a significant long-term impact on a child's life by encouraging parents to speak to their children. Additionally, explaining the role of incidental learning on a child's function may assist parents in understanding the impact of speaking to and around their children.

pass their hearing screening, but did not receive follow-up, ensure that they receive additional testing for hearing loss. Current data suggests that 0.7% of those referred for the newborn hearing screening do not have appropriate follow-up. In the attempt to combat the loss of follow-up, several measures have been taken by the states to empower parents. One such idea is the EHDI 136 website (https://ehdi136.com). This Early Hearing Detection and Intervention website provides parents information about the 1, 3, 6 JCHI guidelines, provides links for information, and allows them to sign up for email reminders. Encouraging parents and empow-ering them to take the control of their child's health care can have a long-term impact on their hearing ability, language success, and overall health. As the SLP, you have the power to help parents navigate the healthcare system; there are many resources available to them and you as their health-care provider.

School Hearing Screening

As an SLP, it may be your job to set up and administer school hearing screenings. According to ASHA, it is within the scope of

---

CLINICAL TIP: Hearing Screening for Children with Hearing Loss

Should you do a hearing screening on those children who already have diagnosed hearing loss? Probably not. Screening is conducted at 20 dB HL, and if a child is diagnosed with a hearing loss, their hearing is worse than that. However, you may consider conducting otoscopy and tympanometry on these children to ensure that they don't have ear wax or middle ear issues. Also, make sure that they are following up with their audiologist for continued care.

---

practice for an SLP to oversee a school hearing screening. We discussed this briefly in Chapter 2, but will provide some additional information here. School hearing screenings are recommended to occur as follows:

- Kindergarten through third grade: every year
- Seventh grade: prior to starting high school
- 11th grade: prior to high school graduation
- Any child new to the school district
- Any child who repeats a grade
- Any child receiving speech and language services
- Any child with behavioral or other concerns

To assist with your screening, you may consider asking the parents for a brief history of ear concerns, history of seeing an ENT, ear tubes, and/or other ear issues. A signed consent form may be required by your state or school district. Screenings may be conducted by anyone that you oversee to ensure that the appropriate protocol is followed. It is common for the screening to be conducted by health-care providers, support personnel, and even volunteers. With appropriate training and supervision, hearing screening program protocols can provide consistent and accurate screening outcomes, referrals, and diagnoses.

Middle ear effusion is the most common cause of transient hearing problems in children. During screenings for children kindergarten through third grade, it may be suggested to obtain input from parents and teachers regarding any history of middle ear issues (note: parents will often refer to this a "middle ear infection" although in many cases it is not). Success for Kids with Hearing Loss developed a History of Ear and Hearing Problems Parents' Checklist that was designed to be completed by a parent during a routine screening (Table 9–1). Using this questionnaire could assist an SLP in a referral for a child who has a routine problem. This questionnaire will help identify those who may be at risk for hearing loss and need additional screening.

Hearing screening should be conducted in a quiet environment free of visual distractions. Screening should consist of otoscopy, tympanometry, and pure-tone air conduction screening.

Otoscopy

Using a lighted otoscope, put a clean specula on the end. Then pull the ear back to straighten out the ear canal and place the tip

Table 9–1. Success for Kids with Hearing Loss—History of Ear and Hearing Problems Parents' Checklist

Parent or guardian, please answer the following questions:	NO	YES
1. Did your child have <u>any</u> ear problems before 12 months of age?		
2. Has your child had an ear problem in the last 6 months?		
3. Has your child ever had a draining ear?		
4. Has your child ever had an ear problem that lasted 3 months or longer?		
5. Does your child tend to have 3 or more ear problems each year?		
6. Approximately how many ear problems has your child had in his or her life? 0–2 _____ 3–5 _____ 6–10 _____ 10 or more _____		
7. Has anyone related to the child had many ear problems (parents, brothers or sisters, cousins)?		
8. Has your child ever been seen by an ear doctor (ENT, otologist)? If yes, at about what age was the child during these visit(s)? _____		
9. Has your child ever had tubes placed in his or her eardrums? If yes, how many times? _____ At about what age(s)? _____		
10. Has anyone related to the child had permanent hearing loss as a child or young adult (blood relatives only)?		
11. Does your child have any permanent hearing loss that you know about?		
12. Have there been times when you have been seriously concerned about your child's hearing?		

Source: Reprinted with permission from http://www.successforkidswithhearingloss.com.

in the ear. Look for the tympanic membrane. If you see excessive ear wax, redness, puss, or inflamed area, refer to a physician for follow-up. Additionally, as noted previously, if you see preauricular tags or pits, refer for follow-up testing. There is a correct way to hold an otoscope—bracing is recommended. The preferred method is shown in Figure 9–6.

Tympanometry

Tympanometry is conducted using a screening tympanometer. This test puts air into the ear and pulls it back out to determine if the tympanic membrane is moving correctly. This will give you the ear canal volume, pressure, and gradient/compliance. See Chapter 2 for a complete description of immittance testing and the expected findings. The screening audiometer values are programmed. However, referral criteria are available in Table 9–2.

There are a few different methods of tympanometry that are currently available. Historically, 226 Hz has been used as the probe tone for testing. However, there are more frequencies that can be tested;

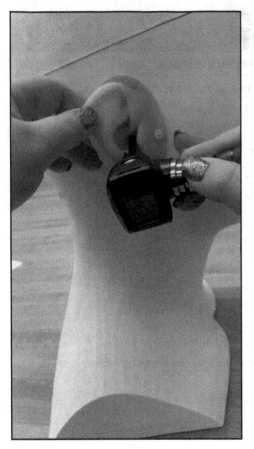

Figure 9–6. Appropriate way to hold an otoscope.

knowing what frequencies were used can help you determine if the test completed is appropriate.

226 Hz Versus 1000 Hz. Tympanograms recorded from normal ears of newborn infants are very different from those obtained from older infants, children, and adults. There are several factors that can influence the results; however, a 226 Hz lower frequency probe tone does not give accurate information about the function of infant ears. If testing tympanometry on infants, a 1000 Hz probe tone should be used. Given the anatomical differences in the infant ear—such as more compliant ear canal wall, smaller ear canal and middle ear space, tympanic-membrane thickening, middle-ear fluid and mesenchyme, and a more horizontal orientation of the tympanic membrane—a 1000 Hz probe tone is recommended. A 1000 Hz probe tone does not have set norms for refer, but we do know that 226 is not valid for measuring middle ear movement. It is suggested that 1000 Hz probe tone be used until the child is 6 to 9 months depending on the size of the child.

Wideband Reflectance. Single frequency tympanometry contrasts with recommendations about multifrequency information collected in other tests of auditory function. All other tests such as behavioral testing, OAE, and ABR use stimuli over a range of frequencies to provide a much more comprehensive analysis. Use of multifrequency tympanometry is not widely accepted in clinical protocols due to the complexity of interpretation. Thus, middle ear function is not currently adequately assessed at the higher frequencies. A relatively new mea-

Table 9–2. Tympanometry Referral Criteria		
	Child Norms	*Adult Norms*
Physical Volume	0.4–1.0 ml	0.6–1.5 ml
Compliance	0.3–0.9 ml	0.3–1.4 ml
Pressure	+50–150 daPa	+50–150 daPa

KEY CONCEPT: Sensitivity Versus Specificity

The efficacy of a screening reflects the extent to which the test is capable of discriminating cases from noncases. A case is a child with the target disorder and a noncase is a child without the disorder. In the simplest version of this discrimination, the screening test yields a binary (pass–refer) result. Not all screening tests are binary, but the tests used in the early hearing detection and intervention context traditionally are used in a binary manner. For any given test on any given child, the disorder might be present or absent and the test might be positive (refer) or negative (pass) for the disorder, so the four outcomes are as follows:

■ Disorder present, test refer: a true positive
■ Disorder present, test pass: a false positive
■ Disorder not present, test refer: a false negative
■ Disorder not present, test pass: a true negative

The performance of any binary screening test is commonly summarized by two numbers: the *sensitivity*, which is the probability of a positive test result when the disorder is truly present; and the *specificity* of the test, which is the probability of the test being negative when the disorder truly is not present. A perfect test, which does not actually exist, has a perfect sensitivity (identifies all children with the disorder) and perfect specificity (does not refer anyone who does not have the disorder). A useless test would miss a large portion of the children with the disorder or refer too many people who do not have it. For example, we could say that everyone with a heartbeat has hearing loss. While this would catch everyone with a hearing loss, it would also refer all others who do not have the disorder. Conversely, we could say that only those with blue eyes have hearing loss; this test would miss everyone with different eye color who also has hearing loss. These examples would not meet good sensitivity and specificity. When choosing a screening protocol, you must be aware of the sensitivity and selectivity of the test chosen so you refer the appropriate people, not missing too many and not overreferring either.

---

surement, wide band reflectance, has been introduced to contrast single-frequency tympanometry. This test uses a similar procedure as typical 226 Hz tympanometry, but is composed of a wide range of frequencies, up to approximately 10 kHz. This newer measurement has the potential to improve clinical diagnosis of infants, children, and adults with middle ear pathology.

Pure-Tone Air Conduction

Supra-aural headphones are suggested to be used for hearing screenings. Devices should be cleaned between children using antimicrobial wipes or cloths. Screening should occur at 1000, 2000, and 4000 Hz and at 20 dB HL. This means that you should set the audiometer at 20 dB and see if the child

---

CLINICAL TIP: Recognizing a Hearing Problem

What does a hearing loss look like? It is often invisible. It can present in a variety of factors:

- Classroom misbehavior
- Not following directions
- Immature social skills
- Unclear or unintelligible speech
- Limited vocabulary or only uses concrete words

- Difficulty with words with ambiguous or multiple meanings (e.g., right)
- Reading or reading comprehension concerns
- Inattention/distractible
- Socially withdrawn/plays alone
- Passivity/shyness (never speaks up)
- Bossiness (controls conversations)

CLINICAL TIP: Tympanometry and Ear Tubes

When conducting tympanometry, it is expected that you would see a large ear canal volume in a child with PE tubes, assuming that they are open. Tubes are placed in the eardrum by a physician to relieve the pressure and allow for drainage of the middle ear space. When tympanometry is conducted, the ear canal volume is measured in the outer and middle ear for children with tubes.

If you visually see a tube, but obtain a normal middle ear volume, this can suggest that the tube has migrated out of the ear. If the eardrum is moving normally, this is a good sign that the tube has fulfilled its job and no referral is needed. If the tube is clogged or not functioning and the ear canal is normal size and the eardrum is not moving, the child should be referred back to the physician.

---

responds. If they do not, no need to turn it up, just move on to the next frequency. If a child does not respond to the sound, try one more time and then refer for follow-up testing. Audiometers should be calibrated yearly to ensure consistent and appropriate function. ASHA guidelines for hearing screening are available in Appendix G.

Other concerns to note should be if the child has any speech or language delays and any behavioral problems or concerns as these can be signs of hearing loss. If you, a teacher, or parent expresses concerns about a child's attention or hearing ability, refer on for further testing.

It should also be noted that sometimes a child may fake a hearing loss. This is also called non-organic hearing loss as discussed in Chapter 3. There is ample evidence that children who present a nonexistent or exaggerated hearing loss are at risk for having psychosocial problems. Beyond determining genuine hearing status, SLPs and audiologists can play a key role in identifying the possibility of psychosocial problems and referring for evaluation of any underlying problem. The child may have normal hearing or may be exaggerating a hearing loss. Rates of false or exaggerated hearing loss in children are unclear; however, older data suggests that it may be around 2% of those children who are screened. Girls outnumber boys by 2:1 and it is most common between 7 and 16 years of age, with exaggeration being most common around 11 years of age. For the most part, losses are reported as consistent across all frequencies and between ears. The most common causes for exaggeration are school difficulties, history of ear disease, seeking attention, and psychosocial problems. Typically, school performance is low despite having normal intelligence.

Describing the Impact of Hearing Loss to Teachers and Parents

While the actual description and impact should come from an audiologist, as an SLP, you may be responsible for reiterating and reinforcing the recommendations and outcomes described by the audiologist. Chapter 10 will discuss the rehabilitation process, including the impact of hearing loss on speech and language development and other educational and social impacts of hearing loss.

Demonstrating the hearing loss may be a way to show the teacher or parent the impact of hearing loss. There are many places and systems that are available to demonstrate hearing loss; however, unlike vision, it is not just removing the auditory information, there are also understanding problems associated with hearing loss, so keep this in mind when describing the hearing loss. Further, ensuring that the family and teacher understand that hearing loss is more than just sounds are not loud enough will set appropriate expectations for hearing aid/cochlear implant and other device use. Success for Kids with Hearing Loss has several simulations available for public use to describe hearing loss, use of cochlear implants, use of hearing aids, and other simulations (http://www.successforkids

withhearingloss.org). Keep in mind, when working with teachers, they are often busy, have a full room of children, and the child with hearing loss is not their only child of concern. When describing the impact, keep it to small chunks of information and under 10 min. Hearing loss can impact the child even more when the family and teacher don't understand the hearing loss. For parents, the exam and explanation may be overwhelming; they may come to you for more information, particularly, how hearing loss impacts their child's speech, language, and educational development. The Early Listening and Function (ELF) questionnaire may be useful in helping the parents reconcile their child's hearing loss with educational function. For older children, the Children's Home Inventory of Listening Difficulties (CHILD) may be useful to help parents and teachers develop a plan for educational success.

Disability Laws Related to Education

The purpose of the Individuals with Education Act (IDEA) is to "ensure that all children with disabilities have available to them a free, appropriate education that emphasizes special education and related services designed to meet their unique needs and prepare them for further education, employment, and independent living." Its purpose is also to ensure that children with disabilities have their right's protected. Schools are tasked with providing a free and appropriate education (FAPE) for all eligible students. The IDEA law of 2004 states that each state must provide any individual child with a disability FAPE regardless of the child's disability, even if the child has not failed or repeated a grade. There are two types of plans that are available to states and school districts

THINGS TO REMEMBER: Turn It to the Left!

An important and often overlooked component of hearing screening programs in school-aged children is education regarding hearing protection and conservation. You have a prime one-on-one opportunity to pass along some advice that might change their life. This component is particularly important for adolescents and teens who are at increased risk for noise-induced hearing loss. Recent evidence suggests a significant increase in noise-induced hearing loss in teens. Loud music and earphone use is likely the culprit for this spike in hearing loss. In a recent study, 46% of teens reported tinnitus, with 1/6 reporting it all the time. While 88% of the teens reported that they knew that their music was often too loud, most of them reported that they would not turn it down unless asked to do so. So tell them to turn it to the left (the volume control that is)! See Figure 9–7 for some examples.

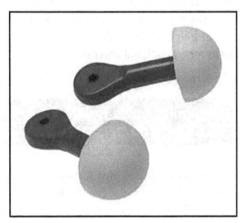

A

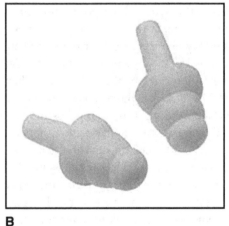

B

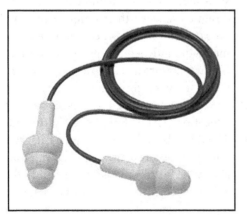

C

Figure 9–7. A–C. Examples of hearing protection. *Source*: Photos courtesy of 3M © 2019. All rights reserved.

KEY CONCEPT: A Poignant Article

The article below was written by a 14-year-old student with a significant hearing loss who uses bilateral hearing aids. He has always been the only student in his school with a hearing loss. His article is titled "The Lone Sounds of Life":

My life as the only student who is hard of hearing in my school can sometimes feel like a bottomless pit of confusion. It is not always that bad, but it is a struggle. I miss a lot of sounds. I often don't even know if I have missed a sound, sometimes at my own expense. My life at school is defined by what I hear, what I don't hear, and how I learn to cope with the differences.

When I meet new people, they do not always notice my hearing aids. They often do not understand why I do things in a different way, and it may seem weird to them. They will shout at me because they think I am doing something wrong, even though it is just the way I do things. Sometimes, even when they do notice my hearing aids, they will still shout at me. They think I am just being "difficult" or I am lying about my hearing loss. They think I am dumb or don't have any "feelings" because I can't hear well.

In school, I struggle with how some teachers act. They cannot seem to adjust to having a student who is hard of hearing. For example, even though my parents and I have asked them not to, they will do things like speak facing the board and not toward the class. The sound just bounces off the board and away from me. I can only hear a bit of what they say. I can't understand those lone bits of sound if they don't talk to me.

Teachers will also sometimes change assignments orally and I will miss what they say. Then, when I turn in the assignment, I get marked down or get an "incompletion" grade, even if I have everything else correct. This makes me feel sad and confused because I try so hard, but I don't seem to meet their standards. It is not that I cannot do the work, but I need to do it my way. It takes a lot of extra energy to do simple things, like listen to a lecture or take notes on a video that is not closed-captioned. If I cannot see the notes or the information the teachers are trying to pass on to me, I find it harder to understand.

I have learned how to cope with the frustrations of being hard of hearing. I spend time with family and friends who understand me. I am also active in sports, like basketball, soccer, and tennis, and that helps, but it is not without problems. Occasionally while playing basketball, I will receive a technical foul because I cannot hear the referee, and once a soccer coach threatened to kick me off the team because I couldn't hear him.

Surprisingly, there are some advantages to being hard of hearing. When I sleep without my hearing aids, noises don't wake me up. I sleep well and have lots of energy when I wake up. The only bad part, of course, is actually having to get up. In school, I find it easy to focus when I take my hearing aids out. Also, I can turn my hearing aids off if my parents are nagging me. Of course that just makes them mad, but, after all, I am a little bit of a teenager (but not too much of one).

There are advantages and disadvantages to being the only student who is hard of hearing in my school. Once I explain my hearing loss, most people understand and treat me fairly. Good teachers, good coaches, and other school officials have helped me thrive. I have challenges to overcome, but so does everyone else, each in their own way. I may be the only kid who is hard of hearing in my school, but as I listen to the lone sounds of my life, they tell me I am not alone.

Source: Volta Voices, May/June 2010.

regarding specialized student instruction. Individualized Education Plans (IEP) and Section 504 (504 plan) provide guidelines for the special education process. Figure 9–8 demonstrates the relationship between traditional education, 504 plans, and IEPs.

If you are an SLP in the education setting, you are likely very familiar with the 504 and IEP process, but how do these relate to hearing loss? In some states, hearing loss alone qualifies a student for an IEP; while in other states, they must also have another disability that is related or unrelated to the hearing loss. Along with the educational audiologist, you may assist with the assessment and evaluation of auditory function and determining if the child qualifies for an IEP or 504 plan. Figure 9–9 demonstrates the differences between an IEP and 504 in children with hearing loss.

In developing the IEP or 504, there are several components that should be considered

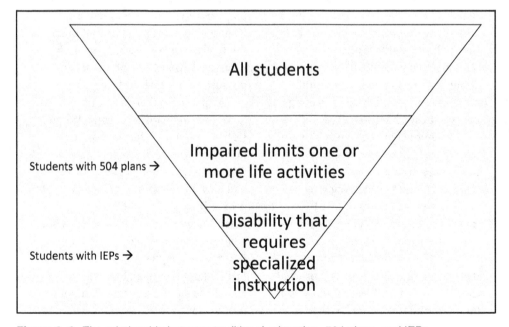

Figure 9–8. The relationship between traditional education, 504 plans, and IEPs.

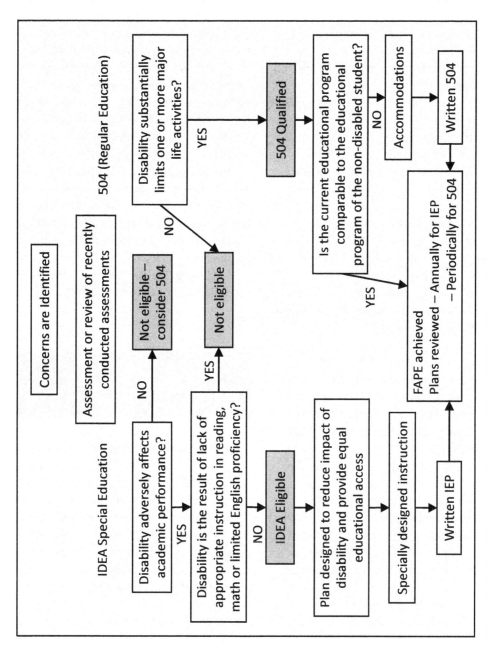

Figure 9–9. The differences between an IEP and 504 in children with hearing loss.

to get the most benefit out of the meeting and meet the needs of the student:

- Strengths of the child
- Concerns of the parents
- Results of any evaluations or interventions
- Academic progress over the last period of the IEP/504
- Developmental and functional needs of the child
- Functional needs of the child
- Available resources
- General education, special education, or other outside instructor abilities

Additionally, there are certain people who must be in an IEP/504 meeting. However, these may be waived by the parent if they choose not to have them involved. The waiver must be in written form. The team members who are mandated to participate include the following:

- Parents/guardians of the child
- At least one regular education teacher
- A representative of the school who is qualified to provide or supervise the specialty instruction or intervention needed by the child
- An individual who can interpret the results of any testing (this may be one of the people previously listed)
- Child (if child is 16 years of age or older)
- Any other institutional representatives or people as desired by the parent or child if they are 16 years of age or older

So what is the difference between an IEP and a 504? Table 9–3 demonstrates the differences; however, the primary differences have to do with funding and legal requirements. Typically, those with more severe disabilities will qualify under IEP requirements, while those with less restrictions to their education will have a 504. To qualify for an IEP, a student must qualify from two different assessments; for example, a student will not qualify based solely upon one single assessment of language ability.

While we have talked about the requirements of access to services for those with disabilities in public schools, the rules are different for parentally placed private schools or parochial schools. Private schools are not required to provide services or accommodations for students with disabilities. Private schools may apply to local school districts to provide funding for special education services based on the proportional amount of federal funding that the school district spends on special education. Because there is not a requirement to provide the services, an agreement is typically put in place as to who will provide the services—the local school district or the private school.

Support Strategies for Self-Advocacy Skills and Health Literacy

On a daily basis you advocate for patients and families. By definition, an advocate seeks support for the rights and well-being of others or the advancement of a cause. By application, you have advocated for intervention, family support, and more. You advocate for appropriate educational setting, extracurricular accommodations, technology, and continuity of care. When our patients reach adolescence, you face a new challenge—transitioning that to empowering the patient to advocate for themselves. In addition to being aware of the laws related to hearing and hearing loss, children and teens will need practice and feedback as they develop communication and interpersonal skills to

Table 9–3. Comparison of IEP and 504 Plans

	IEP	*504*
Cost	Free to children	Free to children
What does it do?	Provides specialized education and related services to meet the needs of the child	Provides list of services and methods of changing instruction to meet the needs of student to be similar to that of other students
Laws	IDEA	Section 504 of Rehabilitation Act 1973
Who is eligible?	1. Has to have one or more of the specified disabilities as listed in IDEA 2. Disability must impact the child's educational performance	1. Any disability (broader definition of disability than IEP) 2. Must interfere with child's ability to learn in general education setting
Who creates the plan?	A team utilizes strict legal criteria	People who are familiar with child and who understand the evaluation data and available services
What's in the plan?	Sets measurable learning goals for a child and describes the services the school will provide	No standard; generally includes specific accommodations or support services
How often is it reviewed?	At least every year, and evaluations must be completed every 3 years to ensure that the child qualifies for the services	Varies by state
Funding	States receive federal funding for eligible students	States do not receive any additional funding; cannot use IDEA funds

effectively explain their rights to others. These rights include acoustic access and nondiscrimination with applying to college, vocational training, and employment. Teens usually receive school-based support in developing these skills, which includes goals such as:

- assume responsibility for one's technology and educational materials;
- develop introductory financial management skills to include health-care-related financial management as,

once they reach adulthood, hearing aids may not be covered by health insurance or other state programs; and

- schedule and attend regular meetings where they will learn to advocate for their needs to hear during these meetings.

There are many resources that are available to you to assist these students in being a self-advocate in difficult situations. An example of a method to empower the student is the Guide to Access Planning (GAP).

Transition Planning in Health Care
A Proposed Three-Stage Model

Early Stage (13-14 yrs)

The Audiologist Will:

- Introduce the concept of transition
- Seek parents' thoughts on transition process
- Discuss eventual, gradual withdraw of parents from appointments
- Introduce concept of confidentiality

Sample Goals/The Patient Will:

- Explain degree, history of hearing loss
- Manage hearing technology
- Identify and repair communication challenges
- Identify support systems

Middle Stage (14-15 yrs)

The Audiologist Will:

- Discuss new thoughts/concerns of parents and patient
- Update transition plan
- Suggest 5 minutes one-on-one with patient, family steps out

Sample Goals/The Patient Will:

- Keep appointment calendar
- Become expert in hearing technology
- Know how to contact help in emergencies
- Be able to provide basic info for case history, family history

Late Stage (16-18 yrs)

The Audiologist Will:

- Update transition plan
- Provide relevant materials, info
- Suggest 10 minutes one-on-one with patient, family steps out

Sample Goals/The Patient Will:

- Maintain a personal health file
- Schedule own appointments
- Fill out health history form
- Explain legal rights and accommodations in health care

Figure 9–10. An example of a transition planning three-stage model. *Source*: From *Comprehensive Handbook of Pediatric Audiology* (2nd ed., p. 882), by A. M. Tharpe and R. Seewald, 2017, San Diego, CA: Plural Publishing. Reprinted with permission.

This checklist provides examples and ideas for areas of improvement for children and teens. This checklist is available in Appendix H. Some examples include the following:

- Hands & Voices is coauthoring information on age-specific development of safety skills with Kidpower
- PACERS's National Bulling Prevention Center
- StopBullying.gov
- Office for Civil Rights and Prohibited Disability Harassment
- Knowledge Is Power (KIP): a program to help students learn about hearing loss

See Figure 9–10 for an example of a transition planning three-stage model.

Beyond self-advocacy, it is important for a child to have good health literacy as they grow into adulthood. Patient education is not inherently easy. Every SLP has those moments when you realize that your patient does not understand you. Sometimes the patient is emotionally distraught and cannot concentrate, and sometime you may unintentionally provide more information than they can process. The ability to process the information provided and have good patient–provider communication is a part of health literacy. Health literacy should not be taken for granted. The National Assessment of Adult Literacy reports that half of the adults in the United States (77 million) have limited health literacy. Persons at or below basic literacy are not able to fully understand how to fill out medical paperwork or follow a calendar. Related to low health literacy, they are more likely to make mistakes in medication usage, have more emergency room visits and hospitalizations, and are at a higher risk of death. This could mean misunderstanding how to use a hearing aid or how to use the devices provided to them. Further, they may misunderstand their rights and the responsibilities related to being a person with a hearing-related disability. As an SLP, you may help the student with understanding medical paperwork, medications, speaking with a health-care provider, and advocating for their needs related to their health care. These skills are essential as they enter adulthood.

Hearing Loss and Learning

Children with hearing loss present a unique challenge in school to a teacher, classroom, and a speech-language pathologist. According to the Centers for Disease Control (CDC), 1.3 out of every 1,000 8-year-olds has hearing loss in both ears of at least 40 dB and at least 14.9% of children between 6 and 19 years of age have at least a minimal hearing loss in both ears. Even hearing loss in one ear can have a tremendous impact on school performance. Research suggests that children with hearing loss in only one ear have a 25% to 35% change of failing at least one grade.

To state the obvious, hearing and learning are connected. As discussed in previous chapters, hearing is essential to the perception of speech and, therefore, is critical to speech and language development. Those who desire to use auditory and spoken communication require auditory input for perception to develop those skills. Hearing loss can cause delay in the development of speech and language skills, and, therefore, can cause learning problems, which results in poor school performance. For those with more severe hearing loss, the lack of intervention leads to lack of progress and many do not progress beyond the third grade. Unfortunately, poor academic performance often leads to behavioral concerns; hearing loss is often misidentified as a learning disability.

Just because a child has a hearing loss does not mean that the child is any less capable of doing well in school than their peers. However, sometimes the classroom environment itself does not support a child with hearing loss. A busy teacher who has many students or does not understand the hearing loss is often unable to alter their teaching style or assist the student with hearing loss during lessons. For example, a teacher may turn their back to the students and the child with hearing loss may struggle without access to visual cues. It typically is at about third grade that you may see a decrease in performance as that is about when teachers begin to give assignments and teaching instruction in auditory-only form as opposed to auditory and physical form. For example, a first grade teacher may take out the book, hold it up, and say, "take out your purple book and turn to page 7," while a third grade teacher will just give the instructions without providing the visual reinforcement.

In addition to the classroom environment, certain subjects are just intrinsically more difficult for a child with hearing loss. While the ability to hear affects all aspects of academic achievement, perhaps the areas most affected are those involving language concepts. Vocabulary, language arts, sentence structure, and idiomatic expressions are extremely difficult for a child affected by hearing loss to grasp.

Frustration and confusion can also play a big part in poor academic performance. Though the child may have perfectly normal speech, a child with only mild hearing loss can still have trouble hearing a teacher from a distance or in the presence of background noise. Imagine the difficulty and confusion of not being able to hear the high-frequency consonants that you as a speech pathologist know are so important to speech understanding.

In addition to academic struggles in school, children with hearing loss can also experience trouble socially. Communication is vital to social interactions and healthy peer to peer relationships; without the ability to communicate effectively, they often report feelings of isolation and unhappiness. If a child with hearing loss is excluded from social interactions or is unwilling to participate in group activities, they may become socially withdrawn, which will lead to additional unhappiness.

As an SLP, there are some areas that should receive special attention when you work with a child with hearing loss. One of the most impactful findings of evidence from the Outcomes of Children with Hearing Loss (https://ochlstudy.org/)is that children who have appropriate wear time (most of the day), hearing aids that are providing appropriate amplification, involved parents, and access to support services as needed will do significantly better than those without one or more of these. The data suggest that those who have auditory access will have better speech perception and production, and will have better educational outcomes. As an SLP, you can have an important impact on the child's outcomes. You can encourage device use and parental involvement. You may be involved in the child's assessments and educational meetings and therefore their outcomes. Directly related to SLP services, concerns related to hearing loss are provided in the following list for your consideration.

- Speech Production
  - Delays in onset of babble increase with increase in amount of hearing loss (Moeller et al., 2007)
  - Some children are at risk for slower transitions from babble to words depending on their hearing loss (Moeller et al., 2007)

- Differences in consonant repertories (McGowen et al., 2008; Moeller et al., 2007)
- Receptive and Expressive Language
  - Grammar is similar to those with normal hearing
  - Grammar understanding is similar to those with normal hearing
  - Wide variability in the literature
- Academic Outcomes
  - Educational success is directly tied to language and communication skills
  - Hearing loss limits development of language and may have a direct impact on education
    - Verbal IQ
    - Speech perception in noise
    - Localization of sounds
- Social Communication
  - More likely to have difficulty making friends, and more likely to be teased or bullied
  - Delayed in the use of advanced language to explain complex cognitive processes and social reasoning skills
  - Social reasoning and narrative discourse skills may be delayed

As an SLP, your ability to work directly on the skills that are typically lacking in children with hearing loss will significantly impact their educational performance. Further discussion on rehabilitation and rehabilitative strategies are in Chapter 10.

Hearing Aids on Little Ears

In Chapter 4, we reviewed all the different hearing aid styles that are available today. In general, we discussed many of the pros and cons that apply to adults, but what about children? Do we normally think of different styles for them? To some degree, that will depend on whether we are talking about infants and toddlers or teenagers.

Infants and Toddlers

Because children grow so quickly in their first years, the style of hearing aid most appropriate is a behind-the-ear. This style of hearing aid is connected to a mold that will be made specifically for the child. This type of hearing aid is used for several reasons.

- The child moves around a lot and the style of hearing aid with a mold will better stay in place when they are less stable, being picked up, and running around.
- The mold may be remade as many times as necessary without having to take away the aid to be remolded. This is done often as they grow. Audiologists might remake an earmold several times in one year for an infant.
  - Acoustic feedback is a significant concern for small ears. Small ears have a higher risk of feedback due to the distance between the microphone and the end of the aid where the sound exits, as well as their fast growth making the mold too small.
- As the child grows, changes may need to be made to the aid more often than with an older child. This style of hearing aid is more flexible and allows for the aid to be changed appropriately

Older Children

Older children may have a wider selection of available styles of hearing aids. Similar to adults, the style of hearing aid depends on physical limitations like dexterity and cognitive function. It is also limited based on audiometric thresholds—the more hearing loss, the more gain needed from the aid, which may drive the style selection. However, style is often left up to older children. One caveat to their selection is that for children enrolled in school, audiologists will want to ensure that the aid has the ability to access FM systems or remote microphones as necessary. For further discussion on FM systems refer to Chapter 8.

Troubleshooting

As previously discussed, hearing aid function should be ensured at the beginning of each therapy session as well as prior to any therapy. There are many things that can go wrong with devices. If there are continued problems, the person should return to see the audiologist for a solution. For example, if the child produces a lot of sweat, there are bands that can be put on the aids to protect them from moisture (Figure 9–11). In many cases, you may be the one to discover or be asked to remedy hearing aid or cochlear implant problems. The following is a list of problems and potential solutions. If these solutions do not work or the person continues to report problems, send them to their audiologist for follow-up.

Hearing aid is not making any sound

- Insert a new battery
- Check if the battery is inserted correctly
- Check to see if the sound channel is blocked; carefully remove any debris
- If rechargeable, does it simply need to be charged?

Cochlear implant is not making any sound as reported by the student

- Insert a new battery
- Ensure device is on

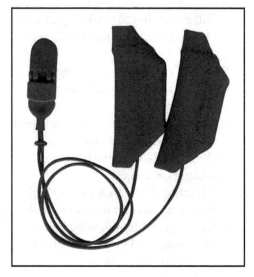

Figure 9–11. An example of sweat bands that can be put on hearing aids to try to protect them from moisture. *Source*: Photo courtesy of Ear Gear Enterprises, Inc.

- Ensure the device is on the correct ear—this is particularly true if the patient has two devices or if they are around another person with a similar device
- Check volume and sensitivity controls

Hearing aid sound is weak

- Check to see if the sound channel is blocked; carefully remove any debris
- Check to make sure that the device microphones are not clogged; carefully remove any debris

Cochlear implant is weak per report of the student

- Check to make sure that the device microphones are not clogged; carefully remove any debris
- Check cable and headpiece for cracks, shorts, or frays
- Check volume and sensitivity controls

Acoustic feedback (whistling)

- Any cracks in the shell of the hearing aid or the earmold will cause whistling; in this case, contact the audiologist
- Poor fit of the earmold will cause whistling. If the earmold no longer fits in the ear properly (the child has grown), a new earmold needs to be made. It is also possible that the person did not put it in correctly or it has become dislodged; reinsert the mold.
- If clothing or any hard surface come in contact with the hearing aid, feedback can occur
- Excessive wax in the ear canal can cause feedback; a qualified professional should remove wax

Intermittent functioning

- Corroded battery contacts; clean the contacts with alcohol
- Defective battery; replace the battery
- Moisture in the tubing; tubing can be removed from the aid and blown out using an air blower or compressed air canister
- Check cable and headpiece for cracks, shorts, or frays

Device sounds "noisy"

- Dirt in battery contacts; clean the contacts with alcohol
- Check to make sure that the device microphones are not clogged; carefully remove any debris

If these solutions don't work

- If this is a hearing aid: contact the audiologist
- If this is a cochlear implant: contact the cochlear implant manufacturer directly

Special Features for Children

There are many features that are available in current hearing aids that can help or hinder the speech, language, and auditory ability of children with hearing loss. Some of the features are automatic and should be verified as discussed in Chapter 6. As discussed in previous chapters, verification of hearing aids is essential to ensure their appropriate function. If you notice that a child is not making progress as you would expect, ask an audiologist to verify the function of the hearing aid. Additionally, you may query as to if these functions are enabled or disabled in the hearing aid.

As discussed in Chapter 5, most modern hearing aids are wide dynamic range compression hearing aids. This means that the aids compress the available auditory signals that are in speech and the world in the reduced dynamic range (softest they can hear to the loudest they can stand) of the child with hearing loss. This provides auditory access to the speech signals; however, there are some consequences of "squishing" the signal into a reduced range. Research suggests that people with hearing loss do better with compression than without because they have audible access; however, they also may struggle with distinguishing minute differences between sounds. This could have an impact on your ability to teach minor differences in speech production or perception.

Directional microphone hearing aids have made a significant impact on improving speech perception in noise. Using advanced technology, the device attempts to determine the desired signal and reduce the gain of the undesired signals. While this is not perfect, research suggests a significant improvement in speech perception in noise. However, how does this impact children? In infants, most learning occurs via incidental learning. If directional microphones cut out signals that are all around the children, it may reduce incidental learning. In school, directional microphones might reduce a child from hearing their classmates during instruction. Directional microphones should be used with caution with infants and young children. For the most part, this should not be a concern, as the directional processing is automatic, and will only activate when the background noise is at a relatively high level—higher than most listening situations for young children. With older children, directional microphone technology may be of significant benefit in noise, and again, the activation will be automatic, although it can be controlled with a smartphone app. It would be difficult today to purchase a hearing aid that does not have directional technology. Environmental manipulations should be discussed so that the child may get the most out of the directional benefit.

For children with significant high frequency hearing loss that cannot be amplified, frequency lowering may be utilized to provide acoustic access to the high frequency speech sounds (see Chapter 5 for in-depth discussion). This means that the hearing aid will take the speech sounds that occur in the unaidable frequency range and place it in a lower range. There are many philosophies and methods of doing frequency lowering and they vary by manufacturer. While the majority of the research on this feature has been conducted using one manufacturer, the research suggests that while people may report that the sound is altered, they tend to do better with identification of speech sounds. As with all amplification features, the frequency lowering should be verified. This is particularly important to ensure that /s/ and /ʃ/ are audible and different from each other.

In Closing

Studies have shown that early intervention is the key to fostering peer-level academic performance as well as healthy social interactions for children with hearing loss. Those children who had greater parental involvement, earlier intervention, and who spent more time reading scored higher on the tests than others. SLPs are in a unique position to help students by arming themselves with the knowledge as to how a student with a hearing loss receives and understands information,

---

CLINICAL NOTE: After-School Activities

Don't forget about after-school activities like drama, sports, music, or speech and debate. In kindergarten through high school, the IEP or 504 can also be used to dictate access to athletics and other after school activities. Special considerations should be made for children with hearing loss to be able to participate fully in after school activities. The state-specific high school activities association regulates the high school sports and may be able to provide information regarding specific policies related to accessibility and activities. Ideas for participation in different athletics can be found in the freely available book *Time Out! I Didn't Hear You High School Edition* and *College Edition* from Palmer et al. (2017), available at https://pitt.app .box.com/v/timeout

as well as comprehensive knowledge of an individual student's capabilities and level of comprehension. Since early intervention is key, signs SLPs and teachers can watch for in the classroom include the following:

- Inattentiveness
- Inappropriate responses to questions
- Daydreaming
- Trouble following directions
- Speech problems

Hearing loss has a significant impact on learning and educational success. Rehabili-tation will be further discussed in Chapter 10 of this book.

As an SLP, you may have a significant influence on the education of a child with hearing loss. The hearing loss has the potential to impact the educational and vocational pursuits of a child. Children who receive intervention early and often are more likely to succeed in traditional educational environments and have access to a wider array of vocational options. For the school-aged child with hearing loss, it is often the SLP who helps them navigate their educational world with their hearing loss.

10 Rehabilitation

First, it should be noted that there are entire texts and volumes of texts devoted to the rehabilitation of hearing loss—so consider our review only a starting point (e.g., Hull, 2014; Montano & Spitzer, 2009; Schow & Nerbonne, 2012; Tye-Murray, 2014).

The rehabilitation of communication function for people with hearing loss has little to do with the actual rehabilitation of hearing and more to do with communication. Very rarely does an audiologist hear that the person wants to "hear the beeps better"—with the exception of people who work with large vehicles with backup beepers. Most people are more concerned with communication ability. While we understand that most hearing devices cannot make communication perfect, the goal of hearing devices is to ensure that the person has good *communication competence*. With that in mind, this chapter will focus on several steps and processes that you can do to help those with hearing loss. In many cases, focused auditory rehabilitation will be with children, but communication competence is also important in adults.

Over the years, the term "aural rehabilitation" has been used to loosely define those activities contributing to the remediation process for persons with hearing loss. The American Speech-Hearing-Language Association released its first position statement in 1984 defining aural rehabilitation as referring to services and procedures for facilitating adequate receptive and expressive communication in individuals with hearing impairment. These services and procedures are intended for those persons who demonstrate a loss of hearing sensitivity, or function in communicative situations as if they possess a loss of hearing sensitivity. (ASHA, 1984)

The Academy of Rehabilitative Audiology, founded in 1966, viewed lipreading and auditory training paradigms as independent of the amplification provided (Alpiner, Kaufman, & Hanavan, 1993). More recently, the term *aural rehabilitation* has been used to refer to those activities or services beyond the diagnostic process, and as a supplement to the use of amplification devices, including hearing aids, cochlear implants, or any assistive listening device. Even more recently, the trend has been to refer to the rehabilitation of hearing loss as rehabilitative audiology.

Many models of adult rehabilitative audiology are available in clinical practice. Some clinicians spend one-on-one time with patients following the fitting of hearing devices and other hearing assistive devices. While those sessions are likely to focus on immediate concerns of the patient, other models include auditory-training based individual sessions and/or counseling-based group efforts. We maintain that, minimally, all hearing device provisions must include the verification, orientation, and validation procedures outlined in the previous chapters of this book. Additional training (individual or group sessions) can be used to enhance long-term outcomes. Face it, it's an acoustically hostile world out there. Any form of this so-called rehabilitative audiology helps to educate hearing-impaired people to manipulate both their situations and their approach to encountering them. Ideal "audiologic rehabilitation" is about empowering patients with accurate knowledge regarding hearing loss, communication strategies, and psychosocial impacts of impairments. It should also help each hearing device user and their families to build the confidence necessary to be active in better communication, no matter the "acoustic" weather.

Regardless of how you provide aural rehabilitation, you will find that three basic principles apply. These were explained quite nicely several years ago by Brian Walden and colleagues, based on their years of experience with the extensive aural rehabilitation program conducted at Walter Reed Army Medical Center. We borrow heavily here from the Walden, Prosek, and Holum-Hardegan (1984) article as we discuss the three principles.

Principle 1. It is unlikely that communication handicaps and the rehabilitation needs of any two patients will be exactly alike.

- A reminder that patients differ in hearing loss, speech recognition ability, personality variables, listening demands, cognitive function, family dynamics, and a variety of other factors that impact success with hearing devices.

- This means that the rehabilitative services offered, whether they be individual or in a group setting, need to be responsive to those personalized factors which bear most importantly on the patient's communication needs.

- This is why a "canned" AR program often has limited success.

Principle 2. Audiologic rehabilitation is a learning experience for the patient.

- Audiologic rehabilitation takes time. A change in communication and perception of communication will not occur until the patient has certain experiences which result in the acquisition of specific skills. The goals of AR must be consistent with the time available, or the time the patient is willing to devote keeping in mind that particularly for a child, time and

---

CLINICAL TIP: Reimbursement for AR

Medicaid, Medicare, and private insurance companies classify audiologists as diagnosing professionals who are not in a position to provide ongoing rehabilitation, and as such, are not reimbursed for their services. However, you as the speech-language pathologist (SLP) *can* be reimbursed. In 2006, CPT codes were introduced to underscore the profession-neutral status of auditory rehabilitation in lieu of audiologic rehabilitation. Audiologists or SLPs would be considered qualified providers under this code. Medicare clarified in 2008 that no provision exists in their reimbursement schedule to compensate audiologists for therapeutic services. Therefore, if a practice or school district would want to be reimbursed for providing aural rehabilitation, they would need to hire you, an SLP, to provide these services.

POINTS TO PONDER: What Does It Mean?

The original definition proffered by ASHA referred to audiologic rehabilitation as those "services and procedures for facilitating receptive and expressive communication in individuals with hearing impairment (ASHA, 1984, p. 38). That sort of covers our whole series of books and several others! How have others defined this elusive AR term?

■ "Audiologic rehabilitation is aimed at restoring or optimizing a patient's participations in activities that have been limited as a result of hearing loss and also may be aimed at benefiting communication partners who engage in activities that include persons with hearing loss." (Gagné, 2000)

■ "Adult audiologic rehabilitation is here defined holistically as the reduction of hearing-loss-induced deficits of function, activity, participation, and quality of life through a combination of sensory management, instruction, perceptual training, and counseling." (Boothroyd, 2007)

■ "Intervention aimed at treating residual problems associated with hearing loss when hearing aids alone do not provide optimal rehabilitation." (Paraphrased from Hawkins, 2005)

■ "If you are an adult, aural/audiologic rehabilitation services will focus on adjusting to your hearing loss, making the best use of your hearing aids, exploring assistive devices that might help, managing conversations, and taking charge of your communication. Services can be individual, in small groups, or a combination of both." (ASHA, n.d.)

■ "Audiologic/aural rehabilitation (AR) is an ecological, interactive process that facilitates one's ability to minimize or prevent the limitations and restrictions that auditory dysfunctions can impose on well-being and communication, including interpersonal, psychosocial, educational, and vocational functioning." (ASHA, n.d.)

■ "Audiologic habilitation/rehabilitation can be defined as those professional interactive processes actively involving the client that are designed to help a person with hearing loss." (Schow & Nerbonne, 2018)

■ "In contemporary terminology, 'rehabilitative audiology' developed as a remediation process to lessen the consequences of hearing loss on an individual's everyday life." (Alpiner and McCarthy, 2000)

commitment of family is one of the largest contributing factors to success.

■ Because it's a learning experience, a fundamental fact is that behavior changes progressively as a function of reinforcements. The concepts of extinction, generalization, and conditions of practice also apply.

■ Learning is driven by motivation. For learning to occur, the patient must first believe that there is a need, and then, the aural rehabilitation provided must significantly improve the perceived problems. In adults, these problems may be problems that were acquired over time and need to be recognized; while for a child, these may be problems that present in the future and need to be realized by the family. Either way, success depends on expectations and appropriate identification of current and future problems.

■ Regardless of the type of AR program employed, it is helpful to reassess the patient and/or parent at periodic intervals to determine if learning has occurred (e.g., objective tests or assessment inventories).

Principle 3. The patient's communication handicap is dynamic.

■ The patient's communication problems change on a short-term basis because of different listening situations, variations in motivation, emotional state, development, and many other factors.

■ The patient's communication problems change on a long-term basis because of changes in hearing impairment, communication skills, cognitive function, development, and overall health.

■ Routine periodic evaluations are important to determine if there has been a change in the communication problems and communication needs.

■ Auditory rehabilitation is an ongoing treatment and is not limited to any given period of concentrated training or therapy.

The Process of Acceptance

Rehabilitation for hearing loss typically begins before the person or family pursues hearing devices. Figure 10–1 demonstrates the factors that interrelate to the use and purchase of hearing devices.

As reviewed by Taylor and Mueller (2011), it is a commonly held belief that people go through a grieving process with a diagnosis of hearing loss. This is true for adults with acquired hearing loss or parents of a child newly-identified with hearing loss. The five stages of grief as described by Kubler-Ross are denial, anger, bargaining, depression, and acceptance. It is helpful with initiating communication with a patient or family member of a person with hearing loss that they may fall into any of these stages. The time it takes a person to move through the five stages is extremely variable; for some patients, it seems to happen in a single afternoon, for others, it may take years. Not everyone goes through all stages or goes through them in a linear fashion. Some stages may not be experienced at all. Because, in most cases, hearing loss is not life-threatening, the stages of anger may not be observed in the adult patient. However, in the parent of a child with hearing loss, these stages may last longer and have a more significant impact on the outcomes; you may have to push through some of the stages to get the child the rehabilitation they need. With the typical patient consideration, the use of hearing device, denial stage is so common it is almost expected. Examples for each stage are provided in Table 10–1.

In some cases, you may see people who are still in the denial phase. It depends on the age of the person with hearing loss as to when you approach them to push them

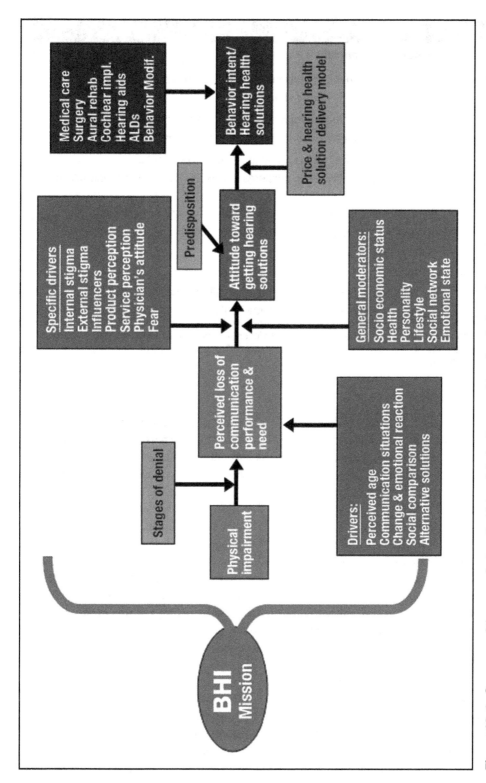

Figure 10–1. Summary of the many factors that interrelate for the use of hearing devices. *Source:* Adapted from Kochkin, 2007. From *Modern Hearing Aids: Pre-Fitting Testing and Selection Considerations* (p. 33), by H. G. Mueller, R. Bentler, and T. A. Ricketts, 2014, San Diego, CA: Plural Publishing. Reprinted with permission.

Table 10–1. Stages of Grief as Described by Kubler-Ross

Stage	What the Patient Might Say
Denial	"I don't have a hearing problem; other people mumble."
	"I hear everything I need to hear."
Anger	To their friends: "Are you purposely talking behind my back?"
	To the professional: "Are you sure you did the testing correctly?"
Bargaining	"Okay, maybe I just wasn't listening. I'll pay more attention."
	"Let's see if I'm still having problems next year, maybe my hearing will get better."
Depression	"It seems like my family avoids me because of my hearing loss."
	"There are things I'll probably never hear again."
	"I'm getting old."
Acceptance	"Wearing hearing aids is really no big deal."
	"My quality of life will probably improve with the use of hearing aids."
	"A lot of people my age have worse health problems than hearing loss."

Source: Adapted from Taylor and Mueller, 2011. From *Modern Hearing Aids: Pre-Fitting Testing and Selection Considerations* (p. 41), by H. G. Mueller, R. Bentler, and T. A. Ricketts, 2014, San Diego, CA: Plural Publishing. Reprinted with permission.

toward solution. If the person with the hearing loss is a child, you may want to push harder for the parents to decide mode of communication and move forward with a solution to this. For parents with normal hearing, initial research suggested that 40% of parents wanted their child to use spoken communication. However, as hearing device technology has improved, more recent evidence suggests that 85% of parents choose spoken communication for their child with hearing loss. (Brown, 2004; Brown, Baker, Rickarts, & Griffin, 2006) In this vein, if a parent chooses for their child to use spoken communication, the earlier they are able to be fit with a hearing device, the better their outcomes and their ability to use spoken communication as their primary means of communication. Also, just because someone has moved toward obtaining hearing devices, does not mean that they are accepting of the hearing loss. You will want to ensure that the person is using the device consistently.

An audiologist may have had the responsibility of diagnosing the hearing loss and describing the effects to a person, but you may have to do it again, and again, and again. Knowing how to describe the audiogram (as discussed in Chapter 2) may be important for you to explain the impact of hearing loss on speech, language, and communication. Keep the following key tips in mind when providing counseling about hearing loss and the effects on communication:

■ The audiogram may not provide the most useful information for the person to decide. The perceived needs of the patient and/or parents are couched more often in terms of the impact of hearing loss, the perceived potential

---

CLINICAL TIP: Allowing a Child to Choose

Keep in mind that allowing a child to "choose" whether or not they want to pursue hearing devices is often making the choice for them. By the time a child can make an informed decision, their window of receiving the most benefit from the device has passed. Evidence suggests that for a child to receive the most benefit from hearing devices, they need to receive access to auditory cues early-on in auditory, speech, and lan- guage developmental process. By fitting them with the appropriate devices early, they are receiving access to the auditory information. If later on the child chooses not to use the device, their previous access will not hinder their ability to use visual communication. However, by not fitting them with the device, they miss the critical period for auditory, speech, and language acquisition; they cannot receive the same benefits later on.

---

impact, and the long-term ramifications of treatment

- Don't provide too much information at one time. At any given appointment, a patient and family can only perceive and remember so much information. Information should be presented gradually, using a variety of formats. Absorbing details about diagnosis, treatment, and implications may be too much for the person and the family to absorb at one time.
- Family-centered care placed our patient in the context of their everyday lives. Many patients and family want to understand how their hearing loss will impact their current and future goals and communication challenges. Focusing on this may help patients and families better understand the hearing loss and the implications.

Erdman (2009) discusses the importance of an empathetic practitioner–patient relationship which can engage the patient and may turn their management of the treat- ment and adherence to the treatment. You have the opportunity to provide patients and families with the opportunity to ask questions and gain a better understanding of the hearing loss and its impact. Part of the role of the SLP may be empathetic listening and the provider of quality educa- tion with a compassionate, understanding ear. Figure 10–2 demonstrates a model for empathetic listening in relation to hearing loss. Through empathetic counseling, you are providing rehabilitation to the patient in relation to hearing loss. You will help people move toward determining what they would like to do with the information.

Mode of Communication

Prior to starting any rehabilitative audiology program in children particularly, it is impor- tant to discuss the parents' desired primary means of communication. As discussed pre- viously, most hearing parents will choose spoken language for their children, but

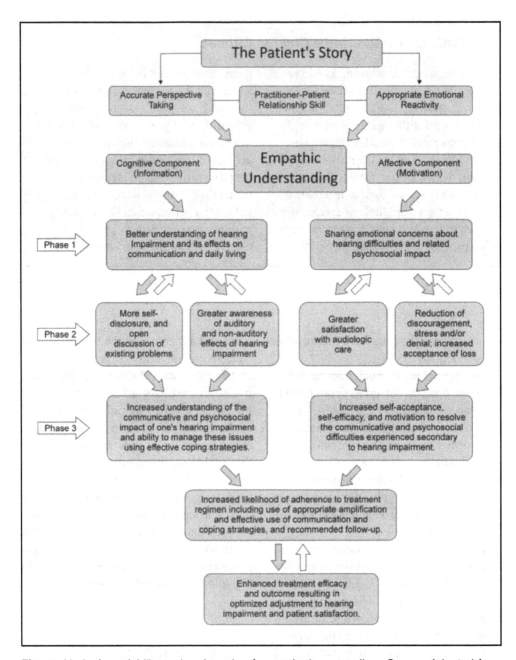

Figure 10–2. A model illustrating the role of empathetic counseling. *Source*: Adapted from Erdman, 2009. From *Modern Hearing Aids: Pre-Fitting Testing and Selection Considerations* (p. 45), by H. G. Mueller, R. Bentler, and T. A. Ricketts, 2014, San Diego, CA: Plural Publishing. Reprinted with permission.

Table 10–2. Communication Approaches and Philosophies (Stredler-Brown, 2009)

Communication Approaches & Philosophies	Definition
Auditory–Verbal Approach	This is an educational approach in which technology is paired with specific techniques and strategies that teach children to listen and understand spoken language. A primary emphasis is placed on access to learning through the auditory modality. This refinement of the auditory–oral approach makes a concerted effort to remove visual cues during therapy sessions so the child can develop the auditory system through directed listening practice. Speechreading is not a primary teaching strategy and this visual information is reduced or eliminated during therapy by covering most of the face while presenting speech stimuli (Estabrooks, 1994).
Auditory–Oral Approach	This approach combines oral spoken language to express oneself and speechreading, accompanied by active listening, to receive information. The use of natural gestures is acceptable.
Sign-Supported Speech and Language	The use of signs to support spoken language development serve as a "bridge" to completely oral communication. Signs may be used as a "backup" in certain situations such as noisy environments or when a hearing device is not in use (Lane et al., 2006).
Simultaneous Communication	This is the use of signs and speech at the same time. In order to provide language in both modes simultaneously, a sign system, rather than a signed language, is used. Pidgin Signed English (PSE), Conceptually Accurate Signed English (CASE), and Manually Coded English (MCE) are examples of sign systems.
Bilingual Model	A person who achieves fluency in American Sign Language and English is bilingual. ASL is often the first language, with English being taught as a second language, to develop literacy skills. English can be taught using a sign system or through print. Spoken English is not included in the bilingual model that is currently promoted by the Deaf Community.
Total Communication	Introduced in the 1960s by Roy Holcomb, this "philosophy" aims to use a number of strategies or modes of communication including sign, oral, auditory, written, and other visual aids. The choice of modalities depends on the particular needs and abilities of the child. The philosophy professes to provide whatever is needed to foster communicative success.

Source: From *Introduction to Aural Rehabilitation* (2nd ed., p. 163), by R. H. Hull, 2014, San Diego, CA: Plural Publishing. Reprinted with permission.

having the discussion and making parents aware of the resources available to them as well as providing information about the Deaf community is an important first step. Table 10–2 discusses communication approaches and philosophies.

Hearing Aid Function

First things first, the person and/or family must understand how to use the device. The audiologist should have explained all of the parts, pieces, and function of the device. However, because there is a lot of information, much of the information may be lost or forgotten. Therefore, your general understanding of the function of the hearing aid, cleaning and checking of the device, and general connectivity may be crucial to the use of the device. As discussed earlier, the best predictor of hearing device success is device use—the person must be able to use the device to be able to wear it consistently.

Realistically, this means that you may have to do troubleshooting on the device. As an SLP, you may have to show parents, teachers, administrators, kids, and adults how to check to ensure the device is working and how to do basic repairs. While discussed in depth in Chapter 9, Table 10–3 provides a list of problems and how to troubleshoot. While this is not exhaustive—it does not cover things like the dog eating the hearing aid—it will cover many of the basic problems and potential solutions. If after you try these and the device still does not work, then the device will likely need to be repaired. In the case of a hearing aid or other assistive device, this will likely mean contacting the audiologist. In the case of an implantable device, you may contact the manufacturer directly; they will walk you through troubleshooting and replacing the problematic parts.

Table 10–3. Troubleshooting Problems and Solutions

Symptom	Cause	Possible Remedy
Hearing instrument has no sound.	Hearing instrument is turned off.	Check to ensure that the hearing instrument is turned on.
	Battery is upside down.	Be sure the battery is in the correct orientation (plus [+] side up for custom instruments).
	Battery is depleted or dead.	Replace the battery.
	Microphone protector is plugged.	Consult your audiologist.
	Hearing instruments, earmolds, slim tubes, and/or domes are blocked with earwax.	Clean earmolds and/or domes. Use cleaning wire to dislodge earwax in slim tubes. Use wax loop to remove wax from the sound outlet. Consult your audiologist.
	Hearing instrument is damaged or defective.	Consult your audiologist.

Table 10–3. *continued*

Symptom	Cause	Possible Remedy
Hearing instrument isn't loud enough.	The volume is set too low.	Turn up the volume. Consult your audiologist for models without a manual volume control or if problem persists.
	Battery is depleted or dead.	Replace the battery.
	Hearing instruments, earmolds, slim tubes, and/or domes are not inserted properly.	Remove and reinsert carefully.
	Hearing instruments, earmolds, slim tubes, and/or domes are blocked with earwax.	Clean earmolds and/or domes. Use cleaning wire to dislodge earwax in slim tubes. Use wax loop to remove wax from the sound outlet. Consult your audiologist.
	Microphone protector is plugged.	Consult your audiologist.
	Your hearing has changed.	Consult your audiologist.
Hearing instruments are whistling.	Noise or whistling when a hand and/or clothing are near ear.	Move hand and/or clothing away from ear.
	Hearing instruments, earmolds, slim tubes, and/or domes are not inserted properly.	Remove and reinsert carefully.
	Hearing instruments, earmolds, slim tubes, and/or domes are blocked with earwax.	Clean earmolds and/or domes. Use cleaning wire to dislodge earwax in slim tubes. Use wax loop to remove wax from the sound outlet. Consult your audiologist.
	Hearing instruments, earmolds, and/or slim tubes are fitting poorly.	Consult your audiologist.
	Battery is depleted or dead.	Replace the battery.
	Microphone protector is plugged.	Consult your audiologist.
Sound is distorted or unclear.	Battery is depleted or dead.	Replace the battery.
	Hearing instruments, earmolds, and/or slim tubes are fitting poorly.	Consult your audiologist.
	Hearing instrument is damaged or defective.	Consult your audiologist.

continues

Table 10–3. *continued*

Symptom	Cause	Possible Remedy
Performance is inconsistent.	Battery is depleted or dead.	Replace the battery.
	Battery contact is dirty.	Consult your audiologist.
Hear beeps.	Battery is depleted or dead.	Replace the battery.
Earmolds, slim tubes, and/or domes are falling out of ear.	Hearing instruments, earmolds, slim tubes, and/ or domes are not inserted properly.	Remove and reinsert carefully.
	Hearing instruments, earmolds, and/or slim tubes are fitting poorly.	Consult your audiologist.
The sound is weak on the telephone.	Hearing instrument requires adjustment.	Consult your audiologist.
	Telephone is not positioned properly.	Move telephone receiver around ear for clearer signal.

Source: Adapted from Unitron, Inc. From *Essentials of Modern Hearing Aids: Selection, Fitting, and Verification* (P. 712–713), by T. A. Ricketts, R. Bentler, and H. G. Mueller, 2019, San Diego, CA: Plural Publishing. Reprinted with permission.

CLINICAL TIP: A Few Hearing Device Tips

1. Avoid temperature extremes—don't leave them in the hot car
2. Avoid moisture when possible
3. Do not use hairspray or hairdryers (while wearing the hearing aids)
4. Do not take apart the hearing device
5. Keep hearing device away from pets—dogs and cats can be drawn to feedback and even the smell of their owner's earwax

---

DID YOU KNOW: Rice Is Not Just for Supper Anymore!

A recent study suggested that rice may be just as effective at removing moisture from an electronic device as a professional drying system. In 2017, Nelson, White, Baker, Hayden, and Bird compared rice with several commercial desiccants. They found that all performed equally as well at removing moisture from hearing devices. So if a hearing device gets wet, try placing it in a bag of uncooked rice overnight. This may revive its function. However, beware! Pieces of rice could become lodged in the hearing device making it nonfunctional. We are a fan of Uncle Ben's, although the article did not identify a specific brand.

What Are the AR Goals?

Rehabilitation depends heavily on when the person became hearing impaired and the method by which the hearing loss occurred. At the onset of any AR, it is important to consider the *real* goals of such an undertaking. If your program involves intensive auditory training for understanding speech in background noise, you could conduct pre- and posttests such as the QuickSIN or HINT to see if there was an improvement. If one wishes to maximize patient satisfaction, we can look to the literature for areas where reasonable benefit has been demonstrated after using one of the types of intervention. If the goal is to improve the auditory skills of a child and catch them up to their normal hearing peers, this is a reasonable goal as well. A number of outcome domains have been studied extensively in terms of auditory rehabilitation in children and adults, and have shown positive benefits for the hearing device user:

- Quality of Life (QOL): Kramer, Allessie, Dondorp, Zekveld, and Kapteyn (2005), Preminger (2009), Preminger and Yoo (2010)
- Hearing handicap: Abrams, Hnath-Chisolm, Guerreiro, and Ritterman (1992), Beynon, Thornton, and Poole (1997)
- Psycho-social status: Chisolm, Abrams, and McArdle (2004), Krikos and Holmes (1996)
- Speech recognition performance: Burke and Humes (2008)
- Performance in noise: Burke and Humes (2007)
- Cortical changes: Gil and Iorio (2010), Kraus (2012)
- Returns for credit: Martin (2007)

- Satisfaction: Brickley, Cleaver, and Bailey (1996), Wayner and Abrahamson (1996)

Counseling as Part of the AR Process

There are several models of AR, and we discuss providing information in AR groups and individual training later. Whether we are considering these specific approaches, the hearing device orientation, or other patient interactions, counseling is an important and integral part of provision of AR. Counseling in this context is meant neither as a psychological or psychiatric intervention, nor a stand-alone approach to accelerating or enhancing hearing aid success. Yet, every interaction the clinician has with the patient will be influenced by the counseling skill of the professional. It is for this reason that counseling training is a part of every audiology and SLP curriculum.

Informational Versus Personal Adjustment Counseling

It is easy for the novice clinician to confuse what is essentially information sharing with personal adjustment counseling. Both are necessary and are intertwined throughout the process of audiologic rehabilitation. From re-explaining the results of an audiogram to the last session of an expanded audiologic rehabilitation program, the patient and parents may/will exhibit needs in both realms and it remains the scope of the SLP to field all but the most pathologic expressions of emotion and adjustment related to hearing impairment (however, in some cases, it is necessary and appropriate to refer a patient to a professional counselor when the counseling issue falls outside your scope of

---

THINGS TO REMEMBER: Being an Effective Counselor

The following are taken from a Bob Margolis article (2004) and provide several key points to remember when conducting counseling with additional notes in italics:

1. Understand and address the patient's (*and parents'*) desires and beliefs
2. Give advice as concrete instructions
3. Use easy to understand language
4. Repeat the most important information
5. Present the most important information first to capitalize on primacy effect
6. Stress the importance of recommendations that you want them to remember
7. State or preview the information that will be shared during the appointment; ask for confirmation of their understanding of this information
8. Present small amounts of information
9. Supplement verbal information with written, graphic, and pictorial information
10. Remember these recommendations are even more important for seniors (*and parents of newly-identified children*)!

---

practice). In general, given a fixed amount of time, most SLPs fill the time with too much informational counseling and too little personal adjustment counseling. Informational counseling easily can be conducted on "cruise control," without a personal involvement with the patient, as the spiel is pretty much the same for everyone. Personal adjustment counseling requires careful thought and needs to be individualized. Both clinician and patient factors impact the success of these efforts.

SLPs are not distinct from other professionals who act in a counseling role in terms of required professional courtesy. The therapeutic alliance built can be undone by consistent failure on the part of the clinician to provide a modicum of politeness and respect for the client. Examples may seem impossibly straightforward: using the last name

with our adult patients, leaning down when speaking with children, avoiding tardiness, making eye contact, maintaining alertness, and so forth; but failure to adhere to these basic rules of professional courtesy can undermine the relationship and cause irreparable damage.

The Ida Institute, a more recent inclusion to our profession, has evolved in an effort to help the field of rehabilitative audiology. You can find a lot of great resources on their website! Their outcome data suggest that those who use their resources are more prepared to work with adults and children with hearing loss across the spectrum of needs. The Institute provides a wide range of tools and trainings to help clinicians at any developmental level improve his or her skills. Especially ubiquitous have been the patient motivation tools to quickly get to

---

TECHNICAL TIP: What Is Remembered?

Regarding informational counseling, as noted earlier, a patient may not remember what we say. As reported by Margolis (2004), we know that about 50% of the information presented to the patient is forgotten immediately and about 50% of the information that the patient *does* remember is incorrect. In one large study, 68% of patients could not remember the diagnosis that was told to them.

---

the heart of a patient's or parent's readiness to seek intervention and ferret out what may be more salient motivations against intervention.

Patient Factors

The patients and families rarely come with an instruction manual. Consequently, we are left to determine which patient needs which intervention. Some clinicians assess personality characteristics in an effort to predict adherence to recommendations. While we agree there is promise in this area related to better serving patients based on personality traits, we believe more work needs to be done before we can recommend evidence-based guidelines for this practice. Cox et al. (2005) have studied the five personality traits of the NEO-FFI[1] (Costa & McCrae, 1992) to quantify personality factors independent of hearing loss: neuroticism, openness, extroversion, agreeableness, and conscientiousness. They found that those seeking hearing devices are lower in openness than the rest of the normal-trait population. The authors suggest that persons who are low in openness are often unable to effectively or creatively fill in gaps in knowledge, thus seeking the help of the clinician. Those same individuals are often not successful at devising alternative strategies to facilitate their communication success. The same investigators have found that persons seeking hearing devices are also lower in neuroticism. It is contended that those high in neuroticism are unwilling to experience communication breakdowns and face embarrassment. They are more prone to worry. Using a tool such as the NEO-FFI might offer insight into the likelihood of any one patient or family benefiting from additional rehabilitation beyond the issuance of the hearing devices. It is also possible to be used when discord is observed between family members or parents when approaching the use of the hearing devices.

There may also be gender differences among those seeking audiologic rehabilitation services as well. Garstecki and Erler (1998) found that females reported less denial and greater problem awareness related to hearing loss than did males. These researchers also found that women place greater importance on social communication than men, which might influence their decision to seek help for their hearing difficulties.

---

[1] NEO stands for Neuroticism, Extroversion, and Openness; FFI refers to the five factors that are assessed in this inventory: neuroticism, extroversion, openness, agreeableness, and conscientiousness.

As far as adjustment to hearing loss, other authors have reported that females report greater use of nonverbal communication strategies, and are more likely to admit to physical and mental disabilities (Erdman & Demorest, 1998; Garstecki & Erler, 1998, 1999; Padgett, 1999). In this vein, you may appeal to the mother of a child more easily than a father. It is possible that the mother may move toward acceptance more quickly than the father and the mother may be your resource to move toward a rehabilitate strategy for a child with hearing loss.

Types of AR Programs

There are two primary means of providing aural rehabilitation, individually or in a group. For most children, you will integrate aural rehabilitation into other therapies and, thus, it will likely occur on a one-on-one basis. Additionally, given the variability between children and their distractibility, it may be impractical to practice group aural rehabilitation. First, we will discuss group rehabilitation, then we will delve into individual therapy programs.

As an addendum here: not all AR programs need to be multisession and include homework! Allen Montgomery (1994), who for many years worked with the audiologic rehabilitation program at Walter Reed Army Medical Center, describes a brief AR course wherein there is only one hour of material presented; this could be in a group or individually. (His mantra: A little bit of AR is better than nothing, which is what happens most of the time.) The program starts with describing lipreading, moves on to specific AR techniques, and ends with consumer education. WATCH is the acronym for the five steps of the model.

W—Watch the talker's mouth, not just the eyes

The patient is encouraged to watch their conversational partner's mouth at all times for speech reading. It may be difficult at first to stop maintaining eye contact. First, have the patient practice the technique when stationary, and then try it while walking around the room. If this is a child, remind the parent that they have to get the child's attention and look at them the entire time. Encourage the patient to practice at home. Inform the patient and/or parent that speech reading is a great way to aid in understanding speech in noisy situations when it is impossible to turn the noise down.

A—Ask specific questions

Patients are encouraged to ask for clarification in more specific ways than by asking, "What?" or "Huh?" or feigning understanding. To practice this technique, the clinician can speak in a lower voice and slur or mumble words. For example, the patient might hear, "We are going to see the movie at 6 o'clock." Instead of asking, "What?" the patient is encouraged to ask, "At what time are we going to the movie?" Another point of this is rephrasing. Instead of repeating back exactly what was said previously, the talker should change the phrase. Instead of repeating the same phrase they could say, "The movie starts at 6 o'clock tonight."

T—Talk about your hearing loss

As discussed previously, self-advocacy is particularly important for successful communication. The patient is informed of the importance of telling conversational partners about their hearing loss. It is important because many sources of communication breakdown (noise, talker clarity, etc.) cannot be compensated for by the hearing devices alone. Therefore, to help themselves out, the patient, and/or parent if the child is very young, must be willing to tell the communication partner about the hearing loss and ask them to turn down the noise, move to a quieter place, move somewhere with better lighting, and to look directly at the person with hearing loss when they are speaking.

C—Change the situation

The clinician and patient discuss where communication breakdowns occur and how to overcome them. When the patient and/or parent is upfront about their hearing loss, they can then more easily make changes when a breakdown occurs. As the breakdown is usually due to auditory or visual interference, if the patient can recognize why it is occurring, they can take steps to change the situation, such as asking a server in a restaurant to stand where facial features are more visible.

H—Health care knowledge

The clinician tells the patient where to obtain hearing health care and hearing loss information. This can be in the form of audiologists, websites, magazines, books, and support groups.

Group AR Programs

For adults, it is common to provide AR in the form of group settings in which persons with hearing loss and their significant others meet with the audiologist for three or four group classes following the provision of the hearing devices. When group AR is provided, it is typically following the individualized counseling and information session that is part of the hearing device fitting/mapping and orientation. Hawkins (2005) notes the major advantages of the counseling-based group model:

- it allows persons with hearing loss to share feelings, problems, and solutions with others and learn alternative ways of dealing with communication breakdown;
- the clinician is able to provide services to more people with hearing loss in the same amount of time; and
- it is (consequently) more financially feasible for the clinician and the persons with hearing loss to provide group AR than individual AR.

While group programs may vary from setting to setting, they share many common features. The ideal group involves four or five couples or families with one or more having a hearing loss. You serve as the leader and facilitator. The group sessions typically span 3 to 6 weeks, with 1 to 2 hr sessions. They are designed to include three types of experiences (Montgomery, 1995):

- Members share feelings, experiences, successes, and failures concerning their hearing loss. They should not feel judged or shamed about their feelings or concerns.
- Structured activities such as communication strategies training and/or assertiveness training, with or without role-playing, are conducted.
- Information relative to the hearing mechanism, hearing disorders, hearing devices options, and other consumer-related topics is imparted.

While group AR sessions are usually a "feel good" thing for both the clinician and the patients attending, the underlying question is: Do these counseling-based group programs result in better *outcomes*? Greater hearing device benefit and satisfaction? This can be difficult to assess as in most clinical situations, the individuals who attend the group sessions are those patients who want to make hearing devices work for them. Because of their motivation and attitude, they probably would have been successful without the help of the group. Those patients who are not motivated to use hearing aids usually are also not motivated to attend group AR. However, evidence does suggest that these group AR programs have improvement in outcomes for people with hearing loss and their families.

Individualized Auditory-Training Based AR

To this point we have primarily talked about counseling-based group AR. But not all AR is carried out in groups. In fact, many clinicians believe individual training sessions serve their practice and purposes better, not to mention the needs of their patients. The earliest efforts regarding individualized programs were those developed to assist the rehabilitation of soldiers who had suffered hearing loss while serving in the military (Carhart, 1947). The program consisted of several stages that followed "the practical instruction of the use and care of the aid" and attempted to establish "an attitude of critical listening" (p. 293). The stages included the following:

- Carefully planned drills in listening and discriminating sound contrast patterns
- Precise and rapid recognition of phonemic elements
- Recognition of significant noises
- Listening under poor acoustical conditions

Despite this early contention that practice in *listening* improved skills in *hearing*, most later approaches to providing audio-logic rehabilitation commonly focused on lipreading or speech reading training alone through organized practice. One could argue that all AR models should include *listening* training. In fact, some clinicians have recently pushed to refocus the individualized approach on both listening and comprehension training. While there are many ways to accomplish auditory training and ways to describe it, we prefer this definition from Sanders (1971, p. 205): "*A systematic procedure designed to increase the amount of information that a person's hearing contributes to his or her total perception.*"

Evidence That Auditory Training Is Beneficial

Auditory-based programs encompass any structured lessons and drills designed to improve ability to accurately detect and perceive speech at the sound, word, and sentence level. There is emerging evidence that such training can help some people. Unfortunately, *strong* scientific evidence in this particular realm is sparse. For that reason, we will review some of the evidence base for individual auditory-based AR training programs here.

Humes et al. (2009) trained patients with easy and hard words hoping to see if they could find generalization to running speech in noise. Patients improved on the trained words in and out of sentences. Performance wavered over time after training, but brief retraining was able to maintain performance. In earlier work, Burke and Humes (2007) found that lexically hard words did not generalize to easier words, but longer training paradigms did improve the generalizability of trained words to sentences.

Other investigators have looked for cortical evidence of change following auditory training exercises. Tremblay and colleagues have demonstrated a variety of cortical changes that take place with auditory training including N1–P2 amplitude increase for detecting voice onset time, asymmetric cortical changes with synthetic speech training for P1 and N1 measurements, and increase in mismatch negativity across generalized stimuli (Tremblay & Kraus, 2002; Tremblay, Kraus, Carrell, & McGee, 1997; Tremblay, Kraus, McGee, Ponton, & Otis, 2001). More recent work from Nina Kraus' lab at Northwestern University suggests that if you spend time actively working on making sound-to-meaning connections (i.e., auditory training tasks), you create a nervous system that is automatically able to respond more consistently, pick up on meaningful sound patterns, and efficiently represent meaningful elements of sound (Slater et al., 2015). Still, it is difficult to draw conclusions about cortical evidence for changes as a result of auditory training, as these studies were completed with normal hearing listeners and the measures assessed a clinical parameter not corroborated with behavioral or subjective improvements in self-perceived difficulty or handicap.

Another area of concern is whether the auditory training that patients undergo actually generalizes to *other* stimuli. Well, those data are mixed as well. An early (pre-computer) program developed by Pat Krikos and Alice Holmes (1996), which trained syllable recognition and communication strategies, indeed generalized to the speech-in-noise outcome measure used in their research. And Rubinstein and Boothroyd (1987) found that their top-down training (on skills such as using linguistic context or practicing auditory working memory) generalized, but that their bottom-up training (training the listener to decode the speech signal by, for example, practicing how to hear the difference between /ba/ and /da/) did not. Sweetow and Sabes (2006) showed that trained skills did seem to transfer or generalize to other stimuli; specifically, they found that after training on a speech-in-babble task, their participants did better on the QuickSIN test than prior to training. On the other hand, Burke and Humes (2008) showed otherwise among a group of older hearing-impaired listeners. They found benefits following training with words, but the skills learned did not generalize to untrained words or untrained keywords in running speech. While it is true that training programs and durations (and compliance!) vary across the studies, the advantages may be very individualized.

KEY CONCEPT: *Theory Underlying Auditory Training*

For the most part, auditory training is based on the concept of brain plasticity. That is, the ability of the auditory cortex to reorganize itself in response to a sensory experience. While brain plasticity is greatest for younger individuals, electrophysiological studies have shown that it's present for older brains too (e.g., Tremblay, Kraus, Carrell, et al., 1997). Brain imaging studies have shown different frequency maps in the auditory cortex of individuals with hearing loss compared to those with normal-hearing. The hope is that increased audibility through hearing devices and repeated stimulation of the previously absent speech sounds will assist in establishing more effective neural pathways for processing these inputs, resulting in better speech recognition for adults and children.

There are a number of computer-based individualized training programs available (Table 10–4). In the following sections, we review in detail a few that are currently popular, including the evidence to date supporting these techniques. Individual auditory training models also have been criticized for neglecting the issues of personal adjustment, real-life communication strategies training, and so on, because there

---

KEY CONCEPT: *Describing Auditory Training*

There are a number of different terms that are used when we describe auditory training. Here is a brief description of some of the more common terminology (adapted from Mark Ross, 2011):

- Analytic training: Involves improving consonant/syllable recognition. In this technique, the focus is on the elements of speech. It attempts to improve a person's ability to identify the various sounds of speech, specifically those with which the person has difficulty. Initially, a person may be required to distinguish between such words as /beer/ and /bore/, which have two vowels that differ considerably. From there, a person may be challenged to distinguish finer and finer vowel differences. In analytic consonant training, the vowel remains the same, but now the target consonant is changed (e.g., beer vs. fear). This training also proceeds from large to finer acoustic distinctions. Analytic training is termed a "bottom-up" approach because the intent is to improve overall speech comprehension by focusing on the finer acoustic components of speech messages. The reasoning is that if someone can reliably distinguish the acoustic elements of speech, then he or she should be better able to comprehend the larger units, such as words and sentences (Ross, 2011).

- Synthetic training: This approach is considerably different from analytic, as it usually employs meaningful sentences as training stimuli. Because understanding sentences in quiet can be quite easy for many individuals with hearing loss, most often the sentences are presented to the listeners in the presence of noise. This also adds face validity to the training. The task of the listener is to focus on comprehending the words and sentences, without specifically attending to specific acoustic elements. The speech or the noise often is altered so that there is not a floor or ceiling effect for a given patient, and the patient is continually challenged during the training session. As opposed to the "bottom-up" approach of the analytic technique, synthetic training is termed "top-down," as it requires listeners to employ their knowledge of language and context to fill in the acoustic/perceptual gaps in the message (Ross, 2011).

- Other terms that have been used include "listening training" and "perceptual training," which could be either analytic or synthetic, or some combination.

Table 10–4. Sample of Available Computer-Based Auditory Training Programs

Name	Developed By	Cost	Design	Time	Delivery Mode
Listening and Communication Enhancement (LACE)	Neurotone	$79 (Web-based) to $99 (PC/DVD-based)	Training Tasks: rapid speech, speech in noise, competing speaker, missing word, word memory, QuickSIN.	5 to 10+ hours	Home computer, Web-based, DVD, mobile
Seeing and Hearing Speech	Sensimetrics	$85	Listening and lip-reading tasks presented with visual cues (in quiet or noise).	N/A	CD-ROM (PC Only)
Read My Quips	Sense Synergy	$99	Speech comprehension training consisting of crossword-type puzzles. The listener uses visual and contextual clues to "unlock" witty quotes and advance to more challenging puzzles.	24+ hours	Web-based
Speech Perception Assessment and Training System for Hearing Impaired (SPATS-HI)	Communication Disorders Technology, Inc.	Varies by clinic pricing model	Speech recognition testing and training addressing both analytic and synthetic components of speech. Emphasis on performance-tracking over times.	N/A	Administered onsite by hearing health-care provider
Angel Sound AKA Computer-Assisted Speech Training (CAST)	Tiger Speech	Free through Emily Fu Foundation as Angel Sound	Adaptive auditory training program featuring audio-visual feedback. Self-testing of functional abilities is an included capability.	N/A	Home computer-based as software download (PC Only), CD-Rom by request
eARena	Siemens/Sivantos	Varies by clinic pricing model	Variety of sound training: loudness scaling, everyday sound perception, analytic and synthetic auditory training, hearing in noise.	10 hours	Home computer, DVD, iPad

Source: From *Modern Hearing Aids: Verification, Outcome Measures, and Follow-Up* (p. 414), by R. Bentler, H. G. Mueller, and T. A. Ricketts, 2016, San Diego: CA, Plural Publishing. Reprinted with permission.

is no support group involved, nor are the individual's specific communication problems typically discussed. Other models of hearing aid orientation and training have been proposed to address those concerns in a time- and cost-efficient manner, including group classes. These classes can be held online or in person, but are typically under the supervision of an audiologist or SLP.

Listening and Communication Enhancement (LACE)

One individualized training program that has been recently studied is the Listening and Communication Enhancement (LACE) Program. LACE is a home- or clinic-based interactive, adaptive computer program designed to engage the adult with hearing impairment in the hearing aid fitting process, provide listening strategies, build confidence, and address cognitive changes characteristic of the aging process. The developers of this program, Robert Sweetow and Jenifer Sabin considered the evidence to support auditory training. What they discovered was that synthetic training materials outperformed analytic training materials. Other factors considered in the development of this computer-driven auditory training (AT) program include the following:

1. It must be cost effective
2. It should be easy, fun, and rewarding for the patient
3. It should be verifiable
4. It should incorporate top-down and bottom-up approaches (synthetic and analytic)
5. It must provide the patient with feedback regarding progress

As a result, the LACE software program is designed to provide a variety of interactive tasks across three areas: comprehension of degraded speech, enhancement of cognitive skills, and improvement of communication strategies (Table 10–5). The LACE training CD provides visual feedback on instructions, tasks, and feedback (Figures 10–3, 10–4, and 10–5). Training exercises include the following tasks:

- Degraded and competing speech
- Speech in babble
- Time compressed speech
- Competing speaker
- Cognitive tasks
- Interactive communication strategies

The evidence to support the use of LACE is mixed. In a multisite study of the effectiveness of a pilot version of LACE, significant improvements were shown both on the training tasks, as well as other standardized outcome measures such as the QuickSIN, Hearing Handicap Scale for the Elderly, and Communication Scale for Older Adults (Sweetow & Sabes, 2006). One feature of this program is that individual patient performance data can be transmitted to a HIPAA-compliant server easily accessible online by the audiologist. Scores, trends, even comparisons to normative bodies of data are easily accessible by the managing clinician.

A more recent investigation of the impact of LACE on long-term outcomes has shown equivocal results (Chisholm et al., 2013). These investigators found no clear impact of intervention. Rather, they found that their placebo group and the LACE group both showed a practice effect.

Another investigation of young adults with normal hearing exposed to LACE training as part of an investigation into neural plasticity showed more promising results (Kraus, 2012). Compared to their pre-LACE testing, the participants increased in their ability to understand speech in noise as

Table 10–5. Tasks Included in LACE Training Exercises	
Degraded and Competing Speech Tasks	Speech in babble. Training is organized into topics (health issues, money matters, exercise, etc.) that are chosen by the listener at the onset. Sentences are presented in multitalker babble, starting at +10 SNR. The listener responds yes/no that he/she comprehends the sentence, and the SNR is adaptively changed, initially using 4-dB step size and decreasing to a 2-dB step size.
	Time compressed speech. Using the same paradigm as above, the time compressed ratio is altered instead of the SNR. The rate of the speech is initially compressed to .85 of average rate (or about four syllables per second). The pitch cues are not altered. The first five iterations are adjusted in steps of .75 time compression; after that, the compression factor is 0.25.
	Competing speaker. The exact same paradigm as speech in babble is used, except that the competition is made up of only one other talker.
Cognitive Tasks	Auditory Memory exercises are used with six levels of difficulty. In this task, the listener is visually presented a target word (TW). Following auditory presentation of a sentence containing the TW, the listener is asked to select via multiple choice the target word. The levels of difficulty include:
	Level 1: TW before the sentence
	Level 2: TW after the sentence
	Level 3: Two TWs before two sentences
	Level 4: Two TWs after two sentences
	Level 5: Three TWs before three sentences
	Level 6: Three TWs after three sentences
	Missing word/speed of processing tasks include the presentation of one sentence at a time in which one word is masked by an environmental noise (e.g., car honking, telephone ringing). The listener is scored both on accuracy of choosing the missing word and the speed of their response.
Interactive Communication Strategies	These "helpful hints" are interspersed throughout the training modules. They include topics such as managing the acoustic environment, assertive listening skill, care and maintenance of the hearing aid, and so on.

Source: From *Modern Hearing Aids: Verification, Outcome Measures, and Follow-Up* (p. 418), by R. Bentler, H. G. Mueller, and T. A. Ricketts, 2016, San Diego: CA, Plural Publishing. Reprinted with permission.

measured using the QUICKSIN and HINT, when compared to an untrained control group of normal hearing young adults.

LACE training is available in a DVD version, and a study by Olson, Preminger, and Shinn (2013) examined the efficacy of this presentation mode for both new and experienced hearing aid users. Adults with hearing loss ($n = 29$) were assigned to one of three groups: new hearing aid user plus training, experienced hearing aid user plus training, or control (new hearing aid user

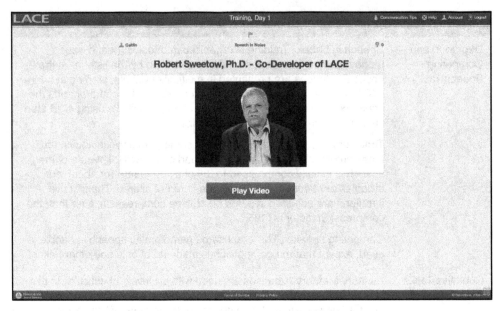

Figure 10–3. Screenshot from LACE software showing the co-originator, Robert Sweetow. *Source*: From *Modern Hearing Aids: Verification, Outcome Measures, and Follow-Up* (p. 416), by R. Bentler, H. G. Mueller, and T. A. Ricketts, 2016, San Diego, CA: Plural Publishing. Reprinted with permission.

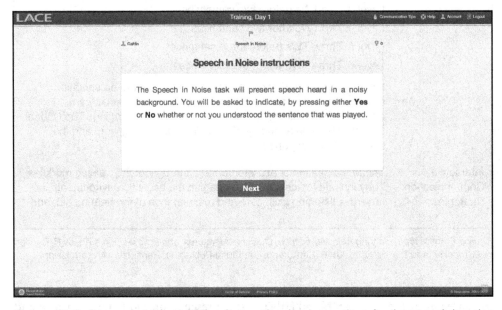

Figure 10–4. Screenshot from LACE software showing instructions for the speech-in-noise module. *Source*: From *Modern Hearing Aids: Verification, Outcome Measures, and Follow-Up* (p. 417), by R. Bentler, H. G. Mueller, and T. A. Ricketts, 2016, San Diego, CA: Plural Publishing. Reprinted with permission.

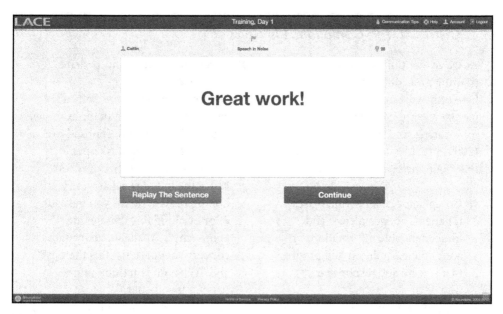

Figure 10–5. Screenshot from LACE software showing reinforcement for session with patient option to repeat or continue training session. *Source*: From *Modern Hearing Aids: Verification, Outcome Measures, and Follow-Up* (p. 417), by R. Bentler, H. G. Mueller, and T. A. Ricketts, 2016, San Diego, CA: Plural Publishing. Reprinted with permission.

with no training). The training groups used the lessons from the LACE DVD program at home over a period of 4 weeks. Several objective listening measures were administered including speech in noise, rapid speech, and competing sentences tasks. Their findings were encouraging: both new and experienced users improved their understanding of speech in noise, understanding of competing sentences, and communication function after training in comparison to the control group—a larger training effect was observed for the new hearing aid users. All current versions of the LACE may be obtained from the Neurotone website.

Seeing and Hearing Speech

Seeing and Hearing Speech was developed by Sensimetrics as a training program in auditory-visual communication for people with hearing loss. Sensimetrics Corporation was founded in 1987 and provides tools for researchers, educators, and clinicians in the field of human communication.

Seeing and Hearing Speech can be ordered from the developer's website in the form of a CD-ROM that can be installed on personal computers. The software is a collection of lessons designed for training in the use of visual and auditory cues for understanding speech. Lessons are organized into four broad groups devoted to different aspects of speech and the speech-reception task:

1. Vowels
2. Consonants
3. Stress, intonation, and length
4. Everyday communication

TECHNICAL TIP: Compliance Is Key

As we've mentioned, the individual training procedures that we discuss here only will be successful if the patient is compliant. This is not a minor issue, and Robert Sweetow (2009) provides some suggestions that might help:

- Compliance generally increases if patients are given clear and understandable information about their condition and progress in a sincere and responsive way
- Simplify a patient's instructions or treatment regimen as much as possible
- Have systems in place to generate patient treatment or appointment reminders

- Listen and respect your patients' concerns
- Determine your patients' attitudes and past experiences. If, for example, your patient is firmly opposed to engaging in therapy, ask open-ended questions such as: "When you came in today, what were you hoping I might do for you instead of prescribing this therapeutic approach?"; "What are your main concerns about doing this therapy?"; and "What do you think might happen if you do it?"
- For home-based training, conducting the first session face to face with the patient, and then having the patient proceed with training at home, can significantly increase compliance rates

---

Within each of these four groups, there are subgroups of lessons that focus on specific aspects of the group. Lessons within a subgroup typically differ in the nature of the speech material used: some lessons use isolated words, some use a short phrase, and others use sentences. Seeing and Hearing Speech lets you choose among three different speech presentation conditions: auditory-visual, auditory-only, and visual-only. Every lesson has buttons on the left side of the computer screen on which a word, phrase, or sentence is printed. On the right side of the screen is the video window, where the video footage of a person speaking is presented. Each button on the left is paired with a speech utterance. For example, in a lesson that uses isolated words,

the button labeled "book" would be paired with an audio/video recording of the talker speaking the word "book." Lessons that use sentences, however, sometimes use a shortened label on the button that pairs it to a sentence. For example, the button labeled "book" might be paired with the sentence, "She wrote it in her book."

Research has shown that Seeing and Hearing Speech training may improve speech-in-noise perception in postlingually deafened CI users (Ingvalson, Lee, Fiebig, & Wong, 2013). There is also evidence that speech reading improves when using Seeing and Hearing Speech Training with normal hearing adults as well; however, these data may differ from how adults or children with hearing loss may benefit from this auditory/

visual training program (Blumsack, Bower, & Ross, 2007). Overall, Seeing and Hearing Speech Training is intended to assist those with hearing loss gain better speech understanding.

Read My Quips (RMQ)

Read My Quips was developed by Harry Levitt with Advanced Hearing Concepts, Inc. (ca. 2005). This speech-reading training is a play-based system for understanding speech in noise with maximum visual cues for both male and female speakers. It was developed to provide a computer-based training tool designed to motivate individual patients to complete the training tasks. RMQ is an online training system that requires the user to have a high-speed Internet connection. It can be obtained or accessed from the Sense Synergy website. RMQ has the following design:

- Following an introductory screen of purpose (Figure 10–6), two screens are displayed to the user: a video feed of a speaker (Figure 10–7) alongside what is essentially a crossword puzzle (Figure 10–8), though the listener is expected to complete words in each square instead of letters.

- Familiar and clever "quips" are recited by the speakers using a relatively high degree of visual cues. Users integrate the auditory information they received with the existing words in the puzzle to complete the sentence.

- RMQ is a computer-based adaptive assessment tool, meaning that success on a quip will lead to more challenging

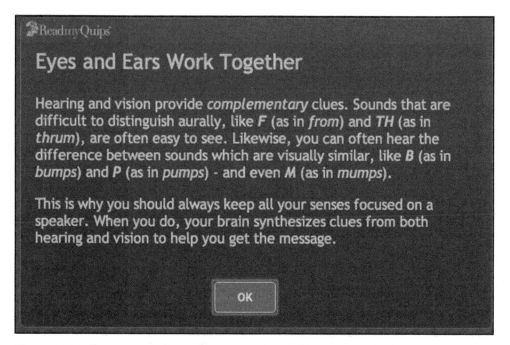

Figure 10–6. Screenshot from software Read My Quips. *Source:* From *Modern Hearing Aids: Verification, Outcome Measures, and Follow-Up* (p. 421), by R. Bentler, H. G. Mueller, and T. A. Ricketts, 2016, San Diego, CA: Plural Publishing. Reprinted with permission.

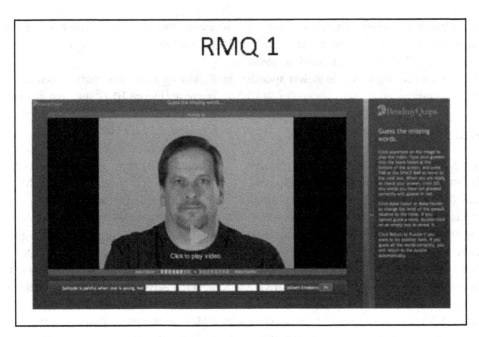

Figure 10–7. Screenshot from software Read My Quips. *Source*: From *Modern Hearing Aids: Verification, Outcome Measures, and Follow-Up* (p. 421), by R. Bentler, H. G. Mueller, and T. A. Ricketts, 2016, San Diego, CA: Plural Publishing. Reprinted with permission.

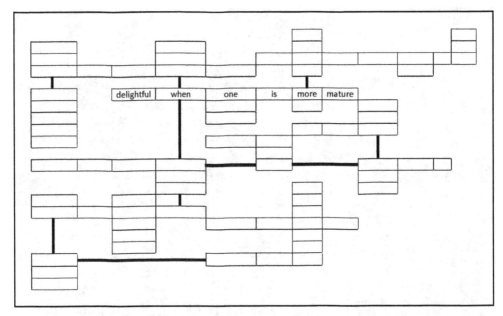

Figure 10–8. Screenshot from software Read My Quips. *Source*: From *Modern Hearing Aids: Verification, Outcome Measures, and Follow-Up* (p. 422), by R. Bentler, H. G. Mueller, and T. A. Ricketts, 2016, San Diego, CA: Plural Publishing. Reprinted with permission.

listening constraints in terms of noise, visual distracters, or fewer initial cue words on subsequent items.

◼ The adaptive nature of the training system also means it could be appropriate for a variety of hearing losses and communication levels.

◼ The phrases are in English and are spoken in a conversational style, which may add increased challenges for nonnative speakers. Preliminary data were compiled with subjects who were native speakers.

Although there are no peer-reviewed data to speak to its effectiveness or generalization to non-computer-based listening-in-noise tasks, preliminary data suggest that there may be a positive effect, and that users were not averse to spending time on the tasks and may even have found it entertaining (Levitt, Oden, Simon, Noack, & Lotze, 2011)! These investigators/designers also found large differences in time-on-task between subjects, with seven of ten subjects showing statistically significant improvements in their listening-in-noise scores; that is, a decrease in signal-to-noise ratio at which 50% of IEEE sentences were recognized (i.e., 4.1 dB average reduction). The subjects showing the largest improvements were those who spent the longest time on the training tasks, an intuitive, but difficult to coerce, concept!

Speech Perception Assessment and Training System (SPATS)

The Speech Perception Assessment and Training System (SPATS) (Miller, Watson, Kewley-Port, et al., 2008a) training module has a slightly different focus. It is designed to sharpen the listener's attentional focus on spectral-temporal properties of syllables, including onsets (single consonants and clusters), nuclei (vowels and vowel-like sounds) and coda (final consonants and clusters). The authors describe this as *constituent* training; the term "syllabic constituents"

POINTS TO PONDER: Should Training Be Fun?

It would make sense that making auditory training fun would be a good idea. Robert Sweetow states that this was one of the goals of LACE, and this notion is also incorporated into Harry Levitt's Read My Quips training. Nancy Tye-Murray et al. (2012) looked at auditory training outcomes in both hearing aid and CI users. They found that subjects reported improvements in their ability to recognize spoken language and in self-confidence as a result of the exercises. But, interestingly, their perceived benefit did not correlate with perceived enjoyment of the task. We have to consider, of course, that compliance tends to be considerably higher when a patient is participating in a research study, so in this case, "fun" probably didn't impact compliance. For your individual patients, however, who might easily tire of doing the training, fun is probably a good thing. For example, Levitt (2014) reports that in his feasibility study, the recommended home training session was 30 min, yet the average duration of actual training was 45 min.

refers to the subgrouping of segments within the syllable. An example would be to divide the syllable into three constituents: onset, nucleus, and coda (Davis, 1988). The onset is a constituent comprising the syllable-initial consonant or consonant cluster; the nucleus consists of the vowel or syllabic consonant and is considered the peak of the syllable; and the coda contains the syllable-final consonant or consonant cluster.

An additional sentence-based module is used in training as well. Developed simultaneously, but independently, a primary difference between the approaches is intermixing of the constituent and sentence training modules in the SPATS, and that the interpretation is provided in percentage improvement rather than SNR improvement, as with the LACE. The SPATS software was designed for use with both hearing aid and cochlear implant recipients.

The SPATS consists of two independent speech-recognition testing and training programs, one for the constituents of speech ("the code") and one for sentences. The authors of this training system suggest five criteria for successful (re)training (from Watson et al., 2008):

- prompt feedback during the training that informs the participant of the nature of the error;
- a large corpus of recorded stimuli which includes older and younger, and male and female talkers;
- syllable training in a variety of phonemic environments, as well as sentence training, which combines top-down and bottom-up recognition skills;
- concentration of the training exercise on specific syllable constituents with which the participant has particular difficulty; and
- a curriculum that guides training in such a way that the participant can

appreciate their improvement over time, and thus be willing to continue their efforts.

In order to train users on syllables, the developers chose 109 elements of English speech perception. Those constituents included 45 onsets, 28 nuclei, and 36 codas. Each constituent group was further broken down into four levels. The first level (Level I) consists of the top 25% of these elements, Level II is made up of the top half, Level III contains the top 75% of these elements, and Level IV has all 109 constituents. By combining onsets with different nuclei and codas with different stems, the developers of SPATS have included 388 different syllables in the training software. Each of the syllables were then recorded by eight different talkers to provide a variety of voices (Miller, Watson, Kewley-Port, et al., 2008a).

During the training sessions, one constituent at a time is played; the listener is encouraged to first repeat what they heard and then choose the letter on the screen that represents the sound. Feedback on the correctness of the choice immediately follows selection. If the listener identifies the wrong element, they are encouraged to "rehear" the correct and incorrect constituents by clicking on them on the screen. The developers call this "post-trial rehearing" and assert that it "speeds perceptual learning" (Miller, Watson, Kewley-Port, et al., 2008a).

Presentation of each constituent is governed by an adaptive algorithm. In the beginning, the algorithm presents constituents "that are moderately difficult for the client and most likely to be learnable" most often. As the client learns to identify the constituents, they are presented less frequently and are replaced by other sounds. This avoids ceiling or floor effects and can reduce participants' frustration (Miller, Watson, Kewley-Port, et al., 2008a).

The SPATS sentence training module contains 1,000 sentences spoken by 10 different talkers that consist of simple, common questions and statements that the clients would use in everyday life. Some examples are "What would you like for dinner?" and "We are under a tornado alert" (Miller, Watson, Kewley-Port, et al., 2008a).

During testing, a sentence is played and then an alphabetical list of words appears on the screen. The listener then clicks on each word they heard. Each correct word has 3 foils. When the correct word is selected, it appears in its position in the sentence at the top of the screen. If the listener selects a foil, the word turns red and the program replays the sentence. This repeats until all of the words in the sentence have been correctly identified (Miller, Watson, Kewley-Port, et al., 2008a). Refer to Figure 10–9 for an example.

To evaluate SPATS, Miller, Watson, Kisler, Preminger, and Wark (2008b) compared hearing aid users ($n = 12$) with and without SPATS training. Two-thirds of the participants received training and the other third served as the control group. All test group participants completed approximately 12 to 24 hr of training. On average, the trained participants showed an average gain of 11% over the control participants, who showed no improvement. After the training,

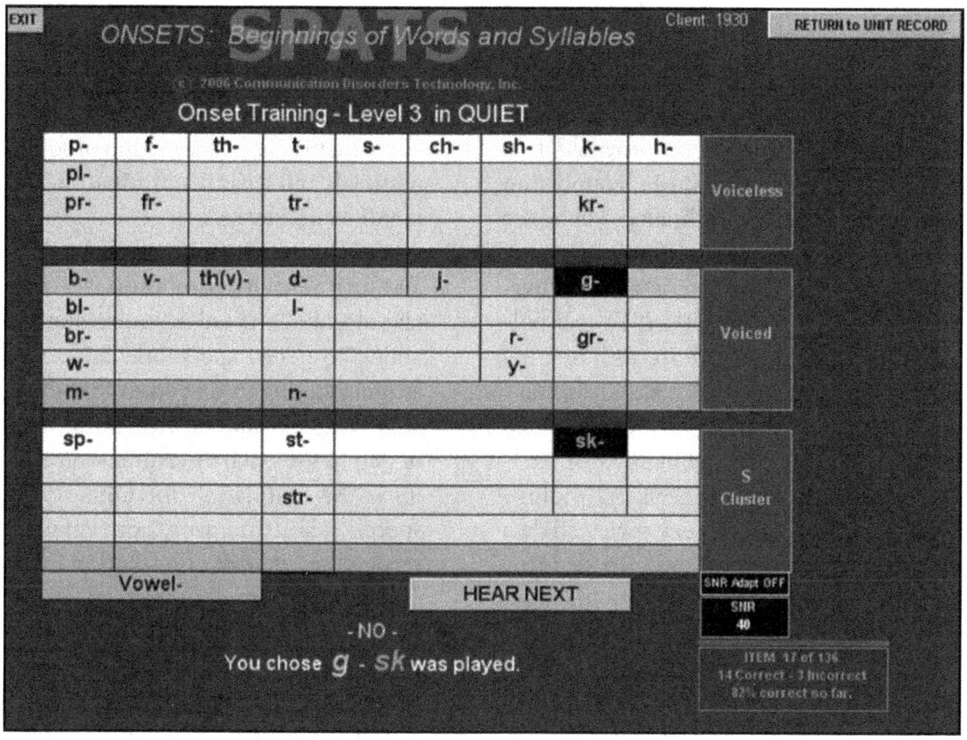

Figure 10–9. A response screen used in SPATS. The listener initiates the trial, imitates the sound heard, and clicks on the appropriate response button. The screen immediately shows the correct response. In this example, an error was made and the correct answer/onset (sk) is shown, as is the error (g). *Source*: From *Modern Hearing Aids: Verification, Outcome Measures, and Follow-Up* (p. 424), by R. Bentler, H. G. Mueller, and T. A. Ricketts, 2016, San Diego, CA: Plural Publishing. Reprinted with permission.

the participants commented that this program aided in understanding their hearing losses. The participants also remarked that it helped them become aware of "their specific problems in the identification of speech sounds" and helped them "attend to the details of sounds and talker differences."

The most obvious differences in the LACE approach and the SPATS approach are the training of syllable constituents and the intermixing of constituent and sentence training. The SPATS system is available through the Communication Disorders Technology, Inc. website.

Angel Sound, a.k.a. Computer Assisted Speech Training (CAST)

Angel Sound software was developed in 2011 by Dr. Qian-Jie Fu and Xiaosong Wang in conjunction with House Research Institute and supported by National Institute of Health. This software is provided free through the Emily Shannon Fu Foundation (formerly TigerSpeech Technology) in honor of Fu and Wang's daughter, Emily.

Angel Sound software is a computer-assisted speech training (CAST) technology designed to benefit those with hearing aid devices, cochlear implants, and auditory processing disorders. It can be downloaded through the Internet or obtained on CD-ROM from the Tiger Speech Technology website. While there are peer-reviewed data on the effectiveness of auditory training and CAST programs for those with hearing impairments (Gagné, Dinon, & Parsons 1991; Picora-Fuller & Benguerel, 1991), there is no information regarding the effectiveness of Angel Sound software.

According to Fu and his personal study for the development of Angel Sound, individuals perceived benefit from the program if they practiced for roughly 1 hr per day, 5 days a week, for one month. This is the equivalent of about 20 hr of use. The program is adaptive, so that the level of difficulty automatically adjusts to match personal developing listening skills. The system provides audio-visual feedback, highlighting areas where the individual can continue to practice. Users can download the software for either English or Mandarin speech. Angel Sound has seven different modules, ranging from easy to difficult training tasks. Each module is developed to train an individual for specific needs.

1. **Basic module:** The basic module targets a very broad range of training tasks, including pure-tone discrimination (basic frequency resolution); environmental sounds; voice genders; as well as vowel, consonant, words, and sentence recognition. This module is suitable for new cochlear implant and hearing aid users so they have the chance to familiarize themselves with all kind of sound materials and basic discrimination and identification tasks.

2. **Auditory resolution module:** The auditory resolution module is a special module targeted at improving the ability to detect the subtle difference among sounds in one specific dimension, such as frequency, temporal, and/or amplitude. Such discrimination ability is the foundation for higher-level speech (phoneme, word, or sentence) recognition. Auditory resolution module is suitable for all users.

3. **Telephone speech recognition module:** This module is exactly the same as the basic module except that all the sound materials are band limited to the frequency range of telephone speech (300–3300 Hz). Anyone who is interested at improving telephone conversation can try this module, after they are familiar with the basic module.

4. **Melodic contour identification module:** This is a simple music module that is targeted at melodic contour identification. The difficulty is controlled by semitone between notes and this module also provides midi sounds from several different instruments. Anyone who is interested at improving music appreciation should try this module first.

5. **Adaptive speech-in-noise module:** This is an advanced module. In general, the user should perform better than 80% in quiet conditions before using this module. All the tasks in this module use an adaptive approach, where the noise level will be adjusted according to the users' response. In general, this module is suitable for good-performing users.

6. **Comprehensive music module:** This is an advanced music module which is targeted at various aspects of music appreciation, including basic note discrimination, melodic contour identification, melodic sequence recognition, chord recognition, polyphonic contour identification, and so forth. Many tasks are very difficult so this module is generally suitable only for good-performing users.

7. **Open-set recognition module:** Most speech conversation is generally open-set since the listener generally does not know the speaker's specific intent. The open-set recognition module is aimed at mimicking real-life conversation where the listener has to recognize the sentences or words without knowing the intended contents or choices made by the speaker. In general, this module is relatively difficult and suitable only for good-performing listeners.

The CAST system has been transformed into commercial products (e.g., "Sound and WAY Beyond" from Cochlear Americas

and "Sound and Beyond" from Cochlear Corporation); however, Angel Sound is not related to Cochlear Corporation. The agreement with Cochlear Corporation has been terminated and they will no longer hold rights to "Sound and WAY Beyond" once all the remaining CDs are distributed. Angel Sound is the latest technology and will be the exclusive product based on the CAST technology in the future. Here are the website addresses http://angelsound.tiger speech.com/angelsound_about.html and http://www.tigerspeech.com/index.html

CASPERSent. Computer-Assisted Speech Perception Testing and Training at the Sentence Level (CASPERSent) is a multimedia program designed by Author Boothroyd. The primary target is perceptual skills training. It is founded on the model of speech perception that includes the following:

- sensory evidence
- contextual evidence
- knowledge skill

CASPERSent is comprised of 60 CUNY sentences representing 12 topics and three sentence types. The principal target of testing is performance in a conversational context. Secondary targets are the effects of talker, perceptual modality, topic knowledge, sentence length, and sentence type. While there is limited evidence as to the effectiveness of CASPERSent, it appears that it could be of use for people with hearing devices.

cLEAR (Customized Learning: Exercises for Aural Rehabilitation). Nancy Tye-Murray and her colleagues at Washington University in St. Louis have developed a customizable, computer-based auditory training program called cLEAR. It is somewhat unique in that it is available to patients only through a licensed professional. The customizable program is subscription-based, thus clinicians can bundle it with the purchase of hearing aids, or offer it as a stand-alone fee-for-service.

Clinicians can tailor the auditory training directly to the needs of the individual. Each clEAR auditory training exercise lasts about 20 minutes and patients are expected to complete two to three exercises per week over a 12 week period. Also, clEAR allows provides instantaneous feedback to the clinician and patient so that progress can be easily tracked. The clEAR program includes a recording and automated editing system that enables patients use the speech of a specific frequent communication partner. In addition, clEAR, which works with either a tablet and laptop computer, employs a game-like format, designed to make the training more fun and engaging. Audiologist report that they are able to customize lesson plans, follow progress and use instant messaging to stay in close contact with patients without requiring burdensome extra office visits.

One of the goals of cLEAR is to make auditory training fun. Not surprising, therefore, are the names of the training games that can be played:

- ARplane
- pokEAR
- TreasEAR Island
- FarmEAR in the Dell
- MountainEAR
- EARonaut
- ShakespEARe
- pEARl Crunch

As mentioned, it can be customized for a given patient. The following are the different lesson plans that are available:

- Lesson Plan for the New Hearing-Aid User

- Lesson Plan for the User Who is Not Yet Ready for Hearing Aids
- Lesson Plan for the User Who Complains of Listening in Noise
- Lesson Plan for the User Who has Difficulty in Hearing Female and Child Voices
- Lesson Plan for the New Cochlear Implant User
- Lesson Plan for the User Who Cannot Tolerate Noise
- Lesson Plan for the User with Central Auditory Processing Disorder
- Lesson Plan for the User Who Wants to Better Understand the Speech of an FCP (Frequent Communication Partner): Plan 1
- Lesson Plan for the User Who Wants to Better Recognize the Speech of an FCP: Plan II

Long-Term Benefit of Individualized Training

We have presented several options for individualized auditory training, either conducted under supervision at the clinic, or more commonly, in the patient's home following the fitting of hearing devices. We've also reported on some research that has supported the use of this training, including the finding of improved speech recognition in background noise. It's important to point out, however, that in most of these studies, the posttraining measures were conducted immediately after the conclusion of the training period. In the practical world of fitting hearing devices, what we are primarily concerned with is the long-term effects of training. Will these reported signal-to-noise ratio benefits still be present a month after training? Three months after training? A year after training? Or, does the patient need to continue the training to experience the benefit? We question

---

CLINICAL NOTE: Looking at the Evidence

The most comprehensive meta-analysis of the benefit of computer-based auditory training (CBAT) has been published by Henshaw and Fergusen (2013). It was not overly positive. They state:

> Individual computer-based auditory training (CBAT) is a time and cost efficient, flexible self-management intervention that has the potential to be delivered to people with hearing loss in their home environment. It is easily accessible to the target population via PCs and the Internet, and can be tailored to individual need. Our findings demonstrate that although

individual CBAT is a feasible intervention for people with hearing loss, published evidence for the efficacy of individual CBAT to improve speech intelligibility, cognition and hearing abilities for adults with hearing loss is neither consistent nor robust. As such, the evidence cannot be used reliably to guide intervention at this time (Henshaw & Fergusen, 2013, p. 16).

Since this review, new methods have emerged; several of them are more engaging, which might increase use and compliance.

---

if many patients would be willing to commit to this. There is limited research that has examined this important question, and the evidence to support the programs is mixed, but promising.

Potential Barriers for AR from the Audiologist's Perspective

- The clinician would need to become familiar with the implementation of the training offered.
- If group training is employed, a meeting room is necessary. Smaller offices might not have these facilities.
- Most hearing devices are sold with a bundled price. The average patient does not have an expectation that auditory training is included.
- Audiologists cannot directly bill for rehabilitative audiology services and

would, therefore, need to contract with you, the SLP, for additional services.
- In the school, the SLP may be seen as only providing speech and language services, not auditory services.

Potential Barriers for AR from the Patient's Perspective

- A lack of computer skills or a general hesitancy to avoid this technology.
- Visual and cognitive limitations.
- Lack of time and motivation.
- The benefits from the training (if present) are subtle, and often are not obvious to the patient (e.g., a significant 2 dB SNR improvement in noise may have no direct impact on the patient's daily communication situations).
- Many patients believe that they have spent enough money on products and professional programming and

have the unrealistic expectation that success should rest solely with the hearing device—the newest, high-tech, multifunction, expensive hearing devices alone should provide optimal benefit, without more effort from the user!

Even More Ways to Obtain AR Programs

Each of the individualized programs is available for clinicians to access or purchase as described previously. But wait! In this era of smartphones and iPads, there are many more that deserve consideration by the interested clinician, not to mention the motivated patient.

Nontraditional AR Methods: Tablet Apps

There is a plethora of tablet and other mobile device apps available to the consumer today. Many of the hearing-related apps are for measurement of hearing rather than for improved hearing (amplification and auditory training), which we have been discussing in this chapter. Several of these apps that are developed by manufacturers serve both as a screening and a marketing tool. This listing is only a sampling of what is available to the patient at the time of the writing of this book. The list does not include the LACE and Read My Quips programs discussed earlier in this chapter, although both are now available on devices using web browsers with Flash.

Hear Coach. Developed by Starkey Laboratories, the manufacturer refers to these games as exercises in "Focused Listening." There are two main sections: Repeater and Word Target. Each has five levels of difficulty,

with 80% or better necessary to advance. Loudness is initially is set based on user preference listening to the Rainbow Passage. Word Target asks the user to choose the correct word heard in a background of increasingly difficult noise. There are 200 training items, with three minimal pairs chosen as foils (these differ by one speech sound in terms of place, manner, and voicing). Noise proceeds from quiet to bus noise to types of music to multitalker babble. See Figures 10–10 through 10–13 for screenshots.

Repeater asks the user to repeat a string of digits. Difficulty increases as the chain of digits grows in length. Some might consider this a working memory task. The user is allowed to hear the target in quiet if guessed wrong initially in background noise. Points are awarded for accuracy and rapidity.

uHear. This app was developed by Unitron. It contains a sensitivity screener, speech-in-noise screener, a questionnaire, results of screening discussion, and a section for the individual to "learn" about hearing loss including healthy hearing tips. The questionnaire is based on the Hearing-Dependent Daily Activities Scale to evaluate impact of hearing loss in older people (Lopez-Torres Hidalgo et al., 2008). How is this a rehabilitative application? The results of the questionnaire are presented with common communication tips for success. This tends to be more of an app for a person with hearing difficulties who has not yet come into an audiologist's office, but could be a handy resource for tips, or a launching point for completion in the waiting room.

"I Hear What You Mean." "I Hear What You Mean" is an additional auditory training program rooted in the philosophy that training that utilizes highly meaningful items will result in more effective generalization than what would take place under the

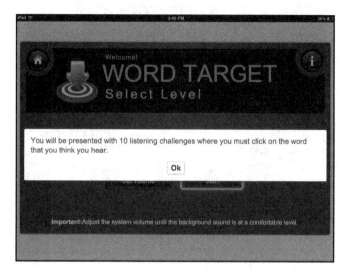

Figure 10–10. Screenshot from Hear Coach. *Source*: From *Modern Hearing Aids: Verification, Outcome Measures, and Follow-Up* (p. 430), by R. Bentler, H. G. Mueller, and T. A. Ricketts, 2016, San Diego, CA: Plural Publishing. Reprinted with permission.

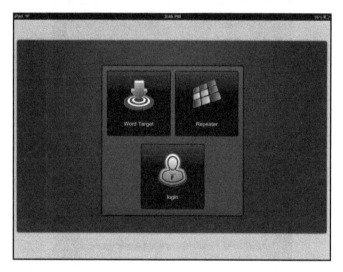

Figure 10–11. Screenshot from Hear Coach. *Source*: From *Modern Hearing Aids: Verification, Outcome Measures, and Follow-Up* (p. 430), by R. Bentler, H. G. Mueller, and T. A. Ricketts, 2016, San Diego, CA: Plural Publishing. Reprinted with permission.

supervision of an audiologist. This software-based AT program was developed by Joe Barcraft and his colleagues at Washington University in St. Louis. Their goal was to identify *meaningful* tasks in the language of psycholinguistics (Barcraft et al., 2011). For a training activity to be meaningful, it must activate and elicit semantic processing. In lieu of repetition, meaning hinges on comprehension and attendance to training

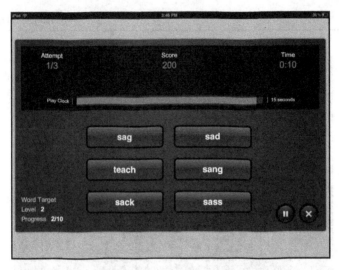

Figure 10–12. Screenshot from Hear Coach. *Source*: From *Modern Hearing Aids: Verification, Outcome Measures, and Follow-Up* (p. 431), by R. Bentler, H. G. Mueller, and T. A. Ricketts, 2016, San Diego, CA: Plural Publishing. Reprinted with permission.

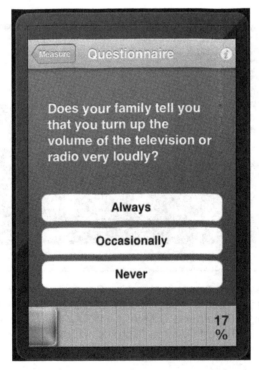

Figure 10–13. Screenshot from Hear Coach. *Source*: From *Modern Hearing Aids: Verification, Outcome Measures, and Follow-Up* (p. 431), R. Bentler, H. G. Mueller, and T. A. Ricketts, 2016, San Diego, CA: Plural Publishing. Reprinted with permission.

materials. Training progresses through five activities, moving from analytic activities to synthetic discourse comprehension:

- Sound identification
- Four-choice discrimination
- Sentence completion
- Contextualized sentences
- Discourse comprehension

Each hour-long lesson incorporates a variety of speakers to theoretically increase generalization and will focus on a theme that is pertinent to an adult listener (e.g., restaurants, travel, sports) and will progress through each of the five types of activities. At present, this computer-assisted software program is only employed in the clinic at Washington University St. Louis, but we're told it is currently being developed for iPad use by the creators.

Nontraditional AR Methods: Other Online Resources

In our era of Internet use, the possibilities of service provision for hearing health care are only beginning to surface. Some clinicians have expressed concern relative to the accuracy of the information that is offered on those sites. This may be a prudent concern, as Laplante-Levesque et al. (2012) found that a relatively small portion of the most commonly returned websites on search engines such as Google provide balanced and accurate information regarding hearing loss and intervention options. Regarding readability of the sites (even the quality ones), they reported it to be rather poor, with an average required reading level of 11 to 12 years. It is typical to target adult training materials at no greater than an eighth-grade reading level. This highlights the need for clinicians to be involved in any

eHealth applications used by their patients. These data also encourage building personal (clinician-based) online resources with quality information and accurate representations of health information including hearing loss. Health on the Net (HON) offers certification schemes for health websites. Very few have it.

Health literacy on and off the web can impact patient's ability to access and make sense of information provided. Health literacy is defined by the National Network of Libraries of Medicine as "the degree to which individuals have the capacity to obtain, process, and understand basic health information and services needed to make appropriate health decisions." People can successfully access health information via the Internet with adequate training and materials designed with them in mind (Czaja et al., 2012).

Nontraditional AR Methods

There are a few other methods that you could use to access patients and their families. In some cases, you may be already doing them. For example, if you are part of birth to 3 services, you may already be seeing patients in their homes. You may be following patients via telecare or other computer-based therapy programs. You may be in e-mail or social media communication with your patients or parents of your patients.

In the Home

Ongoing counseling in the home can be cost effective and lead to significantly expanded hearing device use according to a study by Vuorialho, Karinen, & Sorri (2006). Patients were visited at home by "audiology assistants" in Finland. The results of this project showed improved HHIE-S scores, and the number of regular hearing device users increased. Patients reported improved abilities using the telephone (makes sense as they're in their own home using THEIR telephone), ease of cleaning and maintaining devices, and remembering to place their hearing aids in their ears after follow-up. This is something you can do as part of any in-home therapy you do.

AR by Telehealth

On possible means of conducting AR is via telehealth. In this scenario, you could connect to a patient or their family via a video streaming service. There are several video streaming services that are available that are HIPAA compliant. You then could provide several of the programs or therapies we've discussed. This is of particular use when you are working in a more rural setting or area. You could also use a program in your teletherapy that tracks progress and gives ideas of sentences. One example of this is Computer Assisted Tracking Simulation and Computer Assisted Speech Training (CATS). The CATS program allows the patient and another person, such as a clinician, to interact. It works in the following way: the talker says a sentence or phrase, and the listener repeats verbatim the sentence or phrase. If the sentence is correct, the talker goes on to another sentence or phrase. If it is incorrect, the talker repeats some variation of the utterance until the listener correctly repeats it. The computer-based tracking program makes it easier to score the results of each session and monitor progress.

AR by E-Mail and Social Media

The use of e-mail and social media sites such as Facebook, Instagram, and Twitter for information and communication has become as common as a telephone call for many. Qualitative explorations of individual hearing aid patient's use of e-mail with their audiologist revealed it to be a powerful communication medium to explore the day-to-day experiences of new hearing aid users. Patients were able to obtain answers to simple questions in a timely fashion and could send them along when they were most pressing. Daily e-mails provided an opportunity to emphasize smaller doses of information regarding adjustment to and care for the aids. This of course did not guarantee satisfaction with the hearing aids and some audiologists reported lacking the time to devote to reading and answering a daily e-mail (Laplante-Lévesque, Pichora-Fuller, & Gagné, 2006).

Since the time of this report by Laplante-Lévesque et al. (2006), texting and other forms of social media have increased significantly. We suspect that most SLPs do not want a 24/7 texting arrangement with their patients, but there certainly are ways where this type of technology can be managed and used effectively to improve the rehabilitative process. We know some clinicians who have even set up social media accounts for their patients that can serve as everything from a support group, to an information clearing house, to a group help desk, and beyond.

AR Online

Although many of the training options discussed thus far are programs to be used with a computer or smartphone applications, there are additional options that allow for the use of e-mail as an online intervention option. One program included information, professional guidance, and interaction with peers. The 78 participants were randomly assigned to an online intervention group ($n = 38$) or a control group ($n = 38$). The intervention group "attended" a 5-week intervention program, while the control group was wait-listed. Significant improvements on the HHIE were found for intervention group and the effects were maintained at 3 months follow-up.

No matter how you choose to provide AR to your patients, it is essential that you choose the program that is right for them and that is appropriate for their cognitive level, readiness, and meets their communication needs.

Children with Hearing Loss

There are specific concerns when working with children with hearing loss. As discussed in Chapter 9, hearing loss has a significant impact on speech, language, and social development. When discussing AR in children, there needs to be a distinction between rehabilitation and habilitation. While we have been saying aural rehabilitation, in the case of some children, it is just habilitation. Habilitation refers to providing therapy for something that they never had. This is opposed to rehabilitation which is providing therapy to regain something that was lost. For most children, habilitation is the focus of therapy. While there is a distinction, much of the literature calls habilitation in children rehabilitation.

The most important thing when discussing children with hearing loss whose primary communication mode is spoken language is that they must use their devices consistently and have strong parental and teacher involvement. Figure 10–14 may be used to demonstrate the importance of their impact on parents.

Research shows that children who were identified with hearing loss and started intervention by six months of age had expressive and receptive language within normal limits (within one standard deviation), whereas later-identified children demonstrated significant delays in receptive and expressive language (Mayne, Yashingano-Itano, Sedey, & Carey, 2000; Moeller, 2000; Yoshigano-Itano, 2003). An early start to intervention can mitigate the negative impact of hearing loss—so common years ago—on linguistic, social, emotional, cognitive, and academic development (Calderone, 2000; Moeller, 2000). Early intervention also includes parents. You can enhance carryover in your treatment by encouraging parents to play with their kids, expanding vocabulary, and working on the skills you are working to develop (Figure 10–15). As discussed in Chapters 7 and 9, early identification, advanced hearing device technology, early implantation, and bilateral implantation have provided early access to sounds for children with hearing loss. Better access to the sounds of speech can limit the negative effects of hearing loss on speech and language development. When working with parents, it may be worth providing them with some suggestions on ways to best engage their children. For many, this is not a natural process. Providing them with specific points may assist them with their engagement. It may be worth saying "talk around the clock." This means that they will say out loud everything that they are doing. For example, "Now we are going to bring in all the groceries. Okay, now I need to take them all out and put them away. Oh what is this? An apple? It goes on the counter in the fruit bowl . . . " Some other suggestions include parallel talk, imitation, expansion, recasting, and ensuring that they are asking their children open-ended questions.

How do we integrate what we hear into meaningful speech and learn speech and language? There are 10 auditory processes that we can discuss when looking at auditory skills development. These develop at

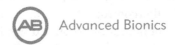

Giving Your Child's Brain the Best Start with Hearing Aids or Cochlear Implants

Be Their First and Best Teacher with These 5 Steps

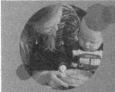

1. Consistent Use:
Put your child's hearing devices on during all waking hours, at least **10 hours** per day, to develop the brain's ability to hear and understand words.

2. Hearing Check Up:
Talk to your child's audiologist to understand how well your child is hearing using their hearing devices. Ask how you can do a daily listening check at home. Bring family members to learn and ask questions.

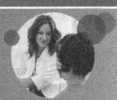

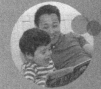

3. Talk in Your Native Language:
Your voice is your best tool! Turn off any distractions in the room, and talk to your child to develop strong auditory pathways to the brain.

4. Sing and Read:
Singing and reading to your child everyday has been shown to have a direct link[2] to successful early brain and language development! Use fun musical activities in the BabyBeats℠ early intervention resource app to develop your baby's listening and language skills.

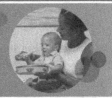

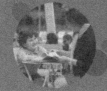

5. You Are Your Child's Best Teacher:
Find a therapist or teacher who is experienced and knowledgeable about hearing loss and auditory brain development. If a therapist or teacher who speaks your primary language is not available, find one who will guide YOU to teach your child.

For more information, contact us at 866.844.HEAR (4327), email us at **hear@AdvancedBionics.com** or visit **AB4kids.com**

Figure 10–14. A sample of a list of things parents can do to enhance communication for children with hearing loss. *Source*: Provided courtesy of Advanced Bionics, LLC © 2019.

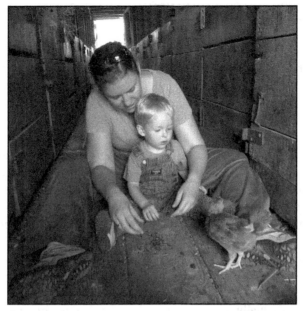

A

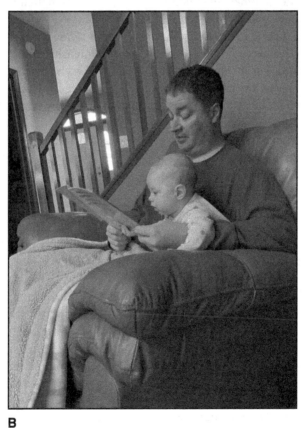

B

Figure 10–15. A–B. The interactions between parent and child provide enhanced speech and language development. *Source*: Photos courtesy of Kyle and Lindsey Jorgensen.

different times during childhood but are all essential for appropriate and quality social and educational communication.

1. Auditory attention
2. Auditory memory
3. Auditory discrimination
4. Auditory integration
5. Auditory feedback
6. Auditory recognition
7. Auditory sequencing
8. Auditory comprehension
9. Auditory retrieval
10. Auditory application

Each of these is equally as important and crucial to the development of children with hearing loss. We will discuss each of these, their role in development, and some suggestions of ways to work on them. You may find that integrating them into other speech therapies may be the best means of addressing them.

1. Auditory attention
   - Selective attention to sounds
   - Active or passive listening
   - Ability to maintain attention to a stimulus over time
   - Ways to improve
     - Practice attending to sounds in different environments
       - In the presence or absence of visual attention or physical attention
     - Young kids—draw attention to it, label it, attend to it, label it
2. Auditory memory
   - Function of short- and long-term memory
   - Individuals need a good auditory memory for remembering
     - Phonemes that make up words
     - Words that comprise phrases and sentences

- Ways to improve
  - Start with familiar sounds
  - Increase length and complexity
  - Practice number sequences
3. Auditory discrimination
   - Same-/different judgements of prosodic and segmental features leading to speech recognition
   - Essential to be able to discriminate
     - Frequency/pitch
     - Intensity/loudness
     - Duration
   - Why are these important?
     - Place of articulation is a frequency cue
     - Manner of articulation has duration, frequency, and intensity cues
     - Voicing has frequency and intensity cues
     - Vowels have frequency cues
     - Sentence-level prosody has duration, intensity, and frequency cues
     - Syllabic and word stress has duration, intensity, and frequency cues
   - Ways to improve
     - Start with material that is highly contrastive and with little acoustic information
       - High frequency beeps versus low frequency beeps
     - Move to less contrastive and ones that contain speech
4. Auditory integration
   - Integrate information from other motor/sensory systems for multisensory meaning, storage, and use of feedback systems
   - Why is this important?
     - Auditory/visual cue integration helps with speech perception, particularly in noise

- Ways to improve
  - Auditory only, visual only, then auditory-visual training
5. Auditory feedback
  - Feedback through hearing and monitoring speech production and environmental sounds
  - Why is this important?
    - May need to adjust speech in the presence of noise
  - Ways to improve
    - Pitch matching through imitation
    - Intensity matching through imitation
    - Singing melodies
    - Working on new multisyllabic words
6. Auditory recognition
  - Associating acoustic events with their reference
    - Environmental sounds
    - Words associated with timed events and quotes
  - Why is this important?
    - Associating sounds with a specific action or thing (e.g., tornado warning or fire truck)
    - Separating speech from environmental sounds
  - Ways to improve
    - Play a sound and pick out from a closed set and move to open set
    - Start with more familiar sounds and move to less familiar sounds with little lexical meaning
    - Start with familiar lexical sounds (e.g., their name) and move to less familiar
7. Auditory sequencing
  - Ability to maintain temporal order of the acoustic sounds
    - Phoneme strings
    - Word combination
    - Sentence sequencing as they are presented

- Why is this important?
  - Story telling
  - Word order in ambiguous sentences (e.g., the big car pulled the little cow; vs. the little cow pulled the big car)
- Ways to improve
  - When working on sentences break them into phrases, pausing between each phrase
  - When working on paragraphs break them into line 1; then 1 and 2; then 1, 2, and 3
8. Auditory comprehension
  - Comprehension of spoken language including semantics, syntax, morphology, phonology, and pragmatics with auditory presented information
  - Why is this important?
    - These kinds of things are important for social interactions
  - Ways to improve
    - Increase vocabulary
    - Understanding
      - Idioms
      - Jokes
      - Puns
      - Slangs
      - Colloquialisms
      - Riddles
9. Auditory retrieval
  - Retrieve and recall stored word images for spontaneous verbal expression
  - Why is this important?
    - Creating new phrases and words
  - Ways to improve
    - Work on events of personal experiences
    - Sequence of events
    - New vocabulary
    - Recall of novel stories
    - Sequence of events
    - New vocabulary

□ Visual imagery to increase comprehension and retrieval
10. Auditory application
   ■ Apply previous nine processes into stories, math, reading, and writing
   ■ Ways to improve
      □ Story problems
      □ Word math problems

Language Development

Even minimal, unilateral, and mild hearing losses can cause delays in communication, speech, and language. As discussed earlier, children with hearing loss often demonstrate academic, social, and behavioral difficulties. These children may demonstrate the inability to hear speech and language adequately in a typical listening situation, which interferes with speech perception (Bess, 1999; Crandell & Smaldino, 2000). An intervention program you may create for children has several purposes: (1) to provide parents with information about the potential impact of hearing loss on development; (2) to conduct ongoing developmental assessments to determine if there are negative consequences of hearing loss; (3) to determine if any other services you are providing may be impacted by hearing loss; (4) to make acoustic accommodations to the environment; and (5) to encourage others around the child, like parents or teachers, to assist the child with the use of hearing devices and help with accommodations.

There may be specific impacts of hearing loss on language that you will need to focus your attention and strategize how to include these auditory developmental milestones. The Outcomes of Children with Hearing Loss study out of Boystown (https://ochl study.org/) has developed the Vocal Development Landmarks Interview (VDLI), a tool for tracking vocal and early verbal milestones for children ages 6 to 21 months. This app can be downloaded in any app store and can be used to assist you with identifying developmental milestones in young children with hearing loss.

KEY CONCEPT:
Looking at Progress

When looking at progress for children with hearing loss, it is essential that you don't just look to see if they are getting better. You want to make sure of two things. First, where the child's development is as compared with their normal-hearing peers. In most cases, you will want to track progress in consistent intervals. You would want to compare their progress to a child with normal-hearing ability. In most cases, you would want to make sure they are making 3-month's progress in 3-month's time—or faster to catch them up.

Semantic Content. Children with hearing loss typically demonstrate delays in vocabulary. Therefore, AR in children may need to work on expanding the vocabulary as these delays may be pervasive throughout adulthood. The understanding of metaphors, idioms, figurative language, and jokes can be particularly challenging. These children generally are challenged by multiple meanings of a word. Therefore, discussing spoken words versus intent and input of nonverbal cues may assist children in developing these skills.

Syntactic Form. To varying degrees, children with hearing loss tend to:

■ Use shorter mean length of utterance (MLU)
■ Use simpler sentence structure

- Overuse the subject-verb-object sentence patterns
- Demonstrate infrequent use of specific word forms (e.g., adverbs, auxiliaries, conjunctions)
- Inappropriate syntactic patterns (i.e., "I want you to go get eat things" to convey the message "I want you to go the store to buy food for dinner")
- Use non-English word order

To work on syntax, you may consider rearranging words in different orders and discussing the changes in meaning, if any. You may consider discussions of adverbs and conjunctions.

Pragmatics. Culberson (2007) reported frequent errors in pragmatic use including restricted use of conversational conventions (e.g., introductions, ending conversations, interrupting) and limited repair strategies (i.e., repeating a message rather than revising it when it is not understood the first time). To work on these difficult concepts, you may consider working on turn-taking and appropriate social etiquette when having a conversation. While the age of the child will determine how much you may expect, a 3-year-old is not so good at turn-taking, you can still start to work on these skills at a young age.

Phonological Development. Speech production is affected; sounds that are not heard, or not heard well, will be misarticulated or omitted from a child's speech. This impacts the speech intelligibility. Although all areas of language are important, many SLP programs focus just on this area when working with kids with hearing loss. It is important to remember all the other areas that may be impacted as well.

Mitigating Language Impact: The Role of the Family. One goal of AR in young children is to teach parents, caregivers, teachers, and other adults to use stimulating, interactive behaviors with young children with hearing loss. The goal applies to young children learning language auditorily, those learning language visually, and those using both modalities.

But access to langue alone does not solve the problem for children with hearing loss. There is a need for specialized intervention; this is YOU. Prescriptive instruction can mitigate the effects of hearing loss on the child's development of language. AR early on teaches parents to provide their children with both direct and indirect language learning. Access to a rich language environment is the goal. Yes, appropriate language use and your one-on-one therapy will likely be the scaffolding, but it is the parents and caregivers who are likely to continue your therapy making it a success. The characteristics of a language-rich environment are described in Table 10–6.

Developing Spoken Language of Children with Hearing Loss

When parents decide that spoken language is their desired form of communication, the first thing you have to stress is the importance of listening. Why do we speak the language we speak? Because that is what we heard. As noted in Figure 10–14, it is important to stress to parents to speak in their desired languages. If they speak multiple languages, they should use them. You will likely have children on your caseload for speech who have hearing loss. Assuming they have appropriately fit hearing devices as discussed at the beginning of this book, there are many effects of hearing loss on the speech, language, social, and educational development of children with hearing loss. You may find yourself working on these skills as part of your speech and language

Table 10–6. Factors Supporting Language-Rich Environments

1. *Capitalize on early development:* Language learning for children with hearing loss is most critical during the first months and years of a child's life (Yoshinaga-Itano et al., 1998). Because this is known, infants and toddlers need to be immersed in an environment that supports language development.

2. *Provide immersion in a language-rich environment:* A language-rich environment is accessible, uses the preferred communication approach of the child and parents, and provides opportunities for active and consistent communication with peers and adults using the selected approach.

3. *Ensure access to language stimulation:* Infants and toddlers with hearing loss may be insulated, to varying degrees, from the sounds and signs of everyday life. In order to compensate for this auditory and/or visual isolation, alternative, supplementary, and/or enhanced methods must be used to help the child access language.

4. *Provide opportunities to learn from peers:* Children learn from one another. It is essential for a child with hearing loss to be in an environment where peers use the same communication system or language.

5. *Make appropriate adaptations to the environment:* The learning environment must facilitate access to auditory and/or visual information. An appropriate acoustic environment promotes language and communication development by minimizing auditory distractions (background noise) and by reducing noise with carpet and other absorptive materials. Equally important are the appropriate environmental adaptations to support visual enhancement of language. This can include appropriate lighting and reduction of visual distractions (e.g., clutter).

6. *Provide parent support:* Early interventionists teach parents about language development, the importance of ongoing, communicative interactions with their child, and specific techniques to promote and enhance their child's language development.

7. *Ensure parents have access to a multidisciplinary team:* The multidisciplinary team of qualified professionals completes evaluations at periodic intervals to assure developmental progress is being made at a satisfactory rate.

Source: From *Introduction to Aural Rehabilitation* (2nd ed., p. 161), by R. H. Hull, 2014, San Diego, CA: Plural Publishing. Reprinted with permission.

KEY POINT: Multilingual Homes and Language Development

Babies are born wired to acquire language—in one or multiple languages. Therefore, children who are exposed to multiple languages early on are more likely to be able to speak those languages. Children under the age of 12 months are able to hear the nuances of speech in different languages. While a bilingual child's vocabulary in each individual language may be smaller than average, his total vocabulary (from both languages) will be at least the same size as a monolingual child. So what does this mean for a child with hearing loss—nothing really. If the child is exposed to multiple languages early on, it will not confuse them. Encourage families to speak to them in their native languages. Use language naturally at home and the child will learn.

therapy. Keep these in mind when working with children with hearing loss.

Hearing loss effects on vocabulary

- Develop vocabulary more slowly
- Use more easily learned concrete words (e.g., cat, run, door, blue) than abstract words (e.g., before, after, angry)
- Have difficulty learning function words (e.g., the, an, are, a)
- Have difficulty understanding words with more than one meaning (e.g., right)
- Hearing loss presents as a barrier to incidental learning
- The gap between the vocabulary of children with hearing loss and children with normal hearing widens with age— unless you provide intervention

Hearing loss effects on sentence structure

- Shorter sentences
- Poorer understanding and writing complex sentences
- Misunderstand and misuse verb tense, polarization, possessives, and demonstrate disagreement between subject and verb

Hearing loss effects on speech production

- Have difficulty producing sounds they do not have auditory access to and therefore may be less intelligible
- Speak loudly or not loud enough
- May speak in unnatural pitch
- May have poor stress, inflection, and rate of speech

Hearing loss effects on other things

- Social and emotional well-being
- Social isolation, poor self-image, feeling as though they are without friends
- Academic achievement
- Difficulty with reading and mathematical concepts
- Difficulty with speech in noise
- Behind peers unless they receive appropriate educational intervention

Developing a Therapy Plan

As an SLP, you are likely versed in therapy plan development and implementation. The first step often includes a needs assessment or questionnaire. The child may fill one out, while others may be obtained from teachers and parents. An example of this may be the CHILD, IT-MAIS, or the HEAR-QL. These questionnaires have been developed for children with hearing loss and will help you assess the family and teacher perception of the child's performance. You may also consider doing your own assessment/ questionnaire. One example of an auditory performance indicator is the Outcomes of Children with Hearing Loss Vocal Development Landmarks Interview (VDLI) app.

Initial assessment will determine where the child is currently functioning. Skills should be addressed in a manner that allows for the child to progress through the skill in a hierarchical manner. First, the child must be able to detect if the stimuli are present. They then can determine if two signals are the same or different. Once they master discrimination, they may be able to correctly identify the signal and then use it in daily communication for comprehension (see Figure 10–16 for hierarchy of skills development). Within each of these key areas, there can be skills that are developed. Figure 10–17 provides ideas for how to address each of these hierarchical skills.

The therapy plan should include each of the domains of aural rehabilitation that we have discussed: auditory skills, language abilities, and general communication

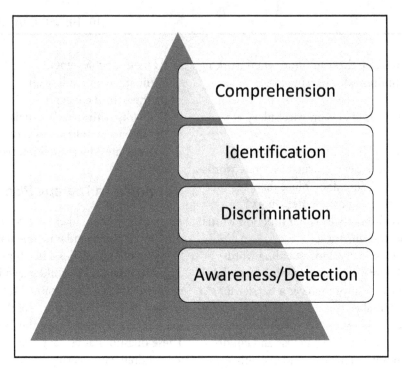

Figure 10–16. Auditory skills development hierarchy.

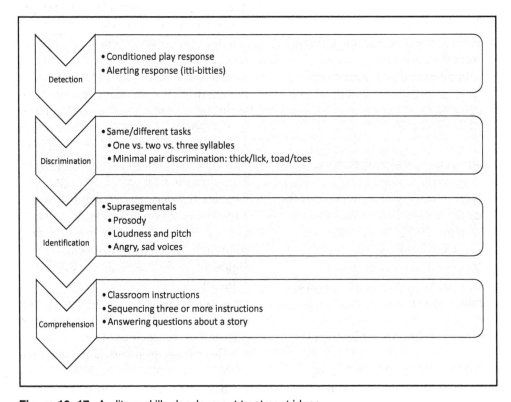

Figure 10–17. Auditory skills development treatment ideas.

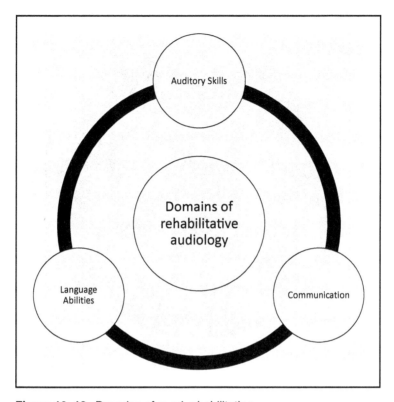

Figure 10–18. Domains of aural rehabilitation.

(Figure 10–18). By having a therapy plan that includes all domains of rehabilitation, you are ensuring effective time management. You may consider addressing several of the 10 auditory processes. As an SLP, you are likely versed in combining varying skills into one therapy session. For example, if you are working on the articulation of the letter /s/, you may also consider working on it in the sense of plurals, discussing the importance of plurals. You may also want to ensure that the child hears the difference and it is not just a visual recognition. Using a speech hoop (Figure 10–19) may help you so that the child can effectively hear you but not see your lips. (A speech hoop is often used when working with children with hearing loss. It allows the sounds go pass through without any obstruction but blocks visual information.)

Using SMART goals, goals should be set and therapy plans generated. SMART goals are goals that are

- Specific—clear and concise goals
- Measurable—can track your progress
- Attainable—challenging yet realistic goals
- Relevant—relevant to your overall plan
- Time based—has a target finish time attached

These goals then are used to develop your overall daily plan for auditory skills development. As stated previously, particularly with children, it is likely that your auditory skills development will be a part of your speech and language goals. However,

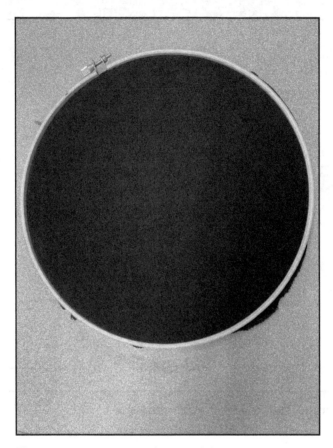

Figure 10–19. A sample of a speech hoop.

when working with kids with hearing loss, it is important that you don't forget that these skills will need to be addressed as well.

What makes a successful habilitation approach? In children, it would include a lot of things that work in conjunction (Figure 10–20) to develop appropriate speech, language, and cognitive skills for quality social and educational performance.

Education Management

There are numerous and complex issues surrounding the education of children with hearing loss. There are varying perspectives in working with these children in the educa-

tional system. These perspectives vary across many professional fields including education, SLP, audiology, and medicine. Professionals from each of these fields approach with different orientations and experiences. The ultimate goal is to ensure the highest educational outcome for children with hearing loss.

Listening Environment. The listening environment may be the most challenging factor affecting children with hearing loss because it is dynamic—constantly changing throughout the day. If children could be individually taught in a sound booth throughout their educational setting, no

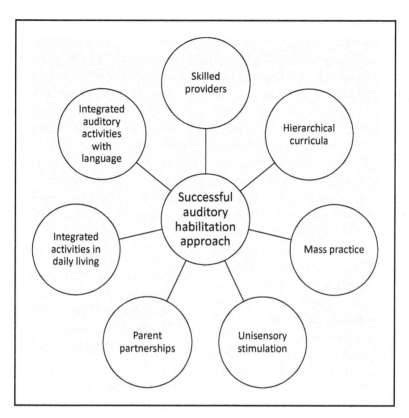

Figure 10–20. Things that go into quality habilitation for children.

child would have language or academic difficulties (although social abilities would certainly be impacted). You along with an audiologist may assess different listening environments and suggest ways to improve acoustic characteristics of the learning environment. Factors include size and shape of a learning space, number of students in the class, noise sources, and the acoustical treatment of the building materials. These factors change every time the child moves to a different room, or when the teacher simply opens a window, leaving the assumption that the child "hears just fine" in question.

Speaking Habits of Adults. Another variable that affects children in the classroom is the speaking habits of the speaker.

Most normal hearing adults can quickly and easily adjust to a wide variety of speaker characteristics. Children, on the other hand, who are still in the early stages of learning rules of speech and language, need special attention paid to the speech model. When talking to children, adults should face the children and focus on speech that is clear, audible, and well-paced. A speaking rate that is appropriate for children is almost tedious to most adults. A good example of an ideal speech rate for children was Mr. Rogers. This is known as "clear speech"; as discussed previously, this is difficult to teach. However, as an SLP, this is something on which you can have a clear and direct impact. Teachers may think that they are providing a quality voice but may benefit from instruction. You may also decrease vocal nodules in the process!

When children are actively engaged in listening, the development of speech and language is optimized. Common sense would tell us that a child with hearing loss needs to have speech presented that is louder. Efforts have been made to train teachers to "just talk louder," but even after continual speech therapy, teachers cannot maintain more than a slight increase in vocal intensity. On the surface, this appears to be a good solution, and possibly is in some listening environments. However, in most classrooms, given poor acoustics and higher noise levels, simply using a louder voice tends to distort the speech signal since the balance between voice and voiceless speech sounds becomes even more discrepant. For example, the vocal tract cannot make a voice vowel sound such as /a/ much louder than a low intensity, high frequency speech sound such as /f/. As such, you as the SLP can make a large impact. Given what we learned in Chapter 8 about remote microphones, using your knowledge and influence, you may be able to instruct the teacher on the need and appropriate use. While not providing direct instruction to the child, this is still part of the habilitation process.

Adults with Hearing Loss

Adults with hearing loss present their own challenges that are different than children. On the surface, you may be dealing with stigma associated with hearing loss that is much different than when working with children. Additionally, while hearing devices may be covered for children, it is unlikely that they will be covered for adults. Therefore, you may be dealing more with the financial impact of recommending audiology for hearing devices. Additionally, on the surface, it seems that most everyone would benefit from aural rehabilitation, and it certainly seems unlikely it could do harm. Yet, overall, aural rehabilitation has received mixed reviews over the years in its application to the adult population.

A variety of factors will influence the pursuit of AR services for adults. One recent investigation examining the motivating factors behind patient choices found the following most influenced the choice (Laplante-Lévesque et al., 2010):

1. Convenience
2. Expected adherence and outcomes
3. Financial costs
4. Self-perceived hearing disability
5. Nature of intervention
6. Preventive and interim solution

Laplante-Levesque et al. (2010) identified convenience as the major factor that will influence the adult patient's choice to pursue or avoid AR. Do the patients drive from far away? Are many in a residential facility and use community resources to access normal appointments? Do patients in the clinic still work outside the home? The type of intervention for each of these cases may be different and the audiologist will be called upon to make individualized recommendations. Expanded AR cannot be a one size fits all approach. The important thing is to offer something and recognize how each type can potentially offer benefit.

Cox et al. (2005) have shown that although those who choose to seek hearing devices (and presumably would be candidates for audiologic rehabilitation) exhibit personality traits within the range of normal, there are statistically significant differences among adults who choose intervention versus those who don't. Among other findings, these authors report that those who present for hearing aids *and* AR may be those who are less able to effectively find strategies to compensate on their own.

Health literacy will also influence any audiologic rehabilitative undertaking. The language used by audiologists, SLPs, and in published materials about hearing devices (such as hearing aid instruction guides) often includes far more jargon than we realize and can create an understanding gap between what we think we are saying and what the average patient is able to understand (Nair & Cienkowski, 2010).

Also contributing to the adult patient's perceived need for audiologic rehabilitative services is the dispensing model used by audiologists that commonly is used today. Approximately 85% of audiologists use a "bundled" model. That is, the patient pays one single price (usually several thousand dollars) for a pair of hearing aids and all related services. Now, one might think that this would encourage people to eagerly return for aural rehabilitative services, as they indirectly have already paid for them. But that doesn't seem to be the case. Rather, the patient thinks of buying hearing aids as if they were buying some other product, and because the product is very expensive, they view the product itself as the ultimate treatment for their problems. Because the "service" from the audiologist is not itemized, it commonly is not viewed as having value. Additionally, unless the audiologist tells the patient about any AR programs, it is unlikely that they will know that they could receive benefit from such a program. Further, unless the audiologist works closely with an SLP and provides compensation through the bundled cost for the time of the SLP, patients may have to pay out of pocket or via insurance for such services from an SLP. They may not realize the benefit of the additional cost of time and money.

Including Spouse or Significant Other (SO)

As discussed earlier, parental involvement has been well studied on the outcomes of children. However, the impact of a spouse or SO on outcomes for adults with hearing loss has been studied much less. When planning for the management of the adult patient with hearing loss, it is important to take in the overall communication picture including those with whom he or she communicates most frequently. He or she may have a lot to offer in terms of functional communication ability of the patient and may be suffering ill effects from the hearing impairment too.

Scarinci, Worrall, and Hickson (2008) qualitatively investigated the effects of hearing loss on the spouses of 10 older hearing-impaired patients, with and without hearing aids. They uncovered a broad scope of emotional effects related to everyday life—need for constant adaptation, acceptance, and aging. Spouses revealed marital discord, feeling burdened by the responsibility, and sadness for the related changes to their social outings and interactions (among many other areas). Such findings underscore the need for rehabilitative audiology to be a process involving both partners as both will be involved in the implementation and AR stands to impact both their psychosocial outcomes. It also demonstrates a need for tools to assess this impact. In another study, they demonstrated that including the significant other in aural rehabilitation significantly improved the overall outcomes of the person with the hearing loss (Figure 10–21).

Preminger (2009) also assessed benefit of participating in a group rehabilitative audiology program for hearing-impaired participants and their significant others. She found that increased use of communication

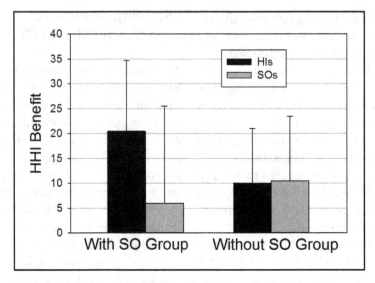

Figure 10–21. Hearing Handicap Index benefit score (pretreatment minus posttreatment): *SO* = significant other; *HI* = Hearing-impaired subject. *Source*: Adapted from Preminger, 2003. From *Modern Hearing Aids: Verification, Outcome Measures, and Follow-Up* (p. 404), by R. Bentler, H. G. Mueller, and T. A. Ricketts, 2016, San Diego, CA: Plural Publishing. Reprinted with permission.

strategies for all participants (participants with and without spouse attending) decreased hearing handicap; however, the greatest reduction occurred when a significant other attended (refer to Figure 10–21). Her overall conclusion from this investigation was that SO participation should be encouraged!

So what should be taught to adults with hearing loss? In many cases, the audiologist may just provide orientation about hearing loss and their hearing device. In other cases, speech reading may be taught. While speech reading may seem like a simple process, the techniques used to teach speechreading are beyond the purview of this text. However, if you desire to engage in speech reading (beyond demonstrating the importance of visual cues), there are many courses and texts available at your disposal. The most important thing that can be taught to an adult in regard to aural rehabilitation is advocacy and good communication techniques.

Good Communication Techniques

Communication is a two-way conversation. It is not very often that people listen to a speaker without giving any input. Usually, the person speaking desires to be heard and will want/need to make an effort to ensure that their message has been heard. Although self-advocacy was discussed in Chapter 9, it is worth noting that this is also part of rehabilitation for people with hearing loss. People with hearing loss will need to advocate for their desire to hear what is being said.

You may first assist a person with hearing loss to identify difficult listening situations. The person may be better able to advocate for themselves if they are able to easily identify when they will struggle to hear what is being said. You may role-play looking at a picture of a restaurant and discussing what situations would make it easier to hear, more difficult, and what parts of the environment may be manipulated. You may discuss where the best place for them to sit would be, how to talk to the server, and how to ask for repetitions. People become better at a skill when it is practiced; you can also include this in any other speech and language treatment in which you engage. As stated previously, communication is a two-way conversation. That means that you may consider engaging with the communication

partner. Some suggestions for a person with hearing loss may be

- Ask the person to move away from the source of noise so that you can understand better
- Ask one of the two people to briefly summarize what has been said before you entered the conversation to give context
- Admit you do not understand and ask for repetition or rephrasing
- Ask for the people to look at you and slow down when speaking

---

KEY CONCEPT: Common Courtesies When Speaking to Someone with Hearing Loss

There are several things you can do when speaking to someone with hearing loss. Additionally, you may find it useful to discuss these points with the family of a person with hearing loss. The following are tips on how family and friends of an individual with hearing loss can help that individual to hear more efficiently:

- Get his or her attention first: This individual may need to prepare himself or herself in order to listen to you.
- Use the individual's name or tap him or her gently on the arm before speaking.
- The individual will only be able to hear one source at a time.
- Slow down: When speaking, speak slowly. This will give the individual time to process what he or she is hearing.
- Face the individual: When facing the individual, he or she will be able

to understand what you are saying better because they are able to see your face.
- Keep your mouth empty: Try to keep your mouth empty (no eating or chewing gum) when speaking with the individual. There is no need to emphasize lip movements when speaking.
- Come closer: Try to stand closer than 3 feet from the person; your voice will be louder and lip reading will be easier.
- Turn it down: The noise levels of devices—such as a TV, dishwasher, or air conditioner—will be more bothersome to those with hearing loss. Turn the volume of these devices down or turn the devices off when speaking to the individual with hearing loss.
- Keep your mouth visible: The individual with hearing loss will struggle less to understand you if your mouth is visible.

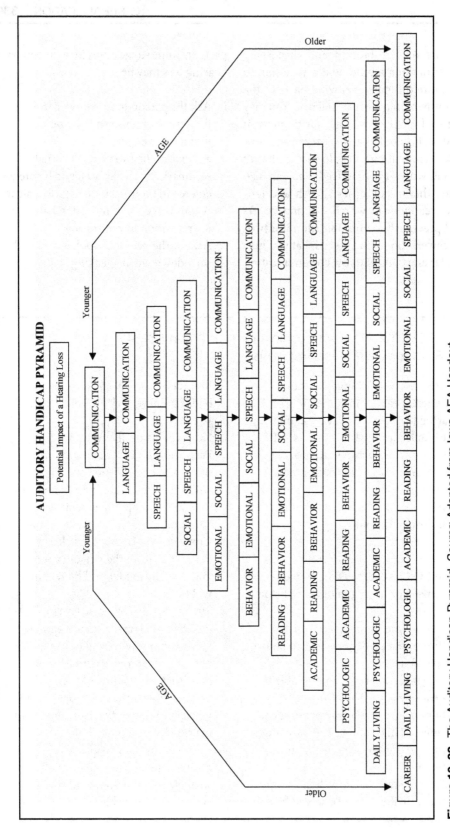

Figure 10–22. The Auditory Handicap Pyramid. *Source:* Adapted from Iowa AEA Handout.

In Closing

A patient is not defined by their hearing loss or communication needs, but by a variety of factors. Thus, there are several concepts and areas that should be considered when developing a plan for a child or adult with hearing loss. Figure 10–22 provides an example of the skills that are built upon each other as the person ages. For each patient or family, these skills may take on a different form or be integrated in a different manner. This under-standing and respect for individuality must begin the moment the patient calls to make the appointment and continue throughout the entire professional relationship with them. The rehabilitation of auditory skills will assist the person to have better communication. As mentioned at the beginning of this chapter, most people communicate with the intent to get their message across, but also to hear what others are saying and engage in conversation. In this respect, rehabilitative audiology will assist a person toward their goal of communication competence.

Appendix A

AAA Scope of Practice

Updated January 2004

Introduction

Development of a Scope of Practice document began in 1990 with the work of an ad hoc committee on Scope of Practice, chaired by Alison Grimes. The document was put into final format by Robert W. Keith in 1992, and revised again in 1996 and 2004.

The Scope of Practice document describes the range of interests, capabilities and professional activities of audiologists. It defines audiologists as independent practitioners and provides examples of settings in which they are engaged. It is not intended to exclude the participation in activities outside of those delineated in the document. The overriding principle is that members of the Academy will provide only those services for which they are adequately prepared through their academic and clinical training and their experience, and that their practice is consistent with the Code of Ethics of the American Academy of Audiology.

As a dynamic and growing profession, the field of audiology will change over time as new information is acquired. This Scope of Practice document will receive regular review for consistency with current knowledge and practice.

Purpose

The purpose of this document is to define the profession of audiology by its scope of practice. This document outlines those activities that are within the expertise of members of the profession. This Scope of Practice statement is intended for use by audiologists, allied professionals, consumers of audiologic services, and the general public. It serves as a reference for issues of service delivery, third-party reimbursement, legislation, consumer education, regulatory action, state and professional licensure, and inter-professional relations. The document is not intended to be an exhaustive list of activities in which audiologists engage. Rather, it is a broad statement of professional practice. Periodic updating of any scope of practice statement is necessary as technologies and perspectives change.

Definition of an Audiologist

An audiologist is a person who, by virtue of academic degree, clinical training, and license to practice and/or professional credential, is uniquely qualified to provide a comprehensive array of professional services related to the prevention of hearing loss and the audiologic identification, assessment, diagnosis, and treatment of persons with impairment of auditory and vestibular function, and to the prevention of impairments associated with them. Audiologists serve in a number of roles including clinician, therapist, teacher, consultant, researcher and administrator. The supervising audiologist maintains legal and ethical responsibility for all assigned audiology activities provided by audiology assistants and audiology students.

The central focus of the profession of audiology is concerned with all auditory impairments and their relationship to disorders of communication. Audiologists identify, assess, diagnose, and treat individuals with impairment of either peripheral or central auditory and/or vestibular function, and strive to prevent such impairments.

Audiologists provide clinical and academic training to students in audiology. Audiologists teach physicians, medical students, residents, and fellows about the auditory and vestibular system. Specifically, they provide instruction about identification, assessment, diagnosis, prevention, and treatment of persons with hearing and/or vestibular impairment. They provide information and training on all aspects of hearing and balance to other professions including psychology, counseling, rehabilitation, and education. Audiologists provide information on hearing and balance, hearing loss and disability, prevention of hearing loss, and treatment to business and industry. They develop and oversee hearing conservation programs in industry. Furthermore, audiologists serve as expert witnesses within the boundaries of forensic audiology.

The audiologist is an independent practitioner who provides services in hospitals, clinics, schools, private practices and other settings in which audiologic services are relevant.

Scope of Practice

The scope of practice of audiologists is defined by the training and knowledge base of professionals who are licensed and/or credentialed to practice as audiologists. Areas of practice include the audiologic identification, assessment, diagnosis and treatment of individuals with impairment of auditory and vestibular function, prevention of hearing loss, and research in normal and disordered auditory and vestibular function. The practice of audiology includes:

Identification

Audiologists develop and oversee hearing screening programs for persons of all ages to detect individuals with hearing loss. Audiologists may perform speech or language screening, or other screening measures, for the purpose of initial identification and referral of persons with other communication disorders.

Assessment and Diagnosis

Assessment of hearing includes the administration and interpretation of behavioral, physioacoustic, and electrophysiologic measures of the peripheral and central auditory systems. Assessment of the vestibular system includes administration and interpretation of behavioral and electrophysiologic tests of equilibrium. Assessment is accomplished using standardized testing procedures and appropriately calibrated instrumentation and leads to the diagnosis of hearing and/or vestibular abnormality.

Treatment

The audiologist is the professional who provides the full range of audiologic treatment services for persons with impairment of hearing and vestibular function. The audiologist is responsible for the evaluation, fitting, and verification of amplification devices, including assistive listening devices. The audiologist determines the appropriateness of amplification systems for persons with hearing impairment, evaluates benefit, and provides counseling and training regarding their use. Audiologists conduct otoscopic examinations, clean ear canals and remove cerumen, take ear canal impressions, select, fit, evaluate, and dispense hearing aids and other amplification systems. Audiologists assess and provide audiologic treatment for persons with tinnitus using techniques that include, but are not limited to, biofeedback, masking, hearing aids, education, and counseling.

Audiologists also are involved in the treatment of persons with vestibular disorders. They participate as full members of balance treatment teams to recommend and carry out treatment and rehabilitation of impairments of vestibular function.

Audiologists provide audiologic treatment services for infants and children with hearing impairment and their families. These services may include clinical treatment, home intervention, family support, and case management.

The audiologist is the member of the implant team (e.g., cochlear implants, middle ear implantable hearing aids, fully implantable hearing aids, bone anchored hearing aids, and all other amplification/signal processing devices) who determines audiologic candidacy based on hearing and communication information. The audiologist provides pre and post surgical assessment, counseling, and all aspects of audiologic treatment including auditory training, rehabilitation, implant programming, and maintenance of implant hardware and software.

The audiologist provides audiologic treatment to persons with hearing impairment, and is a source of information for family members, other professionals and the general public. Counseling regarding hearing loss, the use of amplification systems and strategies for improving speech recognition is within the expertise of the audiologist. Additionally, the audiologist provides counseling regarding the effects of hearing loss on communication and psycho-social status in personal, social, and vocational arenas.

The audiologist administers audiologic identification, assessment, diagnosis, and treatment programs to children of all ages with hearing impairment from birth and preschool through school age. The audiologist is an integral part of the team within the school system that manages students with hearing impairments and students with central auditory processing disorders. The audiologist participates in the development of Individual Family Service Plans (IFSPs) and Individualized Educational Programs (IEPs), serves as a consultant in matters pertaining to classroom acoustics, assistive listening systems, hearing aids, communication, and psycho-social effects of hearing loss, and maintains both classroom assistive systems as well as students' personal hearing aids. The audiologist administers hearing screening programs in schools, and trains and supervises non audiologists performing hearing screening in the educational setting.

Hearing Conservation

The audiologist designs, implements and coordinates industrial and community hearing conservation programs. This includes identification and amelioration of noise-hazardous conditions, identification of hearing loss, recommendation and counseling on use of hearing protection, employee education, and the training and supervision of non audiologists performing hearing screening in the industrial setting.

Intraoperative Neurophysiologic Monitoring

Audiologists administer and interpret electrophysiologic measurements of neural function including, but not limited to, sensory and motor evoked potentials, tests of nerve conduction velocity, and electromyography. These measurements are used in differential diagnosis, pre- and postoperative evaluation of neural function, and neurophysiologic intraoperative monitoring of central nervous system, spinal cord, and cranial nerve function.

Research

Audiologists design, implement, analyze and interpret the results of research related to auditory and balance systems.

Additional Expertise

Some audiologists, by virtue of education, experience and personal choice choose to specialize in an area of practice not otherwise defined in this document. Nothing in this document shall be construed to limit individual freedom of choice in this regard provided that the activity is consistent with the American Academy of Audiology Code of Ethics.

This document will be reviewed, revised, and updated periodically in order to reflect changing clinical demands of audiologists and in order to keep pace with the changing scope of practice reflected by these changes and innovations in this specialty.

Source: Reprinted with permission from American Academy of Audiology (2019). *AAA scope of practice*. Retrieved from https:// www.audiology.org/publications-resources /document-library/scope-practice

Appendix B

ASHA Scope of Practice

Statement of Purpose

The purpose of this document is to define the scope of practice in audiology in order to (a) describe the services offered by qualified audiologists as primary service providers, case managers, and/or members of multidisciplinary and interdisciplinary teams; (b) serve as a reference for health care, education, and other professionals, and for consumers, members of the general public, and policy makers concerned with legislation, regulation, licensure, and third party reimbursement; and (c) inform members of ASHA, certificate holders, and students of the activities for which certification in audiology is required in accordance with the ASHA Code of Ethics.

Audiologists provide comprehensive diagnostic and treatment/rehabilitative services for auditory, vestibular, and related impairments. These services are provided to individuals across the entire age span from birth through adulthood; to individuals from diverse language, ethnic, cultural, and socioeconomic backgrounds; and to individuals who have multiple disabilities. This position statement is not intended to be exhaustive; however, the activities described reflect current practice within the profession. Practice activities related to emerging clinical, technological, and scientific developments are not precluded from consideration as part of the scope of practice of an audiologist. Such innovations and advances will result in the periodic revision and updating of this document. It is also recognized that specialty areas identified within the scope of practice will vary among the individual providers. ASHA also recognizes that credentialed professionals in related fields may have knowledge, skills, and experience that could be applied to some areas within the scope of audiology practice. Defining the scope of practice of audiologists is not meant to exclude other appropriately credentialed postgraduate professionals from rendering services in common practice areas.

Audiologists serve diverse populations. The patient/client population includes persons of different race, age, gender, religion, national origin, and sexual orientation. Audiologists' caseloads include individuals from diverse ethnic, cultural, or linguistic backgrounds, and persons with disabilities. Although audiologists are prohibited from discriminating in the provision of professional services based on these factors, in some cases such factors may be relevant to the development of an appropriate treatment plan. These factors may be considered in treatment plans only when firmly grounded in scientific and professional knowledge.

This scope of practice does not supersede existing state licensure laws or affect the interpretation or implementation of such laws. It may serve, however, as a model for the development or modification of licensure laws.

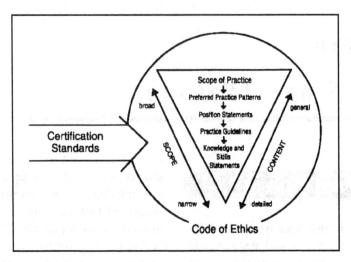

Figure B–1. Conceptual Framework of ASHA Standards and Policy Statements.

The schema in Figure B–1 depicts the relationship of the scope of practice to ASHA's policy documents that address current and emerging audiology practice areas; that is, preferred practice patterns, guidelines, and position statements. ASHA members and ASHA-certified professionals are bound by the ASHA Code of Ethics to provide services that are consistent with the scope of their competence, education, and experience (ASHA, 2003). There are other existing legislative and regulatory bodies that govern the practice of audiology.

Framework for Practice

The practice of audiology includes both the prevention of and assessment of auditory, vestibular, and related impairments as well as the habilitation/rehabilitation and maintenance of persons with these impairments. The overall goal of the provision of audiology services should be to optimize and enhance the ability of an individual to hear, as well as to communicate in his/her every day or natural environment. In addition, audiologists provide comprehensive services to individuals with normal hearing who interact with persons with a hearing impairment. The overall goal of audiologic services is to improve the quality of life for all of these individuals.

The World Health Organization (WHO) has developed a multipurpose health classification system known as the International Classification of Functioning, Disability, and Health (ICF) (WHO, 2001). The purpose of this classification system is to provide a standard language and framework for the description of functioning and health. The ICF framework is useful in describing the role of audiologists in the prevention, assessment, and habilitation/rehabilitation of auditory, vestibular, and other related impairments and restrictions or limitations of functioning.

The ICF is organized into two parts. The first part deals with Functioning and Disability while the second part deals with Contextual Factors. Each part has two components. The components of Functioning and Disability are:

■ **Body Functions and Structures:** Body Functions are the physiological functions of body systems and Body Structures are the anatomical parts of the body and their components. Impairments are limitations or variations in Body Function or Structure such as a deviation or loss. An example of a Body Function that might be evaluated by an audiologist would be hearing sensitivity. The use of typanometry to access the mobility of the tympanic membrane is an example of a Body Structure that might be evaluated by an audiologist.

■ **Activity/Participation:** In the ICF, Activity and Participation are realized as one list. Activity refers to the execution of a task or action by an individual. Participation is the involvement in a life situation. Activity limitations are difficulties an individual may experience while executing a given activity. Participation restrictions are difficulties that may limit an individual's involvement in life situations. The Activity/Participation construct thus represents the effects that hearing, vestibular, and related impairments could have on the life of an individual. These effects could include the ability to hold conversations, participate in sports, attend religious services, understand a teacher in a classroom, and walk up and down stairs.

The components of Contextual Factors are:

■ **Environmental Factors:** Environmental Factors make up the physical, social, and attitudinal environment in which people live and conduct their lives. Examples of Environmental Factors, as they relate to audiology, include the acoustical properties of a given space and any type of hearing assistive technology.

■ **Personal Factors:** Personal Factors are the internal influences on an individual's functioning and disability and are not a part of the health condition. These factors may include but are not limited to age, gender, social background, and profession.

Functioning and Disability are interactive and evolutionary processes. Figure B–2 illustrates the interaction of the various components of the ICF. Each component of the ICF can be expressed on a continuum of function. On one end of the continuum is intact functioning. At the opposite end of the continuum is completely compromised functioning. Contextual Factors (Environmental and Personal Factors) may interact with any of the components of functioning and disability. Environmental and Personal Factors may act as facilitators or barriers to functioning.

The scope of practice in audiology encompasses all of the components of the ICF. During the assessment phase, audiologists perform tests of Body Function and Structure. Examples of these types of tests include otoscopic examination, pure-tone audiometry, tympanometry, otoacoustic emissions measurements, and speech audiometry. Activity/Participation limitations and restrictions are sometimes addressed by audiologists through case history, interview, questionnaire, and counseling. For example, a question such as, "Do you have trouble understanding while on the telephone?" or "Can you describe the difficulties you experience when you participate in a conversation with someone who is not familiar to you?" would be considered an assessment of Activity/Participation limitation or restriction. Questionnaires that require clients to report the magnitude of difficulty that they experience in certain specified settings can sometimes be used to measure aspects

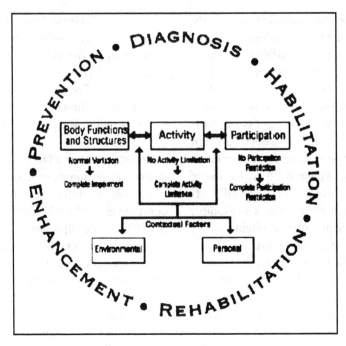

Figure B–2. Application of WHO (2001) Framework to the Practice of Audiology.

of Activity/Participation. For example: "Because of my hearing problems, I have difficulty conversing with others in a restaurant." In addition, Environmental and Personal Factors also need to be taken into consideration by audiologists as they treat individuals with auditory, vestibular, and other related impairments. In the above question regarding conversation in a restaurant, if the factor of "noise" (i.e., a noisy restaurant) is added to the question, this represents an Environmental Factor. Examples of Personal Factors might include a person's background or culture that influences his or her reaction to the use of a hearing aid or cochlear implant. The use of the ICF framework (WHO, 2001) may help audiologists broaden their perspective concerning their role in evaluating a client's needs or when designing and providing comprehensive services to their clients. Overall,

audiologists work to improve quality of life by reducing impairments of body functions and structures, Activity limitations/Participation restrictions and Environmental barriers of the individuals they serve.

Definition of an Audiologist

Audiologists are professionals engaged in autonomous practice to promote healthy hearing, communication competency, and quality of life for persons of all ages through the prevention, identification, assessment, and rehabilitation of hearing, auditory function, balance, and other related systems. They facilitate prevention through the fitting of hearing protective devices, education programs for industry and the public, hearing screening/conservation programs, and research. The audiologist is the professional responsible for the identification of impairments and dysfunction of the auditory, balance, and other related systems. Their unique education and training provides them with the skills to assess and diagnose dysfunction in hearing, auditory function, balance, and related disorders. The delivery of audiologic (re)habilitation services includes not only the selecting, fitting, and dispensing of hearing aids and other hearing assistive devices, but also the assessment and follow-up services for persons with cochlear implants. The audiologist providing audiologic (re)habilitation does so through a comprehensive program of therapeutic services, devices, counseling, and other management strategies. Functional diagnosis of vestibular disorders and management of balance rehabilitation is another aspect of the professional responsibilities of the audiologist. Audiologists engage in research pertinent to all of these domains.

Audiologists currently hold a master's or doctoral degree in audiology from a program accredited by the Council on Academic Accreditation in Audiology and Speech-Language Pathology (CAA) of the American Speech-Language-Hearing Association. ASHA-certified audiologists complete a supervised postgraduate professional experience or a similar supervised professional experience during the completion of the doctoral degree as described in the ASHA certification standards. Beginning January 1, 2012, all applicants for the Certificate of Clinical Competence in Audiology must have a doctoral degree from a CAA-accredited university program. Demonstration of continued professional development is mandated for the maintenance of the Certificate of Clinical Competence in

Audiology. Where required, audiologists are licensed or registered by the state in which they practice.

Professional Roles and Activities

Audiologists serve a diverse population and may function in one or more of a variety of activities. The practice of audiology includes:

A. Prevention

1. Promotion of hearing wellness, as well as the prevention of hearing loss and protection of hearing function by designing, implementing, and coordinating occupational, school, and community hearing conservation and identification programs;
2. Participation in noise measurements of the acoustic environment to improve accessibility and to promote hearing wellness.

B. Identification

1. Activities that identify dysfunction in hearing, balance, and other auditory-related systems;
2. Supervision, implementation, and follow-up of newborn and school hearing screening programs;
3. Screening for speech, orofacial myofunctional disorders, language, cognitive communication disorders, and/or preferred communication modalities that may affect education, health, development or communication and may

result in recommendations for rescreening or comprehensive speech-language pathology assessment or in referral for other examinations or services;

4. Identification of populations and individuals with or at risk for hearing loss and other auditory dysfunction, balance impairments, tinnitus, and associated communication impairments as well as of those with normal hearing;

5. In collaboration with speech-language pathologists, identification of populations and individuals at risk for developing speech-language impairments.

C. Assessment

1. The conduct and interpretation of behavioral, electroacoustic, and/or electrophysiologic methods to assess hearing, auditory function, balance, and related systems;

2. Measurement and interpretation of sensory and motor evoked potentials, electromyography, and other electrodiagnostic tests for purposes of neurophysiologic intraoperative monitoring and cranial nerve assessment;

3. Evaluation and management of children and adults with auditory-related processing disorders;

4. Performance of otoscopy for appropriate audiological management or to provide a basis for medical referral;

5. Cerumen management to prevent obstruction of the external ear canal and of amplification devices;

6. Preparation of a report including interpreting data, summarizing findings, generating recommendations and developing an audiologic treatment/management plan;

7. Referrals to other professions, agencies, and/or consumer organizations.

D. Rehabilitation

1. As part of the comprehensive audiologic (re)habilitation program, evaluates, selects, fits and dispenses hearing assistive technology devices to include hearing aids;

2. Assessment of candidacy of persons with hearing loss for cochlear implants and provision of fitting, mapping, and audiologic rehabilitation to optimize device use;

3. Development of a culturally appropriate, audiologic rehabilitative management plan including, when appropriate:

   a. Recommendations for fitting and dispensing, and educating the consumer and family/caregivers in the use of and adjustment to sensory aids, hearing assistive devices, alerting systems, and captioning devices;

   b. Availability of counseling relating to psycho social aspects of hearing loss, and other auditory dysfunction, and processes to enhance communication competence;

   c. Skills training and consultation concerning environmental modifications to facilitate development of receptive and expressive communication;

   d. Evaluation and modification of the audiologic management plan.

4. Provision of comprehensive audiologic rehabilitation services, including management procedures for speech and language habilitation and/or rehabilitation for persons with hearing loss or other auditory dysfunction, including but not exclusive to speechreading, auditory training, communication stra-

tegies, manual communication and counseling for psychosocial adjustment for persons with hearing loss or other auditory dysfunction and their families/caregivers;

5. Consultation and provision of vestibular and balance rehabilitation therapy to persons with vestibular and balance impairments;

6. Assessment and non-medical management of tinnitus using biofeedback, behavioral management, masking, hearing aids, education, and counseling;

7. Provision of training for professionals of related and/or allied services when needed;

8. Participation in the development of an Individual Education Program (IEP) for school-age children or an Individual Family Service Plan (IFSP) for children from birth to 36 months old;

9. Provision of in-service programs for school personnel, and advising school districts in planning educational programs and accessibility for students with hearing loss and other auditory dysfunction;

10. Measurement of noise levels and provision of recommendations for environmental modifications in order to reduce the noise level;

11. Management of the selection, purchase, installation, and evaluation of large-area amplification systems.

E. Advocacy/Consultation

1. Advocacy for communication needs of all individuals that may include advocating for the rights/funding of services for those with hearing loss, auditory, or vestibular disorders;

2. Advocacy for issues (i.e., acoustic accessibility) that affect the rights of individuals with normal hearing;

3. Consultation with professionals of related and/or allied services when needed;

4. Consultation in development of an Individual Education Program (IEP) for school-age children or an Individual Family Service Plan (IFSP) for children from birth to 36 months old;

5. Consultation to educators as members of interdisciplinary teams about communication management, educational implications of hearing loss and other auditory dysfunction, educational programming, classroom acoustics, and large-area amplification systems for children with hearing loss and other auditory dysfunction;

6. Consultation about accessibility for persons with hearing loss and other auditory dysfunction in public and private buildings, programs, and services;

7. Consultation to individuals, public and private agencies, and governmental bodies, or as an expert witness regarding legal interpretations of audiology findings, effects of hearing loss and other auditory dysfunction, balance system impairments, and relevant noise-related considerations;

8. Case management and service as a liaison for the consumer, family, and agencies in order to monitor audiologic status and management and to make recommendations about educational and vocational programming;

9. Consultation to industry on the development of products and instrumentation related to the measurement and management of auditory or balance function.

F. Education/ Research/ Administration

1. Education, supervision, and administration for audiology graduate and other professional education programs;
2. Measurement of functional outcomes, consumer satisfaction, efficacy, effectiveness, and efficiency of practices and programs to maintain and improve the quality of audiologic services;
3. Design and conduct of basic and applied audiologic research to increase the knowledge base, to develop new methods and programs, and to determine the efficacy, effectiveness, and efficiency of assessment and treatment paradigms; disseminate research findings to other professionals and to the public;
4. Participation in the development of professional and technical standards;
5. Participation in quality improvement programs;
6. Program administration and supervision of professionals as well as support personnel.

Practice Settings

Audiologists provide services in private practice; medical settings such as hospitals and physicians' offices; community and university hearing and speech centers; managed care systems; industry; the military; various state agencies; home health, subacute rehabilitation, long-term care, and intermediate-care facilities; and school systems. Audiologists provide academic education to students and practitioners in universities, to medical and surgical students and residents, and to other related professionals. Such education pertains to the identification, functional diagnosis/assessment, and non-medical treatment/management of auditory, vestibular, balance, and related impairments.

References

American Speech-Language-Hearing Association. (1996, Spring). Scope of practice in audiology. *Asha, 38*(Suppl. 16), 12–15.

American Speech-Language-Hearing Association. (2003). Code of ethics [Revised]. *ASHA Supplement, 23*, 13–15.

World Health Organization. (2001). *ICF: International classification of functioning, disability and health*. Geneva, Switzerland: Author.

Source: Reprinted with permission from American Speech-Language-Hearing Association. *ASHA Scope of Practice in Audiology*. Available from https://www.asha.org/policy /SP2004-00192/

Appendix C

AAA Code of Ethics

Preamble

The Code of Ethics of the American Academy of Audiology specifies professional standards that allow for the proper discharge of audiologists' responsibilities to those served, and that protect the integrity of the profession. The Code of Ethics consists of two parts. The first part, the Statement of Principles and Rules, presents precepts that members (all categories of members including Student Members) effective January 1, 2009 of the Academy agree to uphold. The second part, the Procedures, provides the process that enables enforcement of the Principles and Rules.

Part I. Statement of Principles and Rules

PRINCIPLE 1: Members shall provide professional services and conduct research with honesty and compassion, and shall respect the dignity, worth, and rights of those served.

Rule 1a: Individuals shall not limit the delivery of professional services on any basis that is unjustifiable or irrelevant to the need for the potential benefit from such services.

Rule 1b: Individuals shall not provide services except in a professional relationship and shall not discriminate in the provision of services to individuals on the basis of sex, race, religion, national origin, sexual orientation, or general health.

PRINCIPLE 2: Members shall maintain the highest standards of professional competence in rendering services.

Rule 2a: Members shall provide only those professional services for which they are qualified by education and experience.

Rule 2b: Individuals shall use available resources, including referrals to other specialists, and shall not give or accept benefits or items of value for receiving or making referrals.

Rule 2c: Individuals shall exercise all reasonable precautions to avoid injury to persons in the delivery of professional services or execution of research.

Rule 2d: Individuals shall provide appropriate supervision and assume full responsibility for services delegated to supportive personnel. Individuals shall not delegate any service requiring professional competence to unqualified persons.

Rule 2e: Individuals shall not knowingly permit personnel under their direct or indirect supervision to engage in any practice that is not in compliance with the Code of Ethics.

Rule 2f: Individuals shall maintain professional competence, including participation in continuing education.

PRINCIPLE 3: Members shall maintain the confidentiality of the information and records of those receiving services or involved in research.

Rule 3a: Individuals shall not reveal to unauthorized persons any professional or personal information obtained from the person served professionally, unless required by law.

PRINCIPLE 4: Members shall provide only services and products that are in the best interest of those served.

Rule 4a: Individuals shall not exploit persons in the delivery of professional services.

Rule 4b: Individuals shall not charge for services not rendered.

Rule 4c: Individuals shall not participate in activities that constitute a conflict of professional interest.

Rule 4d: Individuals using investigational procedures with human participants or prospectively collecting research data from human participants shall obtain full informed consent from the participants or legal representatives. Members conducting research with human participants or animals shall follow accepted standards, such as those promulgated in the current Responsible

Conduct of Research by the U.S. Office of Research Integrity.

PRINCIPLE 5: Members shall provide accurate information about the nature and management of communicative disorders and about the services and products offered.

Rule 5a: Individuals shall provide persons served with the information a reasonable person would want to know about the nature and possible effects of services rendered or products provided or research being conducted.

Rule 5b: Individuals may make a statement of prognosis, but shall not guarantee results, mislead, or misinform persons served or studied.

Rule 5c: Individuals shall conduct and report product-related research only according to accepted standards of research practice.

Rule 5d: Individuals shall not carry out teaching or research activities in a manner that constitutes an invasion of privacy or that fails to inform persons fully about the nature and possible effects of these activities, affording all persons informed free choice of participation.

Rule 5e: Individuals shall maintain accurate documentation of services rendered according to accepted medical, legal and professional standards and requirements.

PRINCIPLE 6: Members shall comply with the ethical standards of the Academy with regard to public statements or publication.

Rule 6a: Individuals shall not misrepresent their educational degrees, training, credentials, or competence. Only degrees earned from regionally accredited institutions in which training was obtained in audiology, or a directly related discipline, may be used in public statements concerning professional services.

Rule 6b: Individuals' public statements about professional services, products or research results shall not contain representations or claims that are false, misleading, or deceptive.

PRINCIPLE 7: Members shall honor their responsibilities to the public and to professional colleagues.

Rule 7a: Individuals shall not use professional or commercial affiliations in any way that would limit services to or mislead patients or colleagues.

Rule 7b: Individuals shall inform colleagues and the public in an objective manner consistent with professional standards about products and services they have developed or research they have conducted.

PRINCIPLE 8: Members shall uphold the dignity of the profession and freely accept the Academy's self-imposed standards.

Rule 8a: Individuals shall not violate these Principles and Rules nor attempt to circumvent them.

Rule 8b: Individuals shall not engage in dishonesty or illegal conduct that adversely reflects on the profession.

Rule 8c: Individuals shall inform the Ethical Practices Committee when there are reasons to believe that a member of the Academy may have been in noncompliance with the Code of Ethics.

Rule 8d: Individuals shall fully cooperate with reviews being conducted by the Ethical Practices Committee in any matter related to the Code of Ethics.

Part II. Procedures for the Management of Alleged Noncompliance

Introduction

Members of the American Academy of Audiology are obligated to uphold the Code of Ethics of the Academy in their personal conduct and in the performance of their professional duties. To this end, it is the responsibility of each Academy member to inform the Ethical Practice Committee of possible noncompliance with the Ethics Code. The processing of alleged noncompliance with the Code of Ethics will follow the procedures specified below in an expeditious manner to ensure that behaviors of noncompliant ethical conduct by members of the Academy are halted in the shortest time possible.

Procedures

1. Suspected noncompliance with the Code of Ethics shall be reported in letter format, giving documentation sufficient to support the alleged noncompliance. Letters must be addressed to:

   American Academy of Audiology
   Chair, Ethical Practices Committee
   11480 Commerce Park Dr. Suite 220
   Reston, VA 20191

2. Following receipt of a report of suspected noncompliance, at the discretion of the Chair, the Ethical Practices Committee will request a signed Waiver of Confidentiality from the complainant indicating that the complainant will allow the Ethical Practice Board to disclose his/her name and complaint details should this become necessary during investigation of the allegation.

   a. The Committee may, under special circumstances, act in the absence of a signed Waiver of Confidentiality. For example, in cases where the Ethical Practice Committee has received information from a state licensure board of a member having his or her license suspended or revoked, then the Ethical Practice Committee will proceed without a complainant.

   b. The Chair may communicate with other individuals, agencies, and/or programs for additional information as may be required for Committee review at any time during the deliberation.

3. The Ethical Practice Committee will convene to review the merit of the alleged noncompliance as it relates to the Code of Ethics.

   a. The Ethical Practice Committee shall meet to discuss the case, either in person, by electronic means, or by teleconference. The meeting will occur within 60 days of receipt of the Waiver of Confidentiality, or of notification by the complainant of refusal to sign the waiver. In cases where another form of notification brings the complaint to the attention of the Ethical Practice Committee, the Committee will convene within 60 days of notification.

   b. If the alleged noncompliance has a high probability of being legally actionable, the case may be referred to the appropriate agency. The Ethical Practice Committee will postpone member notification and further deliberation until the legal process has been completed.

4. If there is sufficient evidence that indicates noncompliance with the Code of Ethics has occurred, upon majority vote, the member will be forwarded a Notification of Potential Ethics Concern.

   a. The circumstances of the alleged noncompliance will be described.

   b. The member will be informed of the specific Code of Ethics principle(s) and/or rule(s) that may conflict with member behavior.

   c. Supporting AAA documents that may serve to further educate the member about the ethical implications will be included, as appropriate.

   d. The member will be asked to respond fully to the allegation and submit all supporting evidence within 30 calendar days.

5. The Ethical Practices Committee will meet either in person or by teleconference:

   a. within 60 calendar days of receiving a response from the member to the Notification of Potential Ethics Concern to review the response and all information pertaining to the alleged noncompliance, or

   b. within sixty (60) calendar days of notification to member if no response is received from the member to review the information received from the complainant.

6. If the Ethical Practice Committee determines that the evidence supports the allegation of noncompliance, the member will be provided written notice containing the following information:

   a. The right to a hearing in person or by teleconference before the Ethical Practice Committee;
   b. The date, time, and place of the hearing;
   c. The ethical noncompliance being charged and the potential sanction;
   d. The right to present a defense to the charges.
   e. At this time the member should provide any additional relevant information. As this is the final opportunity for a member to provide new information, the member should carefully prepare all documentation.

7. Potential Rulings.

   a. When the Ethical Practices Committee determines there is insufficient evidence of ethical noncompliance, the parties to the complaint will be notified that the case will be closed.
   b. If the evidence supports the allegation of Code noncompliance, the Code(s)/Rule(s) will be cited and the sanction(s) will be specified.

8. The Committee shall sanction members based on the severity of the noncompliance and history of prior ethical noncompliance. A simple majority of

voting members is required to institute a sanction unless otherwise noted. Sanctions may include one or more of the following:

   a. Educative Letter. This sanction alone is appropriate when:
      i. The ethics noncompliance appears to have been inadvertent.
      ii. The member's response to Notification of Potential Ethics Concern indicates a new awareness of the problem and the member resolves to refrain from future ethical noncompliance.
   b. Cease and Desist Order. The member signs a consent agreement to immediately halt the practice(s) that were found to be in noncompliance with the Code of Ethics.
   c. Reprimand. The member will be formally reprimanded for the noncompliance with of the Code of Ethics.
   d. Mandatory continuing education
      i. The EPC will determine the type of education needed to reduce chances of recurrence of noncompliance.
      ii. The member will be responsible for submitting documentation of continuing education within the period of time designated by the Ethical Practices Committee.
      iii. All costs associated with compliance will be borne by the member.
   e. Probation of Suspension. The member signs a consent agreement in acknowledgement of the Ethical Practice Committee decision and

is allowed to retain membership benefits during a defined probationary period.

   i. The duration of probation and the terms for avoiding suspension will be determined by the Ethical Practice Committee.

   ii. Failure of the member to meet the terms for probation will result in the suspension of membership.

f. Suspension of Membership.

   i. The duration of suspension will be determined by the Ethical Practice Committee.

   ii. The member may not receive membership benefits during the period of suspension.

   iii. Members suspended are not entitled to a refund of dues or fees.

g. Revocation of Membership. Revocation of membership is considered the maximum consequence for noncompliance with the Code of Ethics.

   i. Revocation requires a two-thirds majority of the voting members of the EPC.

   ii. Individuals whose memberships are revoked are not entitled to a refund of dues or fees.

   iii. One year following the date of membership revocation the individual may reapply for, but is not guaranteed, membership through normal channels, and must meet the membership qualifications in effect at the time of reapplication.

9. The member may appeal the Final Finding and Decision of the Ethical Practice Committee to the Academy Board of Directors. The route of Appeal is by letter format through the Ethical Practice Committee to the Board of Directors of the Academy. Requests for Appeal must:

a. be received by the Chair of the Ethical Practice Committee within 30 days of the Ethical Practice Committee notification of the Final Finding and Decision,

b. state the basis for the appeal and the reason(s) that the Final Finding and Decision of the Ethical Practice Committee should be changed,

c. not offer new documentation.

   i. The EPC chair will communicate with the Executive Director of the Academy to schedule the appeal at the earliest feasible Board of Director's meeting.

   ii. The Board of Directors will review the documents and written summaries and deliberate the case.

   iii. The decision of the Board of Directors regarding the member's appeal shall be final.

10. In order to educate the membership, upon majority vote of the Ethical Practice Committee, the circumstances and nature of cases shall be presented in Audiology Today and in the Professional Resource area of the AAA website. The member's identity will not be made public.

11. No Ethical Practice Committee member shall give access to records, act or speak independently, or on behalf of the Ethical Practice Committee, without the expressed permission of the members then active. No member may impose the sanction of the Ethical Practice Committee or interpret the findings of the EPC in

any manner that may place members of the Ethical Practice Committee or Board of Directors, collectively or singly, at financial, professional, or personal risk.

12. The Ethical Practice Committee Chair and Staff Liaison shall maintain electronic records that shall form the basis for future findings of the Committee.

Confidentiality and Records

Confidentiality shall be maintained in all Ethical Practice Committee discussion, correspondence, communication, deliberation, and records pertaining to members reviewed by the Ethical Practice Committee.

1. Complaints and suspected noncompliance with the Code of Ethics are assigned a case number.
2. Identity of members involved in complaints and suspected noncompliance cases and access to EPC files is restricted to the following:

   a. EPC members
   b. Executive Director
   c. Agent/s of the Executive Director
   d. Other/s, following majority vote of EPC

3. Original records shall be maintained at the Central Records Repository at the Academy office in a locked cabinet.

   a. One copy will be sent to the Ethical Practice Committee Chair or member designated by the Chair.

   b. Redacted copies will be sent to members.

4. Communications shall be sent to the members involved in complaints by the Academy office via certified or registered mail, after review by Legal Counsel, as needed.

5. When a case is closed,

   a. The Chair will forward all documentation to the Staff Liaison to be maintained at the Academy Central Records Repository.
   b. Members shall destroy all material pertaining to the case.

6. Complete records generally shall be maintained at the Academy Central Records Repository for a period of 5 years.

   a. Records will be destroyed five years after a member receives a sanction less than suspension, or five years after the end of a suspension, or after membership is reinstated.
   b. Records of membership revocations for persons who have not returned to membership status will be maintained indefinitely.

Source: Reprinted with permission from American Academy of Audiology. (2019). *AAA code of ethics*. Retrieved from https://www.audiology.org/sites/default/files/about/membership/documents/Code%20of%20Ethics%20with%20procedures-REV%202018_0216.pdf

Appendix D

SII 2010 Revision of the 1990 Mueller and Killion Count-the-Dots Audiogram

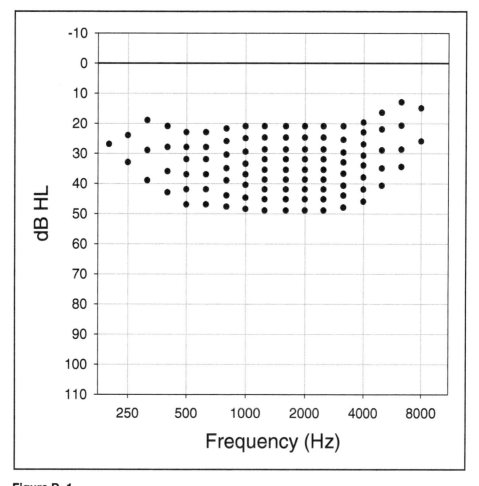

Figure D–1.

Source: Reprinted from Killion, M., and Mueller, H. (2010). Twenty years later: A NEW Count-the-Dots method. *The Hearing Journal*, *63*(1). Copyright 2010 by Wolters Kluwer Health, Inc.

Appendix E

Abbreviated Profile of Hearing Aid Benefit (APHAB)

NAME: _____ ☐ Male ☐ Female TODAY'S DATE: __/__/__

    Last   *First*

INSTRUCTIONS: Please circle the answers that come closest to your everyday experience. Notice that each choice includes a percentage. You can use this to help you decide on your answer. For example, if a statement is true about 75% of the time, circle "C" for that item. If you have not experienced the situation we describe, try to think of a similar situation that you have been in and respond for that situation. If you have no idea, leave that item blank.

A **Always (99%)**
B **Almost Always (87%)**
C **Generally (75%)**
D **Half-the-time (50%)**
E **Occasionally (25%)**
F **Seldom (12%)**
G **Never (1%)**

	Without Hearing Aids	With Hearing Aids
1. When I am in a crowded grocery store, talking with the cashier, I can follow the conversation.	A B C D E F G	A B C D E F G
2. I miss a lot of information when I'm listening to a lecture.	A B C D E F G	A B C D E F G
3. Unexpected sounds, like a smoke detector or alarm bell are uncomfortable.	A B C D E F G	A B C D E F G
4. I have difficulty hearing a conversation when I'm with one of my family at home.	A B C D E F G	A B C D E F G
5. I have trouble understanding the dialogue in a movie or at the theater.	A B C D E F G	A B C D E F G
6. When I am listening to the news on the car radio, and family members are talking, I have trouble hearing the news.	A B C D E F G	A B C D E F G
7. When I'm at the dinner table with several people, and am trying to have a conversation with one person, understanding speech is difficult.	A B C D E F G	A B C D E F G

continues

Abbreviated Profile of Hearing Aid Benefit (APHAB) *continued*

A **Always (99%)**
B **Almost Always (87%)**
C **Generally (75%)**
D **Half-the-time (50%)**
E **Occasionally (25%)**
F **Seldom (12%)**
G **Never (1%)**

	Without Hearing Aids	With Hearing Aids
8. Traffic noises are too loud.	A B C D E F G	A B C D E F G
9. When I am talking with someone across a large empty room, I understand the words.	A B C D E F G	A B C D E F G
10. When I am in a small office, interviewing or answering questions, I have difficulty following the conversation.	A B C D E F G	A B C D E F G
11. When I am in a theater watching a movie or play, and the people around me are whispering and rustling paper wrappers, I can still make out the dialogue.	A B C D E F G	A B C D E F G
12. When I am having a quiet conversation with a friend, I have difficulty understanding.	A B C D E F G	A B C D E F G
13. The sounds of running water, such as a toilet or shower, are uncomfortably loud.	A B C D E F G	A B C D E F G
14. When a speaker is addressing a small group, and everyone is listening quietly, I have to strain to understand.	A B C D E F G	A B C D E F G
15. When I'm in a quiet conversation with my doctor in an examination room, it is hard to follow the conversation.	A B C D E F G	A B C D E F G
16. I can understand conversations even when several people are talking.	A B C D E F G	A B C D E F G
17. The sounds of construction work are uncomfortably loud.	A B C D E F G	A B C D E F G
18. It's hard for me to understand what is being said at lectures or church services.	A B C D E F G	A B C D E F G

Abbreviated Profile of Hearing Aid Benefit (APHAB) *continued*

A Always (99%)
B Almost Always (87%)
C Generally (75%)
D Half-the-time (50%)
E Occasionally (25%)
F Seldom (12%)
G Never (1%)

	Without Hearing Aids	With Hearing Aids
19. I can communicate with others when we are in a crowd.	A B C D E F G	A B C D E F G
20. The sound of a fire engine siren close by is so loud that I need to cover my ears.	A B C D E F G	A B C D E F G
21. I can follow the words of a sermon when listening to a religious service.	A B C D E F G	A B C D E F G
22. The sound of screeching tires is uncomfortably loud.	A B C D E F G	A B C D E F G
23. I have to ask people to repeat themselves in one-on-one conversation in a quiet room.	A B C D E F G	A B C D E F G
24. I have trouble understanding others when an air conditioner or fan is on.	A B C D E F G	A B C D E F G

Please fill out these additional items.

HEARING AID EXPERIENCE	DAILY HEARING AID USE	DEGREE OF HEARING DIFFICULTY (without wearing a hearing aid)
☐ None	☐ None	☐ None
☐ Less than 6 weeks	☐ Less than 1 hour per day	☐ Mild
☐ 6 weeks to 11 months	☐ 1 to 4 hours per day	☐ Moderate
☐ 1 to 10 years	☐ 4 to 8 hours per day	☐ Moderately-Severe
☐ Over 10 years	☐ 8 to 16 hours per day	☐ Severe

Appendix F

Expected Consequences of Hearing Aid Ownership (ECHO)

NAME _____ GENDER M F DATE OF BIRTH __/__/__ TODAY'S DATE __/__/__

<table>
<tr><td>

INSTRUCTIONS

Listed below are statements about hearing aids. Please circle the letter that indicates the extent to which you agree with each statement. Use the list of words to determine your answer.

</td><td>

A Not At All

B A Little

C Somewhat

D Medium

E Considerably

F Greatly

G Tremendously

</td></tr>
</table>

How much do you agree with each statement?

1. My hearing aids will help me understand the people I speak with most frequently.	A B C D E F G
2. I will be frustrated when my hearing aids pick up sounds that keep me from hearing what I want to hear.	A B C D E F G
3. Getting hearing aids is in my best interest.	A B C D E F G
4. People will notice my hearing loss more when I wear my hearing aids.	A B C D E F G
5. My hearing aids will reduce the number of times I have to ask people to repeat.	A B C D E F G
6. My hearing aids will be worth the trouble.	A B C D E F G
7. Sometimes I will be bothered by an inability to get enough loudness from my hearing aids without feedback (whistling).	A B C D E F G
8. I will be content with the appearance of my hearing aids.	A B C D E F G
9. Using hearing aids will improve my self-confidence.	A B C D E F G
10. My hearing aids will have a natural sound.	A B C D E F G
11. My hearing aids will be helpful on most telephones without amplifiers or loudspeakers. (If you hear well on the telephone *without* hearing aids, check here ☐)	A B C D E F G

continues

Expected Consequences of Hearing Aid Ownership (ECHO) *continued*

A Not At All
B A Little
C Somewhat
D Medium
E Considerably
F Greatly
G Tremendously

How much do you agree with each statement?

12. The person who provides me with my hearing aids will be competent.	A B C D E F G
13. Wearing my hearing aids will make me seem less capable.	A B C D E F G
14. The cost of my hearing aids will be reasonable.	A B C D E F G
15. My hearing aids will be dependable (need few repairs).	A B C D E F G

Please respond to these additional items.

LIFETIME HEARING AID EXPERIENCE (includes all old and current hearing aids)	DAILY HEARING AID USE	DEGREE OF HEARING DIFFICULTY (without wearing a hearing aid)
☐ None	☐ None	☐ None
☐ Less than 6 weeks	☐ Less than 1 hour per day	☐ Mild
☐ 6 weeks to 11 months	☐ 1 to 4 hours per day	☐ Moderate
☐ 1 to 10 years	☐ 4 to 8 hours per day	☐ Moderately Severe
☐ Over 10 years	☐ 8 to 16 hours per day	☐ Severe

Source: Reprinted with permission from Hearing Aid Research Lab. (2019). *Expected Consequences of Hearing Aid Ownership (ECHO)*. Retrieved from http://www.harlmemphis.org/files/8213/4625/3211/echo15 .pdf Copyright 1999 by University of Memphis.

Appendix G

ASHA Guidelines for Childhood Hearing Screening

Overview

A **hearing screening** is used to identify individuals who may require a more comprehensive hearing assessment and/or medical management. Hearing screenings for children may take place in early childhood settings, school settings, community settings, audiology clinics, medical settings, and/or home settings.

As of 2011, 97.9% of babies born in the United States were screened for hearing loss shortly after birth (Centers for Disease Control and Prevention [CDC], 2013). Minimal, frequency-specific, late-onset, or progressive hearing losses may not be identified during newborn hearing screenings. By school age, close to 15% of children in the U.S. exhibit some level/type of hearing loss of at least 16 dB HL (Niskar et al., 1998).

Hearing screenings during childhood are vital for early identification and management of hearing loss. "Failure to detect congenital or acquired hearing loss in children may result in lifelong deficits in speech and language acquisition, poor academic performance, personal-social maladjustments, and emotional difficulties" (Harlor & Bower, 2009, p. 1253). Hearing loss does not have to be severe in order to impact a student's access to auditory-based classroom instruction. Educationally significant hearing loss can be unilateral, bilateral, minimal

in degree, high frequency, or long-standing conductive.

Key Issues

Roles and Responsibilities

Audiologists

Audiologists, by virtue of academic degree, clinical training, and license to practice, are qualified to provide guidance, development, implementation, and oversight of hearing screening programs. See ASHA's Scope of Practice in Audiology (ASHA, 2018).

Appropriate roles and responsibilities for audiologists include:

- selecting screening protocols appropriate for the setting, population, and personnel;
- selecting, upgrading, and calibrating screening equipment;
- completing hearing screenings;
- training screening personnel and monitoring the competencies of screening personnel;
- selecting and/or developing educational materials for families;
- monitoring key indicators (pass/fail rates, miss rates, adherence to follow-up protocol, etc.);

- developing and implementing written policies and procedures—
  - ☐ infection control procedures,
  - ☐ screening techniques and process,
  - ☐ documentation of screening results (per state/district/program policies);
- communicating screening results to families, appropriate program and/or school representatives, state public health agencies (e.g., Early Hearing Detection and Intervention [EHDI]), primary care physicians, and diagnostic audiology centers as indicated;
- providing counseling and education;
- completing rescreenings and diagnostic evaluations as indicated;
- referring for medical and/or other professional services as indicated;
- collaborating with health and education professionals to ensure appropriate follow-up and outcomes;
- remaining informed of research in the area of childhood hearing screenings and childhood hearing loss.

As indicated in the Code of Ethics (ASHA, 2016a), audiologists who work in this capacity should be specifically educated and appropriately trained to do so.

Speech-Language Pathologists

Speech-language pathologists (SLPs) play a role in the screening, speech/language/communication assessment, and rehabilitation of individuals with hearing loss and the referral of individuals suspected of having hearing loss to an audiologist as appropriate. See ASHA's Scope of Practice in Speech-Language Pathology (ASHA, 2016b).

Appropriate roles for speech-language pathologists include:

- collaborating with audiologists in the development of screening protocols,

equipment selection, and quality improvement;
- performing hearing screenings;
- referring children who do not pass screenings for audiologic, medical, and/or other professional services as indicated;
- referring children who are difficult to test to an audiologist;
- communicating screening results to families, including recommendations for timely follow-up;
- sharing screening results with appropriate program and/or school representatives, state public health agencies, state EHDI programs for children under 3 years, primary care physicians, and diagnostic audiology centers as indicated;
- providing counseling and education for families, educators, and other service providers;
- collaborating with audiologists, school nurses, teachers, physicians, and/or other professionals to ensure appropriate follow-up and outcomes.

As indicated in the Code of Ethics (ASHA, 2016a), SLPs who serve this population should be specifically educated and appropriately trained to do so.

Considerations for Target Populations

Early Childhood

Periodic screening of all children will help to identify those who were either lost to follow-up or not identified during the newborn period or those who developed hearing loss after the newborn period. Such screening includes the following:

- Ongoing surveillance and hearing screening beyond the newborn period, per the American Academy of Pediatrics (AAP; Harlor & Bower, 2009).

- Children ages 6 months to 3 years typically require screening with automated technology (i.e., otoacoustic emissions [OAEs]).
- Although OAEs are considered an acceptable screening tool, pure-tone screening remains the gold standard and is ideally accomplished by the time the child is 5 years old.
- Children who cannot complete a pure-tone screening prior to kindergarten may be considered for an audiologic referral.

- Mandated hearing, vision, and comprehensive developmental screening within 45 days of entry into Early Head Start and Head Start programs (U.S. Department of Health and Human Services [HHS], 2015a, 2015b).
- Targeted, careful monitoring of children who are at high risk for delayed-onset hearing loss based on Joint Committee on Infant Hearing (JCIH) risk indicators (JCIH, 2007).
- Screening of child's hearing in response to a concern raised by the parent/guardian/caregiver or by a teacher/service provider.
- Inclusion of hearing screening as part of any comprehensive speech-language evaluation.

School Age

Screening for school-age children may include:

- screening of child's hearing upon initial entry or transfer into school and every year in Grades K–3 and 7 and 11 (ASHA, 2006);

- hearing screening as part of educational monitoring for home-schooled or privately educated children;
- annual risk assessment (and follow-up as needed) each year that the child's hearing is not screened or assessed, per the AAP (Hagan, Shaw, & Duncan, 2008);
- screening of adolescents with an adapted protocol (e.g., one that includes 6000/8000 Hz, threshold testing, the use of otoacoustic emissions [OAEs]) for increased likelihood of identifying early high-frequency hearing loss/noise-induced hearing loss (Meinke & Dice, 2007; Sekhar et al., 2014);
- required/mandated hearing screenings, per state;
- screening of child's hearing upon notice of any parent/guardian/caregiver or teacher/school staff concern;
- hearing screening as part of any comprehensive speech-language evaluation.

Screening Equipment and Protocols

The selection and implementation of hearing screening protocols and equipment will be guided by the specific goals of the individual hearing screening program. The target population, available personnel, and type of hearing loss to be included—as well as program-specific needs and/or limitations—are important considerations. Pure tone audiometry, OAE technology, and tympanometry may all be appropriate options for inclusion in hearing screening programs. Automated versions of hearing screening tools are available and can be utilized by trained support personnel. Evidence has been compiled regarding commonly used screening tools (Prieve, Schooling, Venediktov, & Franceschini, 2015).

Otoscopy/Visual Inspection

Otoscopy completed by a trained examiner allows for visualization of the tympanic membrane and inspection of the external ear canal for drainage, foreign bodies, impacted cerumen, infection, or structural abnormalities. A screener who is not trained in otoscopy can perform a general visual inspection of the outer portion of the ear and make note of any abnormalities. The information obtained during visual inspection or otoscopy may have an important impact on screening results and/or call for the discontinuation of screening and referral to medical personnel.

Pure Tone Screening

Pure tone screening is typically accomplished with the use of a pure tone audiometer. Pure tone stimuli at octave-band frequencies are routed through TDH supraaural earphones or insert earphones. With younger children, pulsed or warble tone stimuli may be presented instead of pure tones. Some screening audiometers limit the screening frequencies and presentation levels. These audiometers will not provide the flexibility of a single channel audiometer in regard to adapting protocols for different populations (Johnson & Seaton, 2012).

Factors to Consider

- Personnel may include an audiologist, SLP, nurse, or other trained lay or volunteer screener.
- Noise contamination in the screening environment may prohibit screening in any or all frequency ranges.
- It may not be possible to complete pure tone screenings in the low frequency range, even in a quiet environment, due to physiologic noise from the child or poor acoustics.
- In order for pure tone screening to be accurate, the child must be able to reliably respond to stimuli (i.e., by raising his or her hand when the stimuli are presented). For younger students or students with developmental, cognitive, or motoric challenges and/or delays, conditioned play techniques can also be effective (Harlor & Bower, 2009; Johnson & Seaton, 2012). The cognitive requirements to respond accurately and appropriately to the pure tone tasks may preclude participation by certain groups, such as the very young pediatric population and those with developmental delays.

Pure Tone Screening Procedure

- Condition the child to respond appropriately using suprathreshold (e.g., 40 dB HL) stimuli prior to initiation of screening. Administer a minimum of two conditioning trials to ensure that the child understands the task.
  - Play audiometry may be more appropriate for children ages 2–4 years (Harlor & Bower, 2009). This type of pure tone screening requires screeners who are specially trained in conditioned play audiometry techniques.
- Present pure tones (typically presented at 1000, 2000, 4000 Hz in each ear at 20 dB HL).
- Note: Some screening programs may choose to add 500 Hz at 25 dB HL.
- Note: Some screening programs for older students may choose to add 6000 Hz at 20 dB HL in order to identify possible high-frequency

hearing loss consistent with damage from noise exposure.

- Limit testing to no more than four presentations per frequency to reduce false positive responses (American Academy of Audiology [AAA], 2011).
- If the child does not respond at one or more frequencies, reinstruct, reposition earphones, and rescreen within the same screening period.
- Follow-up may include referral to a health care provider for evaluation of ear canal obstruction and/or middle ear dysfunction.

Pure Tone Screening Results

Pass—appropriate response to all presentation stimuli at screening levels in both ears

Fail—lack of response to any test frequency at screening levels in either ear

Could Not Screen—lack of cooperation, inability to be conditioned to the response task, etc.

Otoacoustic Emissions (OAE)

Otoacoustic emissions (OAEs)—either transient-evoked OAEs (TEOAEs) or distortion product OAEs (DPOAEs)—are measured using a sensitive probe microphone inserted into the ear canal. OAEs are a direct measure of outer hair cell and cochlear function in response to acoustic stimulation and yield an indirect estimate of peripheral hearing sensitivity. OAEs do not technically test an individual's hearing, but rather OAE results reflect the performance of the inner ear mechanics. OAEs are not sensitive to disorders central to the outer hair cells, such as auditory neuropathy spectrum disorder (ANSD), which is a neural hearing loss that leaves cochlear (outer hair cell) function intact.

Factors to Consider

- Personnel may include an audiologist, SLP, nurse, or other trained volunteer screener. Equipment can be automatic with no decision making required regarding equipment parameters or pass/fail criteria.
- "The involvement of a pediatric audiologist is essential in selecting OAE screening equipment, developing and implementing an appropriate screening and follow-up protocol, and providing training and technical assistance to screeners and other professionals" (Eiserman et al., 2008, p. 190).
- The use of OAE technology may be appropriate for screening children who are difficult to test using pure-tone audiometry (those who cannot respond to traditional pure tone or conditioned play techniques; Stephenson, 2007).
- Screening in quiet environments typically reduces the amount of time needed to complete an OAE hearing screening. A reasonable amount of noise may be present without interrupting the OAE screening process. OAE equipment may indicate when the screening environment is too noisy.
- It may not be possible to complete OAE screenings in the low frequency range, even in a quiet environment, due to physiologic noise from the child or poor acoustics.
- With OAE protocols taking less time than pure tone protocols, more children may be screened on a given day (Kreisman, Bevilacqua, Day, Kreisman, & Hall, 2013).

- OAEs will usually be absent when there is outer or middle ear dysfunction.
- OAEs may miss some cases of educationally significant mild and mild-moderate hearing loss or ANSD (AAA, 2011).
- OAE protocols may result in refer rates that are higher than those of pure tone and OAE/tympanometry protocols. Multiple OAE screenings may be needed/used to limit false positive findings and medical referrals for children who fail the initial OAE screen, but who do not actually need treatment (Eiserman et al., 2008).

OAE Screening Procedure

- Complete otoscopic or visual inspection to determine presence or absence of impacted cerumen, drainage, foreign bodies, infection, or structural abnormalities of the pinna, canal, or tympanic membrane. Make note of abnormalities to inform decisions related to follow-up recommendations (Johnson & Seaton, 2012). Follow-up may include referral to a health care provider for evaluation of ear canal obstruction and/or middle ear dysfunction.
- Place small probe in the ear canal to deliver the sound stimuli.
- Read results. Automated OAE screening units will analyze the emission and provide a result of either "pass" or "fail/refer." Diagnostic units will require interpretation of the findings by audiologists. Screeners other than audiologists should not independently change the parameters of the test equipment or provide interpretation of findings.

TEOAEs: Clicks or tone bursts are used as the stimuli at one level—for example, 80 dB SPL. Normal distributions for this condition for normal hearing are documented in the literature (Hussain, Gorga, Neely, Keefe, & Peters, 1998).

DPOAEs: Pure tones are used as the stimuli. Normal distributions for this condition for normal hearing are documented in the literature (Gorga et al., 1997).

OAE Screening Results. Screening programs that use OAE equipment often use the manufacturer's pre-set stimulus and pass/fail parameters, which will vary. This allows for participation by screeners who do not have the background or knowledge to adjust or interpret result parameters. When automated equipment is used, findings will be recorded as either "pass" or "fail/refer." For children who could not complete screening due to lack of cooperation, internal or external noise, or other reasons, the findings are recorded as "could not screen."

Tympanometry

Tympanometry can be added to the protocols of either pure tone or OAE testing to measure the mobility of the tympanic membrane and the status of the middle-ear transmission system. During tympanometry, a probe is fit snuggly into the ear canal. Pressure between the probe and eardrum is varied between +200 dB PA and –400 dB PA. Reflected sound from the probe tone is recorded across the pressure range, and a tympanogram is created. Tympanogram results convey the status of the middle ear system and suggest conditions that may need medical attention, such as eustachian tube dysfunction, middle ear fluid, or perforated eardrum.

Factors to Consider

- Personnel may include an audiologist, SLP, nurse, or other trained volunteer screener. Automated equipment may be used.

- Because younger children are at increased risk of failing the pure tone screen due to middle ear fluid (i.e., otitis media with effusion [OME]), consideration may be made to incorporate tympanometry in screening of children ages preschool through first grade (AAA, 2011). "Children with chronic OME may develop structural changes of the tympanic membrane, hearing loss, and speech and language delay" (American Academy of Otolaryngology–Head and Neck Surgery, 2013, p. S15).

- Tympanometry can better target the need for a rescreening or an immediate referral for medical or audiologic evaluation.

- "Combining office-based otoacoustic emission screening with tympanometry allows the physician to monitor transient conductive hearing loss (CHL) associated with middle ear effusion in the office setting and refer to audiology only those patients with concerns for more persistent CHL or sensorineural hearing loss (SNHL)" (Bhatia, Mintz, Hecht, Deavenport, & Kuo, 2013).

- It is appropriate to immediately refer a child for audiologic assessment if he/she passes tympanometry, but fails pure tone screening.

Tympanometry Screening Procedure

- Complete otoscopic or visual inspection to determine presence or absence of impacted cerumen, drainage, foreign bodies, infection, or structural abnormalities of the pinna, canal, or tympanic membrane. Make note of abnormalities to inform decisions related to follow-up recommendations (Johnson & Seaton, 2012). Make note of the presence or absence of PE tubes. Follow-up may include referral to a health care provider for evaluation of ear canal obstruction and/or middle ear dysfunction.

- Place probe in ear canal to deliver tones and vary the air pressure between positive and negative.

- Tympanogram is created.

- Note: A 220 Hz probe tone is appropriate for the 6 month–18-year-old population (Margolis, Bass-Ringdahl, Hanks, Holte, & Zapala, 2003).

Tympanometry Screening Results

- Automated equipment will report results as "pass" or "fail/refer."

- When nonautomated equipment is used, the recommended referral criteria is >250 da Pa tympanometric width for children 3–12 years of age and >275 da Pa tympanometric width for children below age 3. If the use of tympanometric width is not possible, <0.2 mmhos static compliance is recommended (AAA, 2011).

- Note: Ear canal volume of >1.0 cm3 and flat tympanogram can indicate either patent PE tubes or tympanic membrane perforation.

- Lack of cooperation and/or other factors may result in inability to screen.

Note: The presence of PE tubes may lead to a "refer" result; however, this result must be confirmed with otoscopy by a trained examiner. The presence of patent PE tubes is not differentiated from a perforated tympanic membrane with the use of tympanometry alone.

Screening Protocols

The choice of protocol for a hearing screening program is based on factors such as the type(s) of hearing loss to be included, available technology, population to be screened, and staffing/audiology resources. State regulations must also be considered, as they vary. Obtaining informed parent/legal guardian permission is a recommended part of the protocol; however, extant state statutes/regulations or institutional policies supersede this recommendation.

Decision trees [PDF] for four screening protocols are provided. These decision trees represent examples of the decision-making process that is undertaken during childhood hearing screenings. While processes may vary between screening programs, they should be documented and consistent within a given program.

- Pure Tone Screening Only
- Pure Tone and Tympanometry
- OAE Screening Only
- OAE and Tympanometry

Considerations for Screen/ Rescreen Timelines

- Timelines for referral and rescreening must be determined on a case-by-case basis, with consideration given to the child's overall health, otoscopic examination findings, and individualized educational concerns.
- When a pure tone or pure tone and tympanometry protocol is used, the rationale for the 6- to 8-week timeline between initial failed screen and rescreening is based on the timeline for spontaneous recovery of middle ear effusions and the prevalence of middle ear effusions in children. The

AAP (2004) indicates that a child with otitis media with effusion (OME) and no other significant risk can be managed with watchful waiting for up to 3 months from the date of onset or diagnosis. OME after untreated acute otitis media (AOM) had 59% resolution by 1 month and 74% resolution by 3 months (Rosenfeld & Kay, 2003).

- The 6- to 8-week timeline also allows the clinician to provide information about the persistence of possible middle ear effusion to the primary care provider or other medical professional. "When children with OME are referred by the primary clinician for evaluation by an otolaryngologist, audiologist, or speech-language pathologist, the referring clinician should document the effusion duration . . . and provide additional relevant information such as history of AOM and developmental status of the child" (Rosenfeld et al., 2004, p. S96).
- Some school districts choose to use a shorter 2- to 4-week timeline, which has the benefit of earlier assessment and management of those children with undiagnosed permanent hearing loss. A drawback of a shorter timeline is possible over-referral of children who may have a middle ear effusion in the process of resolution. Otitis media is among the most common health care concerns prompting childhood visits to a doctor.

Program Management

There are many factors that must be considered by administration and/or appropriate staff prior to initiation of a childhood hearing screening program. When a childhood hearing screening program is developed, it is important to include procedures related to appropriate and timely follow-up. Consideration of the resources necessary to provide appropriate services and to maintain ongoing communications with children and their families is vital.

Equipment Calibration

Audiometric equipment must meet applicable specifications of ANSI/ASA S3.6-2010 (ANSI, 2010) and/or manufacturer recommendations to ensure accurate results. Exhaustive electroacoustic calibrations should be performed annually using instrumentation traceable to the National Institute of Standards and Technology. Functional inspection, performance checks, and bioacoustic checks should be conducted to verify equipment performance prior to each use (American National Standards Institute [ANSI], 2010). Visual inspection may be completed to check for any obvious equipment damage. All calibration activities should be conducted by a trained audiologist or an external company/individual who is properly trained in performing such tasks.

Currently, there are no ANSI standards for the calibration of OAE equipment. For this reason, there may be differences in signal calibration, calculation of the noise floor, and response determination algorithms between manufacturers. These differences could impact the level of hearing loss that can be detected during screening.

Personnel Training

Screening programs with supervision provided by an educational audiologist use more uniform protocols that "should result in more accurate screening results, a better system for referrals, and proper diagnoses" (Richburg & Imhoff, 2008, p. 41). All screeners receive thorough initial training and refresher training as needed to maintain screening skills and knowledge. It may be beneficial for the results of new screeners to be validated by experienced screeners until novices become more comfortable with the equipment and screening process. While it is beneficial for screening programs to be flexible and adaptive to meet their specific personnel needs, adherence to stated or written policies/procedures that were chosen or developed for their specific program is essential.

Screening Environment

Test environments for pure tone screening should meet the specifications detailed in Maximum Permissible Ambient Noise Levels for Audiometric Test Rooms (ANSI, 2003).

- Based on a 20 dB HL screening level, the allowable ambient noise, if an individual has 0 dB HL hearing threshold, is 50, 58, and 76 dB SPL respectively for 1000, 2000, and 4000 Hz (ANSI, 2003).
- An alternative approach is to use a biologic noise level check prior to the commencement of hearing screening. This has been defined as the ability to establish hearing thresholds at least 10 dB below the screening level (e.g., 10 dB HL for screening conducted at 20 dB HL) at all frequencies for a person with known normal hearing. If these thresholds cannot be established, the area must not be used for screening (Minnesota Department of Health, 2006). Results of this approach may not necessarily reach ANSI standards.
- The screening environment is free from visual distractions and interruptions.
- There are currently no ANSI standards regarding the OAE screening environment.

Universal Precautions

It is important to ensure that adherence to universal precautions and appropriate infection control procedures are in place during screenings. Instrumentation that comes into physical contact with the patient must be cleaned and disinfected after each use (and per manufacturer's instructions), and clinician hand washing between patients should be routine (Siegel, Rhinehard, Jackson, Chiarello, & the Healthcare Infection Control Practices Advisory Committee, 2007). Disposable equipment, such as probe tips, should be discarded after each use. See Occupational Safety and Health Administration (OSHA) standards relating to occupational exposure to bloodborne pathogens and the Centers for Disease Control and Prevention's universal precautions for preventing transmission of bloodborne infections.

Follow-Up and Referral Procedures

Appropriate follow-up for screening programs includes the rescreening of those children who did not pass the initial screen and the screening of children who were absent during the initial screen, as well as proper referrals for medical, audiologic, or educational evaluations as appropriate (Johnson & Seaton, 2012).

Documentation and Recommendations. Screening documentation generally includes identifying information, comprehensive results, and recommendations, including the need for rescreening and appropriate referrals (ASHA, 2006).

Notification. Local, state, and federal regulations may vary with regard to parent/guardian notification and permission for a child to participate in hearing screening.

Parents/guardians may be informed in writing prior to the screening date to give them the opportunity to express any preference for their child not to be screened, to request that they provide any important background information regarding the child's hearing, and to inform them of the type of follow-up communication they can expect. Parent/guardian notification materials may include basic information about the process and purpose of hearing screening, as well as information about the educational impact of hearing impairment.

Screening and Rescreening Forms. Recordkeeping methodology will be determined, in part, by the setting and/or material availability. Options include student-specific paper forms, classroom-specific paper forms, or computer database entry, among others. Screening form use and type may be determined by the policies of each program/school/district with respect to the compilation and maintenance of child/student health records.

Result Reporting. Proper documentation of screening results may include reporting to the program/school, reporting to the parents/guardians, and receiving information back regarding follow-up recommendations (Johnson & Seaton, 2012). When providing results to parents/guardians whose child is referred for medical or audiologic follow-up, the screener may give the parents/guardians a feedback form to give to the provider and then return to the program/school. Providing screening results to program/school personnel (e.g. health specialists, nurses, teachers, administrators, SLPs) will facilitate the proper follow-up and/or accommodations appropriate for the student. It may be beneficial to notify the parents/guardians after any failed screening, even if a rescreening is planned, so that they can be involved in any decision making regarding next steps.

Program Evaluation

In determining the effectiveness of the screening program, various quality indicators can be used. It is important to collect data, such as the number of children screened, the number of children who did not pass the initial screen and/or rescreening, the number of children referred for medical or audiologic follow-up, the number of children seen for professional follow-up, and the number of children diagnosed with and/or treated for hearing disorders. Other quality indicators may include how quickly children move through the recommended protocol and the number of provider reports returned following referral, as well as parent/guardian satisfaction. Such data "can help document need for the hearing screening program, identify over or under referrals that can target equipment or training needs, help track loss to follow-up, and clarify other issues that impact the efficiency and effectiveness of a hearing screening program in the schools" (AAA, 2011, p. 46).

Laws and Regulations

▨ Most states have hearing screening requirements pertaining to newborns and school-age children. It is important to check with your state for the most current information on its policies and regulations.

▨ Local Head Start/Early Head Start programs must comply with the Head Start Performance Standards (45 CFR Parts 1300–1311) and are monitored by the Administration for Children and Families under HHS.

▨ The Early Periodic Screening, Diagnosis, and Treatment (EPSDT) Program is the child health component of Medicaid. EPSDT provides access to screening, diagnostic, and treatment services for low-income children.

▨ The Individuals with Disabilities Education Act (IDEA) Part B (34 CFR 300) includes hearing screening in the audiology services provided. IDEA Part C requires that audiologists and SLPs who identify hearing loss or language delays in children younger than age 3 initiate a referral to the Part C program "as soon as possible," but not more than 7 calendar days after identification.

References

American Academy of Audiology Task Force. (2011). *Childhood hearing screening guidelines*. Retrieved from http://www.audiology.org/publications-resources/document-library/pediatric-diagnostics

American Academy of Otolaryngology–Head and Neck Surgery. (2013). Clinical practice guideline: Tympanostomy tubes in children. *Otolaryngology—Head and Neck Surgery, 149* (S1), S1–S35.

American Academy of Pediatrics. (2004). Otitis media with effusion. *Pediatrics, 113*(5), 1412–1429.

American National Standards Institute. (2003). *Maximum permissible ambient noise levels for audiometric test rooms* (Rev. ed.) (ANSI S3.1-1999). New York, NY: Author.

American National Standards Institute. (2010). *Specification for audiometers* (ANSI S3.6-2010). New York, NY: Author.

American Speech-Language-Hearing Association. (2006). *Preferred Practice Patterns for the Profession of Audiology* [Preferred practice patterns]. Available from http://www.asha.org/policy

American Speech-Language-Hearing Association. (2016a). *Code of ethics* [Ethics]. Available from http://www.asha.org/policy

American Speech-Language-Hearing Association. (2016b). *Scope of practice in speech-language pathology* [Scope of practice]. Available from http://www.asha.org/policy

American Speech-Language-Hearing Association. (2018). *Scope of practice in audiology* [Scope of practice]. Available from http://www.asha.org/policy

Bhatia, P., Mintz, S., Hecht, B. F., Deavenport, A., & Kuo, A. A. (2013). Early identification of young children with hearing loss in federally qualified health centers. *Journal of Developmental and Behavioral Pediatrics, 34*(1), 15–21.

Centers for Disease Control and Prevention. (2013). *Summary of 2011 national EHDI data.* Retrieved from www.cdc.gov/ncbddd/hearing loss/2011-data/2011_ehdi_hsfs_summary_a.pdf

Eiserman, W. D., Shisler, L., Foust, T., Buhrmann, J., Winston, R., & White, K. (2008). Updating hearing screening practices in early childhood settings. *Infants & Young Children, 21*(3), 186–193.

Gorga, M. P., Neely, S. T., Ohlrich, B., Hoover, B., Redner, J., & Peters, J. (1997). From laboratory to clinic: A large scale study of distortion product otoacoustic emissions in ears with normal hearing and ears with hearing loss. *Ear and Hearing, 18*(6), 440–455.

Hagan, J. F., Shaw, J. S., & Duncan, P. M. (Eds.). (2008). *Bright Futures: Guidelines for health supervision of infants, children, and adolescents* (3rd ed.). Elk Grove Village, IL: American Academy of Pediatrics.

Harlor, A. D., Jr., & Bower, C. (2009). Hearing assessment in infants and children: Recommendations beyond neonatal screening. *Pediatrics, 124*(4), 1252–1263.

Hussain, D. M., Gorga, M. P., Neely, S. T., Keefe, D. H., & Peters, J. (1998). Transient evoked otoacoustic emissions in patients with normal hearing and in patients with hearing loss. *Ear and Hearing, 19*(6), 434–449.

Johnson, C. D., & Seaton, J. B. (2012). *Educational Audiology Handbook* (2nd ed.). Clifton Park, NY: Delmar.

Joint Committee on Infant Hearing. (2007). Year 2007 position statement: Principles and guidelines for early hearing detection and intervention programs. *Pediatrics, 120*(4), 898–921.

Kreisman, B. M., Bevilacqua, E., Day, K., Kreisman, N. V., & Hall, J. W. (2013). Preschool hearing screenings: A comparison of distortion product otoacoustic emission and puretone protocols. *Journal of Educational Audiology, 19*, 48–57.

Margolis, R. H., Bass-Ringdahl, S., Hanks, W. D., Holte, L., & Zapala, D. A. (2003). Tympanometry in newborn infants—1kHz norms. *Journal of the American Academy of Audiology, 14*(7), 383–392.

Meinke, D. K., & Dice, N. (2007). Comparison of audiometric screening criteria for the identification of noise-induced hearing loss in adolescents. *American Journal of Audiology, 16*, S190–S202.

Niskar, A. S., Kieszak, S. M., Holmes, A., Esteban, E., Rubin, C., & Brody, D. J. (1998). Prevalence of hearing loss among children 6 to 19 years of age. *Journal of the American Medical Association, 279*(14), 1071–1075.

Prieve, B. A., Schooling, T., Venediktov, R., & Franceschini, N. (2015). An evidence-based systematic review on the diagnostic accuracy of hearing screening instruments for preschool- and school-age children. *American Journal of Audiology, 24*, 250–267.

Richburg, C. M., & Imhoff, L. (2008). Survey of hearing screeners: Training and protocols used in two distinct school systems. *Journal of Educational Audiology, 14*, 31–46.

Rosenfeld, R. M., Culpepper, L., Doyle, K. J., Grundfast, K. M., Hoberman, A., Kenna, M. A., . . . Yawn, B. (2004). Clinical practice guideline: Otitis media with effusion. *Otolaryngology–Head and Neck Surgery, 130*(5), S95–S118.

Rosenfeld, R. M., & Kay, D. (2003). Natural history of untreated otitis media. *The Laryngoscope, 113*(10), 1645–1657.

Sekhar, D. L., Zalewski, T. R., Ghossaini, S. N., King, T. S., Rhoades, J. A., Czarnecki, B., . . . Paul, I. M. (2014). Pilot study of a high-frequency school-based hearing screen to detect adolescent hearing loss. *Journal of Medical Screening, 21*(1), 18–23.

Siegel, J. D., Rhinehart, E., Jackson, M., Chiarello, L., & the Healthcare Infection Control Practices Advisory Committee. (2007). *Guideline for isolation precautions: Preventing transmission of infectious agents in healthcare settings.* Retrieved from http://www.cdc.gov/ncidod /dhqp/pdf/isolation2007.pdf

Stephenson, M. (2007). The effect of classroom sound field amplification and the effectiveness of otoacoustic emission hearing screening in school-age children. *New Zealand Health Technology Assessment Technical Brief, 6*(3), 1–60.

U.S. Department of Health and Human Services. (2015a). *Head Start Program Performance Standards*; 45 CFR, §1304.20 (b)(1). Retrieved from http://eclkc.ohs.acf.hhs.gov/hslc/standards /hspps/1304/1304.20%20Child%20health %20and%20developmental%20services.htm

U.S. Department of Health and Human Services. (2015b). *Head Start Program Performance Standards*; 45 CFR, §1308.6 (b). Retrieved from http://eclkc.ohs.acf.hhs.gov/hslc/stan dards/hspps/1308/1308.6%20%20Assessment %20of%20children.htm

Content Disclaimer: The Practice Portal, ASHA policy documents, and guidelines contain information for use in all settings; however, members must consider all applicable local, state and federal requirements when applying the information in their specific work setting.

Source: Reprinted with permission from American Speech-Language-Hearing Association. (2019). *Childhood hearing screening.* Retrieved from https://www.asha.org/PRPSpecificTopic.aspx?fol derid=8589935406&section=Overview

Appendix H

Self-Advocacy Competency Skills Checklist

Self-advocacy means "understanding and seeking support for one's personal rights"[1]. Development of these skills should begin early so that you are able to start taking responsibility for your own communication accommodations at a very young age. It is expected that you will be personally responsible for your needs and actions just the same as any other teen or young adult. The *Self-Advocacy Competency Skills Checklist*[2] contains suggested skills in the areas of personal health and medical information, hearing and other assistive technology use, and accommodations and consumer awareness.

To complete the checklist, check the boxes of the skills you feel that you know.

Once completed, you can use this checklist to track the development of your self-advocacy skills. Talk with your audiologist, teachers or parents if you need assistance completing any of the items.

Once you have completed the checklist, you should make a list of skills that you may still need to learn. These are skills that should be included in your *IEP* if you are under age 16, in your *IEP Transition Plan* if you are 16 and have not graduated, or into your *Transition Planner* or *Self-Assessment Planner* (located in the Assessment section) if you have already graduated from high school.

I CAN...

Personal Health/ Medical Information	Concepts of hearing and hearing loss I can... ☐ describe how the ear works and common disorders of hearing loss ☐ describe pitch and loudness characteristics of the audiogram ☐ describe my hearing loss (type, degree and configuration) ☐ describe cause of my hearing loss if known ☐ describe basic communication implications of my hearing loss

continues

	☐ describe basic hearing loss prevention strategies
	☐ develop and rehearse a script for disclosing my hearing loss information and required accommodations
	<u>Access to hearing health professionals</u>
	I can...
	☐ identify pertinent medical and health specialists, their supporting roles, and how to locate them (audiology, otology, genetics, mental health/counseling)
	☐ identify my medical/health support persons
Hearing and Other Assistive Technology Use	<u>Responsibility for equipment</u>
	I can...
	☐ manage all operational components of my personal and assistive technology
	☐ troubleshoot my hearing and hearing assistance technology (HAT) and follow pre-determined procedures for getting equipment serviced
	☐ transport equipment to and from various school environments
	☐ notify the speaker or responsible person (my instructor, employer, audiologist) when my devices are not working properly
	☐ explain the various uses of my devices and demonstrate their flexibility (i.e., ability to couple to audio devices-computers, TV, PA system)
	<u>Use of individual amplification devices</u>
	I can...
	☐ describe the basic parts and functioning of personal and HAT devices including
	☐ program options in HA/CI/bone conduction device
	☐ limitations of technology
	☐ describe the benefits and limitations of my technology in various situations including those outside of school
	☐ utilize the devices in different environments (i.e. lectures, small groups, pass around)
	☐ assist in training staff on my equipment

	☐ describe how to manipulate technology in difficult listening situations
	☐ describe how to connect my equipment into other audio devices
	Use of assistive technologies
	I can...
	☐ describe and demonstrate features of various assistive technologies to accommodate hearing loss (for example: telephone, captioning, alerting, text messaging devices)
	Use of resources
	I can...
	☐ demonstrate use of the web to locate information and resources about hearing instruments and HAT
	☐ identify various funding options for hearing, HAT and other assistive technologies
Accommodations and Consumer Awareness	Strategies to address learning and communication challenges
	I can...
	☐ describe my communication challenges
	☐ identify the accommodations that are helpful to me to address my communication and learning needs
	☐ discuss my Personal Profile and Accommodations Letter (PPAL) with instructors, employers, disability coordinators, VR counselors and use in my community
	☐ develop alternative strategies/solutions when accommodations not provided/available
	☐ describe my educational history (educational test scores, learning styles, communication abilities) and explain the skills that are my strengths and those that are challenges
	☐ identify the academic supports that I need when necessary
	If high school:
	☐ formulate present levels of functioning for my *IEP* & develop my *IEP* goals
	☐ describe my achievements and performance levels for my **Transition Plan** and my **Summary of Performance**

continues

Self-Advocacy Competency Skills Checklist *continued*

	☐ describe and differentiate IDEA, 504, ADA as it relates to hearing loss including eligibility criteria
	☐ demonstrate that I have met with the office of disabilities services to identify my available services for higher education or human resource office for employment
	If post-high school:
	☐ use 504 & ADA to obtain accommodations
	☐ access disability support services when pursing higher education or accommodations for employment.

[1]English, K. (1997). *Self-Advocacy for Students who are Deaf or Hard of Hearing.* Austin, Texas: Pro-Ed.
[2]Adapted from Transition Competency Checklist for Individuals with Hearing Loss, Kate Salathial, 2008.

Source: Reprinted with permission from Phonak. (2019). *Self-advocacy competency skills checklist.* Retrieved from https://www.phonak.com/content/dam/phonak/HQ/en/support/children-and-parents/gap /SelfAdvocacy_Competency_Checklist_FORM.pdf

Glossary

Adapted with permission from *Comprehensive Dictionary of Audiology: Illustrated* (3rd ed.), by B. A. Stach, 2019, San Diego, CA: Plural Publishing.

AAA: American Academy of Audiology; professional association of audiologists founded in 1988

AAS: American Auditory Society; multidisciplinary association of professionals in audiology, otolaryngology, hearing science, and the hearing industry; formerly, American Audiology Society

Abbreviated Profile of Hearing Aid Benefit: APHAB; self-assessment questionnaire used for evaluating benefit received from amplification, consisting of four subscales—the aversiveness scale, background noise scale, ease of communication scale, and reverberation scale

ABR: auditory brain stem response; auditory evoked potential, originating from cranial nerve VIII and auditory brain stem structures, consisting of five to seven identifiable peaks that represent neural function of auditory pathways and nuclei

AC audiometry: air conduction audiometry; measurement of hearing in which sound is delivered via earphones, thereby assessing the integrity of the outer, middle, and inner ear mechanisms; COM: bone conduction audiometry

acclimatization, auditory: systematic change in auditory performance over time due to a change in the acoustic information available to the listener; for example, an ear becoming accustomed to processing sounds of increased loudness following introduction of a hearing aid

acoustic admittance: Ya; total acoustic energy flow through a system determined by both in-phase (resistive) and out-of-phase (reactive) components; reciprocal of acoustic impedance

acoustic feedback: sound generated when an amplification system goes into oscillation, produced by amplified sound from the receiver reaching the microphone and being reamplified; COL: hearing aid squeal

acoustic gain: 1. increase in sound output; 2. in a hearing aid, the difference in dB between the input to the microphone and the output of the receiver

acoustic immittance: global term representing acoustic admittance (total energy flow) and acoustic impedance (total opposition to energy flow) of the middle ear system

acoustic impedance: total opposition to energy flow of sound through the middle ear system; reciprocal of acoustic admittance

acoustic muscle reflex: reflexive contraction of the tensor tympani and stapedius muscles in response to sound; SYN: acoustic reflex

acoustic neurinoma: cochleovestibular schwannoma

acoustic reflex: AR; reflexive contraction of the intra-aural muscles in response to loud sound, dominated by the stapedius muscle in humans; SYN: acoustic stapedial reflex

acoustic reflex, contralateral: crossed acoustic reflex

acoustic reflex arc: pathway of the auditory periphery and brainstem through which the acoustic stapedial reflex courses, from Cranial

Nerve VIII through the superior olivary complex to Cranial Nerve VII

acoustic reflex threshold: ART; lowest intensity level of a stimulus at which an acoustic reflex is detected

acoustic stapedial reflex: reflexive contraction of the stapedius muscle in response to loud sounds; SYN: acoustic reflex

acoustic trauma: 1. damage to hearing from a transient, high-intensity sound; 2. long-term insult to hearing from excessive noise exposure

acoustically modified earmold: ear coupler with adjustments made to the bore, tubing, or vent that results in changes in sound transmission

active feedback control: in hearing aids, digital algorithms designed to minimize feedback by inducing phase reversal of the oscillating signal

acute: of sudden onset and short duration; ANT: chronic

acute diffuse external otitis: diffuse reddened, pustular lesions surrounding hair follicles in the ear canal—usually due to gram-negative bacterial infection during hot, humid weather, and often initiated by swimming; COL: swimmer's ear

acute otitis media: AOM; inflammation of the middle ear having a duration of fewer than 21 days

adaptive compression: hearing aid circuit technique that incorporates output-limited compression with automatically variable release time; SYN: variable compression

adaptive directional microphone: microphone designed to be differentially sensitive to sound from a focused direction that is activated automatically in response to the detection of noise

adaptive frequency response: AFR; hearing aid circuitry technique in which frequency response changes as input level changes

adaptive noise canceller: ANC; multiple microphone instrument that attempts to reduce background noise by changing the hearing aid microphone's directionality adaptively

admittance: Y; total energy flow through a system, expressed in mhos; reciprocal of impedance

adult-onset auditory deprivation: the apparent decline in word-recognition ability in the unaided ear of an adult fitted with a monaural hearing aid following a period of asymmetric stimulation; SYN: late-onset auditory deprivation

advantage, binaural: the cumulative benefits of using two ears over one, including enhanced threshold and better hearing in the presence of background noise

AI: articulation index or audibility index; measure of the proportion of speech cues that are audible; SYN: speech intelligibility index

aided gain, real-ear: REAG; measurement of the difference, in decibels as a function of frequency, between the SPL in the ear canal and the SPL at a field reference point for a specified sound field with the hearing aid in place and turned on

aided response, real-ear: REAR; probe-microphone measurement of the sound pressure level, as a function of frequency, at a specified point near the tympanic membrane with a hearing aid in place and turned on; expressed in absolute SPL or as gain relative to stimulus level

aided threshold: lowest level at which a signal is audible to an individual wearing a hearing aid

air-bone gap: ABG; difference in dB between air conducted and bone conducted hearing thresholds for a given frequency in the same ear, used to describe the magnitude of conductive hearing loss

air conduction audiometry: AC audiometry; measurement of hearing in which sound is delivered via earphones, thereby assessing the integrity of the outer, middle, and inner ear mechanisms; COM: bone conduction audiometry

air conduction threshold: absolute threshold of hearing sensitivity to pure-tone stimuli delivered via earphone

ALD: assistive listening device; hearing instrument or class of hearing instruments, usually with a remote microphone for improving signal-to-noise ratio—including FM systems, personal amplifiers, telephone amplifiers, television listeners

ambient noise: surrounding sounds in an acoustic environment

American Academy of Audiology: AAA; professional association of audiologists founded in 1988

amplification, bilateral: use of a hearing aid in both ears

amplification, linear: hearing aid amplification in which the gain is the same for all input levels until the maximum output is reached

amplification, nonlinear: amplification in which gain is not the same for all input levels

amplification, sound field: amplification of a classroom or other open area with a public address system or other small-room system to enhance the signal-to-noise ratio for all listeners

amplification system, loop: assistive listening device in which a microphone/amplifier delivers signal to a loop of wire encircling a room; the signals are received by the telecoil of a hearing aid via magnetic induction

analog-to-digital conversion: ADC; the process of turning continuously varying (analog) signals into a numerical (digital) representation of the waveform

anechoic chamber: room designed for acoustic research with sound-absorbing material on all surfaces designed to enhance sound absorption and reduce reverberation

antihelix; anthelix: auricular ridge of cartilage anterior and parallel to the helix

APHAB: Abbreviated Profile of Hearing Aid Benefit; self-assessment questionnaire consisting of four subscales used for evaluating benefit received from amplification

ART: acoustic reflex threshold; lowest intensity level of a stimulus at which an acoustic reflex is detected

articulation index: AI; early term for the numerical prediction of the quantity of speech signal available or audible to the listener, based on speech importance weightings of various frequency bands; SYN: audibility index; speech intelligibility index

assistive listening device: ALD; hearing instrument or class of hearing instruments, usually with a remote microphone for improving signal-to-noise ratio—including FM systems, personal amplifiers, telephone amplifiers, television listeners

assistive listening device, FM: an assistive listening device designed to enhance signal-to-noise ratio in which a remote microphone/transmitter worn by a speaker sends signals via FM to a receiver worn by a listener

assistive listening device, infrared: assistive listening device consisting of a microphone/transmitter placed near the sound source of interest that broadcasts over infrared light waves to a receiver/amplifier, thereby enhancing the signal-to-noise ratio

asymmetric hearing loss: condition in which hearing loss in one ear is of a significantly different degree than in the other ear

attack time: latency of a compression circuit from detection of a signal to engagement to its steady-state value

attention deficit disorder: ADD; attention deficit hyperactivity disorder

attention deficit hyperactivity disorder: ADHD; cognitive disorder involving reduced ability to focus on an activity, task, or sensory stimulus characterized by restlessness and distractibility

attenuate: to reduce in magnitude; to decrease

AuD: doctor of audiology; designator for the professional doctorate degree in audiology

audibility index: AI; measure of the proportion of speech cues that are audible; SYN: articulation index, speech-intelligibility index

audibility threshold: threshold of hearing sensitivity

audible range: audible frequency range

audiogram: graphic representation of threshold of hearing sensitivity as a function of stimulus frequency

audiogram, baseline: initial audiogram obtained for comparison with later audiograms to quantify any change in hearing sensitivity

audiogram, behavioral: audiogram obtained by means of behavioral audiometry

audiogram, cookie bite: colloquial term referring to the audiometric configuration characterized by a hearing loss in the middle frequencies and normal or nearly normal hearing in the low and high frequencies

audiogram, corner: audiometric configuration characterized by a profound hearing loss with measurable thresholds only in low-frequency region

audiogram, flat: audiogram configuration in which hearing sensitivity is similar across the audiometric frequency range

audiogram, pure-tone: graph of the threshold of hearing sensitivity, expressed in dB HL, as determined by pure-tone air conduction and bone conduction audiometry at octave and half-octave frequencies ranging from 250 Hz to 8000 Hz

audiogram configuration: audiometric configuration

audiologist, dispensing: an audiologist who dispenses hearing aids

audiometer: electronic instrument designed for measurement of hearing sensitivity and for calibrated delivery of suprathreshold stimuli

audiometric zero: lowest sound pressure level at which a pure tone at each of the audiometric frequencies is audible to the average normal hearing ear, designated as 0 dB hearing level

audiometry, air conduction: AC audiometry; measurement of hearing in which sound is delivered via earphones, thereby assessing the integrity of the outer, middle, and inner ear mechanisms; COM: bone conduction audiometry

audiometry, behavioral: pure-tone and speech audiometry involving any type of behavioral response, in contrast to electrophysiologic or electroacoustic audiometry

audiometry, behavioral observation: BOA; pediatric assessment of hearing by observation of a child's unconditioned responses to sounds

audiometry, behavioral play: method of hearing assessment of young children in which the correct identification of a signal presentation is rewarded with the opportunity to engage in any of several play-oriented activities

audiometry, bone conduction: BC audiometry; measurement of hearing in which sound is delivered via a bone vibrator, thereby bypassing the outer and middle ears and assessing the integrity of inner ear mechanisms; COM: air conduction audiometry

audiometry, conditioned play: behavioral play audiometry

audiometry, COR: conditioned orientation reflex audiometry

audiometry, diagnostic: measurement of hearing to determine the nature and degree of hearing impairment

audiometry, play: behavioral method of hearing assessment of young children in which the correct identification of a signal presentation is rewarded with the opportunity to engage in any of several play-oriented activities

audiometry, sound field: measurement of hearing sensitivity to signals presented in a sound field through loudspeakers; used especially in pediatric assessment

audiometry, visual reinforcement: VRA; audiometric technique used in pediatric assessment in which a correct response to signal presentation, such as a head turn toward the speaker, is rewarded by the activation of a light or lighted toy

auditory acclimatization: systematic change in auditory performance over time due to a change in the acoustic information available to the listener; for example, an ear becoming accustomed to processing sounds of increased loudness following introduction of a hearing aid

auditory brain stem response: ABR; auditory evoked potential, originating from cranial nerve VIII and auditory brain stem structures, consisting of five to seven identifiable peaks that represent neural function of auditory pathways and nuclei

auditory brain stem response audiometry: ABR measure used to predict hearing sensitivity and to assess the integrity of cranial nerve VIII and auditory brain stem structures

auditory deprivation: diminution or absence of sensory opportunity for neural structures central to the end organ, due to a reduction in auditory stimulation resulting from hearing loss

auditory deprivation effect: systematic decrease over time in auditory performance associated with the reduced availability of acoustic information; SYN: late-onset auditory deprivation, acquired suprathreshold asymmetry

auditory disorder, peripheral: functional disorder resulting from diseases of or trauma to the external ear, middle ear, cochlea, and cranial nerve VIII

auditory dysynchrony, auditory dys-synchrony: auditory disorder that appears to disrupt synchronous activity of the auditory nervous system, characterized by normal cochlear outer hair cell function, abnormal auditory brain stem response, absent acoustic reflexes, and threshold and suprathreshold hearing disorder of varying degrees; SYN: auditory neuropathy

auditory neuropathy: auditory dysynchrony; auditory disorder that appears to disrupt synchronous activity of the auditory nervous system, characterized by normal cochlear outer hair cell function, abnormal auditory brain stem response, absent acoustic reflex, and threshold and suprathreshold hearing order of varying degrees

auditory neuropathy spectrum disorder: ANSD; auditory disorder that disrupts transmission of sound from the cochlea to the auditory nervous system through disruption of the cochlear inner hair cells, the synapse of hair cells with nerve fibers, or the synchronous activity of the auditory nerve; SYN: auditory neuropathy, auditory dysynchrony

auditory processing disorder, central: CAPD; disorder in function of central auditory structures, characterized by impaired ability of the central auditory nervous system to manipulate and use acoustic signals, including difficulty understanding speech in noise and localizing sounds

auditory rehabilitation: program or treatment designed to restore auditory function following adventitious hearing loss

auditory trainer: electronic amplification device used in the classroom to supplement conventional hearing aid use

auditory trainer, FM: classroom amplification system in which a remote microphone/transmitter worn by the teacher sends signals via FM to a receiver worn by the student

auditory training: aural rehabilitation methods designed to maximize use of residual hearing by structured practice in listening, environmental alteration, hearing aid use, and so forth

auricle: external or outer ear, which serves as a protective mechanism, as a resonator, and as a baffle for directional hearing of front-versus-back and in the vertical plane; SYN: pinna

autoimmune hearing loss: auditory disorder characterized by bilateral, asymmetric, progressive, sensorineural hearing loss in patients who test positively for autoimmune disease

automatic gain control: AGC; nonlinear hearing aid compression circuitry designed to automatically change gain as signal level changes or limit output when signal level reaches a specified criterion; SYN: automatic volume control

automatic gain control—input: AGCI; circuitry of a hearing aid in which the volume control follows the AGC

automatic gain control—output: AGCO; circuitry of a hearing aid in which the AGC follows the volume control

automatic signal processing: ASP; process in which hearing air circuitry adjusts some parameter of the amplified output automatically or adaptively as the input signal reaches a certain criterion

average, pure-tone: PTA; average of hearing sensitivity thresholds to pure-tone signals at 500 Hz, 1000 Hz, and 2000 Hz

AzBio Sentence Test: speech recognition measure designed to evaluate the speech perception abilities of patient with hearing loss, and to determine candidacy for and performance with cochlear implants

azimuth: direction of a sound source measured in angular degrees in a horizontal plane in relationship to the listener; for example, 0° azimuth is directly in front of the listener, 180° azimuth is directly behind

BAEP: brain stem auditory evoked potential; SYN: auditory brain stem response

BAER: brain stem auditory evoked response; SYN: auditory brain stem response

BAHA: bone anchored hearing aid; bone conduction hearing aid in which a titanium screw is anchored in the mastoid and is attached percutaneously to an external processor, designed primarily for single-sided deafness or conductive hearing loss secondary to intractable middle ear disorder or severe atresia

barrel effect: perception by a hearing aid user of annoying increase in vocal loudness when the outer ear is occluded with an earmold or a hearing aid

baseline audiogram: initial audiogram obtained for comparison with later audiograms to quantify any change in hearing sensitivity

bass increases at low levels: BILL; type of automatic signal processing in a hearing aid that uses level-dependent control of the frequency response, reducing low frequencies in response to high-intensity input

battery door: opening to the battery compartment of a hearing aid

battery drain: amount of electrical current being drawn from a battery

battery pill: device used in a hearing aid analyzer in place of a hearing aid battery, designed to represent the constant load of a hearing aid when measuring battery drain

BC: bone conduction; transmission of sound to the cochlea by vibration of the skull

BC-HIS: Board-Certified in Hearing Instrument Sciences; credential awarded to qualifying hearing instrument specialists by the National Board for Certification in Hearing Instrument Sciences

behavioral audiogram: audiogram obtained by means of behavioral audiometry

behavioral observation audiometry: BOA; pediatric assessment of hearing by observation of a child's unconditioned responses to sounds

behavioral play audiometry: method of hearing assessment of young children in which the correct identification of a signal presentation is rewarded with the opportunity to engage in any of several play-oriented activities

behavioral response: volitional motor response to a stimulus

behind-the-ear hearing aid: BTE hearing aid; a hearing aid that fits over the ear and is coupled to the ear canal via an earmold; SYN: postauricular hearing aid

Bell's palsy: acute unilateral facial paralysis due to facial nerve disorder of idiopathic origin

BICROS: bilateral contralateral routing of signals; a hearing aid system with one microphone contained in a hearing aid at each ear; the microphones lead to a single amplifier and receiver in the better hearing ear of a person with bilateral asymmetric hearing loss

bilateral: pertaining to both sides, hence to both ears

bilateral amplification: use of a hearing aid in both ears; SYN: binaural amplification

bilateral contralateral routing of signals: BICROS; a hearing aid system with one microphone contained in a hearing aid at each ear; the microphones are connected to a single amplifier and receiver in the better ear of a person with bilateral asymmetric hearing loss

bilateral hearing loss: hearing sensitivity loss in both ears

BILL: bass increases at low levels; type of automatic signal processing in a hearing aid that uses level-dependent control of the frequency response, reducing low frequencies in response to high-intensity input; COM: TILL

binaural localization: use of two ears for locating sounds in space

binaural squelch: improvement in speech intelligibility in noise of two ears over one because of interaural phase and intensity cues

binaural summation: cumulative effect of sound reaching both ears, resulting in enhancement in hearing with both ears over one ear, characterized by binaural improvement in hearing sensitivity of approximately 3 dB over monaural sensitivity

bisyllabic: having two syllables

Bluetooth: wireless technology protocol for exchanging data over short distances via short wavelength ultra-high-frequency radio waves

Bluetooth, low-energy: advanced Bluetooth protocol used to convey information over shorter distances using much less power than conventional Bluetooth technology

bone-air gap: difference in dB between bone conducted and air conducted hearing thresholds for a given frequency in the same ear, used to describe the condition in which bone conduction is paradoxically poorer than air conduction

bone anchored hearing aid: BAHA; bone conduction hearing aid in which a titanium screw is anchored in the mastoid and is attached percutaneously to an external processor, designed primarily for single-sided deafness or conductive hearing loss secondary to intractable middle ear disorder or severe atresia

bone conduction: BC; method of delivering acoustic signals through vibration of the skull; COM: air conduction

bone conduction audiometry: BC audiometry; measurement of hearing in which sound is delivered through a bone vibrator, thereby bypassing the outer and middle ears and assessing the integrity of inner ear mechanisms; COM: air conduction audiometry

bone conduction hearing aid: hearing aid, used most often in patients with bilateral atresia in which amplified signal is delivered to a bone vibrator placed on the mastoid, thereby bypassing the middle ear and stimulating the cochlea directly

bone conduction implant: bone conduction hearing aid with an implanted transducer in the mastoid that is attached to an external processor either percutaneously or transcutaneously, designed primarily for conductive hearing loss secondary to intractable middle ear disorder or severe atresia

bone conduction receiver: vibrator or oscillator used to transmit sound through vibration of the bones of the skull

bone conduction threshold: absolute threshold of hearing sensitivity to pure-tone stimuli delivered via bone conduction oscillator

boot, audio: device used with a behind-the-ear hearing aid for coupling with direct audio input cord

boot, FM: small boot-like device containing a frequency modulation (FM) receiver that attaches to the bottom of a behind-the-ear hearing aid

bore, earmold: hole in an earmold through which amplified sound is directed into the ear canal; SYN: sound bore

bore, horn: tapered bore in an earmold that is widest in diameter at its medial aspect, designed to enhance high-frequency amplification

bridge: original term for an immittance meter, when the instrumentation was based on a bridge circuit

broadband noise: BBN; sound with a wide bandwidth, containing a continuous spectrum of frequencies, which equal energy per cycle throughout the band

BSER: brain stem evoked response

BTE: behind-the-ear hearing aid; a hearing aid that fits over the ear and is coupled to the ear canal via an earmold; SYN: postauricular hearing aid

canal earmold: type of earmold that uses only the canal portion of the ear impression with the helix and concha areas removed

canal hearing aid: hearing aid that fits mostly in the external auditory meatus with a small portion extending into the concha; SYN: ITC hearing aid; in-the-canal hearing aid

canal-lock earmold: canal earmold with a fingerlike projection along the bottom of the concha to retain the earmold in place

canal mold: colloquial term for canal earmold

cardioid response: heart-shaped pattern of response of a directional microphone

Carhart's notch: patterns of bone conduction audiometric thresholds associated with otosclerosis, characterized by reduced bone conduction sensitivity predominantly at 2000 Hz

carrier phrase: in speech audiometry, phrase preceding the target syllable, word, or sentence to prepare the patient for the test signal

CCC-A: Certificate of Clinical Competence in Audiology; certification awarded by the American Speech-Language-Hearing Association to individuals who have met specified entry-level academic and clinical requirements to become audiologists

central auditory disorder: CAD; functional disorder resulting from diseases of or trauma to the central auditory nervous system

central auditory dysfunction: auditory processing disorder, characterized by impaired ability of the central nervous system to manipulate and use acoustic signals; SYN: central auditory processing disorder

central auditory processing disorder: CAPD; disorder in function of central auditory structures, characterized by impaired ability of the central auditory nervous system to manipulate and use acoustic signals, including difficulty understanding speech in noise and localizing sounds

cerumen: waxy secretion of the ceruminous glands in the external auditory meatus; COL: earwax

cerumen, impacted: cerumen that causes blockage of the external auditory meatus

cerumen management: extraction of excessive or impacted cerumen from the external auditory meatus

cholesteatoma: tumorlike mass of squamous epithelium and cholesterol in the middle ear that may invade the mastoid and erode the ossicles, usually secondary to chronic otitis media or marginal tympanic membrane perforation

CIC: 1. completely-in-the-canal hearing aid; 2. commissure of the inferior colliculus

circuit noise: unwanted signal in the output of a circuit created by the functioning of the circuit

circuitry: the system or components of an electric circuit

classroom accommodation: adjustment or adaptation of a classroom environment to ensure accessibility for persons with disabilities

classroom acoustics: features of sound characteristic of a classroom environment

classroom amplification: assistive listening devices or free-field amplification systems designed to provide enhanced signal-to-noise ratio in the classroom

click: rapid-onset, short-duration, broadband sound, produced by delivering an electric pulse to an earphone; used to elicit an auditory brain stem response and transient-evoked oto-acoustic emissions

Client Oriented Scale of Improvement: COSI; widely used self-assessment scale in which the patient defines and rank orders areas of perceived communication difficulties with and without hearing aid amplification

clinical audiometer: diagnostic audiometer; wide-range audiometer

COAT: Characteristics of Amplification Tool; short, 9-item self-assessment questionnaire

to determine a patient's communication needs and expectations related to hearing devices

cochlea: auditory portion of the inner ear, consisting of fluid-filled membranous channels within a spiral canal around a central core

cochlear echo: low-level sound emitted by the cochlea in response to an auditory stimulus that resembles an echo of that stimulus; SYN: evoked otoacoustic emission

cochlear hydrops: excessive accumulation of endolymph within the cochlear labyrinth, resulting in fluctuating sensorineural hearing loss, tinnitus, and a sensation of fullness; SYN: cochlear Ménière's disease

cochlear implant: device that enables persons with profound hearing loss to perceive sound, consisting of an electrode array surgically implanted in the cochlea, which delivers electrical signals to cranial nerve VIII and an external amplifier, which activates the electrode

cochlear implant mapping: representation of the threshold and suprathreshold parameters for each electrode or electrode combination in an individual cochlear implant user's sound coding program

cochlear nerve: auditory branch of cranial nerve VIII, arising from the spiral ganglion of the cochlea and terminating in the cochlear nuclei of the brain stem

cochlear nucleus: CN; cluster of cell bodies of second-order neurons on the lateral edge of the hindbrain in the central auditory nervous system at which fibers from cranial nerve VIII have an obligatory synapse

cochlear reserve: ability of the inner ear to function; functionality of the cochlea at suprathreshold levels

cognition: the processes involved in knowing, including perceiving, recognizing, conceiving, judging, sensing, and reasoning

collapsed canal: condition in which the cartilaginous portion of the external auditory meatus narrows, usually in response to pressure from a supra-aural earphone against the pinna, resulting in apparent high-frequency conductive hearing loss

comfortable loudness, range of: difference, in decibels, between threshold of audibility and loudness discomfort level for a specified acoustic signal

comfortable loudness level: intensity level of a signal that is perceived as comfortably loud

compensated tympanometry: acoustic immittance measures adjusted by removal of ear canal contributions

completely-in-the-canal hearing aid: CIC hearing aid; small amplification device, extending from 1 mm to 2 mm inside the meatal opening to near the tympanic membrane, which allows greater gain with less power due to the proximity of the receiver to the membrane

compliance, static: static acoustic immittance

compression: 1. in acoustics, portion of the sound-wave cycle in which particles of the transmission medium are compacted; ANT: expansion; 2. in hearing aid circuitry, nonlinear amplifier gain used either to limit maximum output (compression limiting) or to match amplifier gain to an individual's loudness growth (dynamic range compression)

compression, adaptive: hearing aid circuit technique that incorporates output-limiting compression with automatically variable release time; SYN: variable compression

compression, curvilinear: hearing aid compression in which the compression ratio increases as input level increases, providing dynamic-range compression for low-level and midlevel inputs, and compression limiting for high-level input

compression, full-dynamic-range: wide dynamic-range compression

compression, high-level: compression-limiting process of a hearing aid, characterized by a high threshold, high ratio, and long release time

compression, input: process in which a hearing aid compresses a signal before it reaches the volume control, resulting in a constant dynamic range with a change in maximum output as gain is increased or decreased by the volume control

compression, limiting: method of limiting maximum output of a hearing aid with compression circuitry

compression, linear: in hearing aids, amplifier gain that is linear at input levels that exceed the compression knee point

compression, low-level: hearing aid compression circuitry that is activated in response to low-intensity input, such as wide-dynamic-range compression

compression, output: process in which a hearing aid compresses a signal after it has passed the volume control, resulting in an expanded dynamic range for low-gain settings and a lower knee point for high-gain settings

compression, syllabic: hearing aid compression algorithm that incorporates a low threshold of activation, short attack and release times, and a low compression ratio, resulting in a reduction of the dynamic range of input

compression, wide-dynamic range: hearing aid compression that is activated throughout most of the dynamic range, typically resulting in greatest gain for soft sounds and least gain for loud sounds

compression knee point: the minimum input decibel level at which compression circuitry is activated in a hearing aid; SYN: compression threshold

compression limiting: limiting of maximum output in a hearing aid by use of compression circuitry

compression ratio: the decibel ratio of acoustic input to amplifier output in a hearing aid; for example, a hearing aid with a compression ratio of 2:1 will increase output by 1 dB for every 2 dB increase in input

compression threshold: the minimum input decibel level at which compression circuitry is activated in a hearing aid; SYN: compression knee point

conditioned play audiometry: method of hearing assessment of young children in which the correct identification of a signal presentation is rewarded with the opportunity to engage in any of several play-oriented activities

conductive hearing loss: reduction in hearing sensitivity, despite normal cochlear function, due to impaired sound transmission through the external auditory meatus, tympanic membrane, and/or ossicular chain

conductive mechanisms: that portion of the auditory system, comprised of the outer and middle ear, which conducts airborne sound to the cochlea

congenital: present at birth

congenital atresia: absence or pathologic closure at birth of a normal anatomical opening, such as the external auditory meatus

congenital hearing loss: reduced hearing sensitivity existing at or dating from birth, resulting from pre- or perinatal pathologic conditions

consonant-nucleus-consonant: CNC; a word or syllable used in speech-recognition testing, consisting of a vowel or diphthong (nucleus) between two consonants; SYN: consonant-vowel-consonant

contraindication: a condition that renders the use of a treatment or procedure inadvisable

contralateral: pertaining to the opposite side of the body: SYN: heterolateral

contralateral acoustic reflex: acoustic reflex occurring in one ear as a result of stimulation of the other ear; SYN: crossed acoustic reflex

control, remote: handheld unit that permits volume and/or program changes in a programmable hearing aid

control, volume: VC; manual or automatic control designed to adjust the output level of a hearing instrument

cortex, auditory: primary auditory area of the cerebral cortex located on the transverse temporal gyrus (Heschl's gyrus) of the temporal lobe

COSI: Client Oriented Scale of Improvement; widely used self-assessment scale in which the patient defines and rank orders areas of perceived communication difficulties with and without hearing aid amplification

count-the-dots procedure: a method for calculating audibility of speech in which dots corresponding to weighted speech information are plotted on the audiogram; aided responses super-imposed on the audiogram reveal the proportion of speech information that is audible

coupled FM system: personal FM amplification receiver coupled to a hearing aid wirelessly

coupler, HA-1: standard 2-cc coupler used to connect a hearing aid to an electroacoustic analyzer; the HA-1 device allows direct coupling or an earmold or an in-the-ear hearing aid, with putty used to seal the earmold or shell into the device

coupler, HA-2: standard 2-cc coupler used to connect a hearing aid to an electroacoustic analyzer, the HA-2 device has an earmold simulator and is used for testing earphones with nubs, such as an external receiver of a body aid

coupler gain: the amount of hearing aid gain measured in a coupler

CPA tumor: cerebellopontine angle tumor; most often a cochleovestibular schwannoma located or growing outside the internal auditory canal at the juncture of the cerebellum and pons

CPT codes: Current Procedural Terminology codes; numeric codes assigned to diagnostic and treatment procedures, used primarily for billing purposes

Cranial Nerve VIII: CVIII; C8; CN-VIII; auditory nerve, consisting of a vestibular and a cochlear branch; SYN: vestibulocochlear nerve

CROS: contralateral routing of signals; hearing aid configuration designed for unilateral hearing loss in which a microphone is placed on the poorer ear and the signal is routed to a hearing aid on the better ear

cross-check principle: in pediatric audiology, the concept that no single test obtained during pediatric assessment should be considered valid until an independent cross-check of validity has been obtained

crossed acoustic reflex: acoustic reflex occurring in one ear as a result of stimulation of the other ear; SYN: contralateral acoustic reflex

crossover: the process in which sound presented to one ear through an earphone crosses the head via bone conduction and is perceived by the other ear; SYN: contralateralization, cross hearing

custom hearing aid: ITE, ITC, or CIC hearing aid made for a specific individual from an ear impression

damped ear hook: behind-the-ear hearing aid ear hook containing damping material or filter to decrease amplitude selectively

daPa: decaPascal; unit of pressure in which 1 daPa equals 10 pascals

dB gain: decibels of gain; the difference between the input intensity and the output intensity of an amplifier or hearing aid

dB HL: decibels hearing level; decibel notation used on the audiogram that is referenced to audiometric zero

dB HTL: decibels hearing threshold level; decibel notation used to refer to a patient's threshold of hearing sensitivity

dB nHL: decibels normalized hearing level; decibel notation referenced to behavioral thresholds of a sample of normal-hearing persons, used most often to describe the intensity level of click stimuli used in evoked potential audiometry

dB SPL: decibels sound pressure level; dB SPL equals 20 times the log of the ratio of an observed sound pressure level to the reference sound pressure level of 20 microPascals (or 0.0002 dyne/cm^2, 0.0002 microbar, 20 micro newtons/meter^2)

dBA: decibels expressed in sound pressure level as measured on the A-weighted scale of a sound-level-meter-filtering network, used in the measurement of environmental noise in the workplace

dead ear: colloquial term referring to an ear with a profound hearing loss from which no response can be measured

dead regions: portions along the basilar membrane without apparent function of the inner hair cells or response of innervated neurons

decaPascal: daPa; unit of pressure in which 1 daPa equals 10 pascals

decibel meter: an electronic instrument designed to measure sound intensity in decibels in accordance with an accepted standard; SYN: sound level meter

delayed-onset auditory deprivation: the apparent decline in word-recognition ability in the unaided ear of a person fitted with a monaural hearing aid, resulting from asymmetric stimulation; SYN: late-onset auditory deprivation

dementia: progressive deterioration of cognitive function

deprivation, auditory: diminution or absence of sensory opportunity for neural structures central to the end organ, due to reduction in auditory stimulation resulting from hearing loss

deprivation effect, auditory: systematic decrease over time in auditory performance associated with the reduced availability of acoustic information; SYN: late-onset auditory deprivation, acquired suprathreshold asymmetry

desired sensation level: DSL; number of decibels above behavioral threshold required to amplify the long-term speech spectrum to a prescribed level across the frequency range

Desired Sensation Level prescriptive procedure: DSL prescriptive procedure; method of choosing gain and frequency response of a hearing aid so that the long-term spectrum of speech is amplified to the desired sensation levels, estimated across the frequency range from audiometric thresholds

DI: directivity index; quantification of the directional properties of a hearing aid microphone, expressed as the decibel improvement in signal-to-noise ratio over that expected for an omnidirectional microphone

differential diagnosis: DDx; determination of a disease or disorder in a patient from among two or more diseases or disorder with similar symptoms or findings

diffuse field: sound field containing many reflected waves of random incidence so that the average sound pressure obtained throughout the room is nearly uniform

digital hearing aid: hearing aid that processes a signal digitally; SYN: DSP hearing aid

digital signal processing hearing aid: DSP hearing aid; hearing aid that converts microphone output from analog to digital form, uses software algorithms to manipulate gain characteristics, and converts the signal back to analog form for delivery to the loudspeaker

digital-to-analog conversion: DAC; the process of turning numerical (digital) representation of a waveform into a continuously varying (analog) signal

direct audio input: DAI; direct input of sound into a hearing aid by means of a hard-wire or wireless connection between the hearing aid and an assistive listening devices or other sound source

directional: having the characteristic of being more sensitive to sound from a focused directional range; COM: omnidirectional

directional hearing aid: hearing instrument that contains a directional microphone

directional microphone: microphone with a transducer that is more responsive to sound from a focused direction; in hearing aids, the microphone is designed to be more sensitive to sounds emanating from the front than from the back

directional microphones, adaptive: microphone designed to be differentially sensitive to sound from a focused direction that is activated automatically in response to the detection of noise

directivity: the tendency of a source to radiate, or of a microphone to receive, sound more efficiently in one direction

directivity index: DI; quantification of the directional properties of a hearing aid microphone, expressed as the decibel improvement in signal-to-noise ratio over that expected for an omnidirectional microphone

directivity pattern, polar: expression of the directional characteristics of a hearing aid microphone, usually displayed in a polar plot that depicts the relative amplitude output of a hearing aid as a function of angle of sound incidence

disarticulation, ossicular: detachment or break in the bones of the ossicular chain

discomfort level: intensity level at which sound is perceived to be uncomfortably loud; SYN: loudness discomfort level

discrimination: in speech audiometry, generic term for word-recognition ability

discrimination score: DS; early term for word recognition score, expressed as the percentage of words correctly perceived and identified

dispensing audiologist: an audiologist who dispenses hearing aids

distortion, amplitude: inaccurate reproduction of sound when the limits of an amplifier are exceeded and the output is no longer proportional to the input; SYN: harmonic distortion, nonlinear distortion

distortion, harmonic: frequency distortion of a signal in the form of additional harmonic components

Dmic: directional microphone; microphone that is more responsive to sound from a focused direction

DSP hearing aid: digital signal processing hearing aid that converts microphone output from analog to digital form, uses software algorithms to manipulate amplification characteristics, and converts the signal back to analog form for delivery to the loudspeaker

dual-time-constant compression: output-limiting technique in some hearing aids in which the release time of a compression circuit varies as a function of the duration of the input signal

dynamic range: 1. amplitude range over which an electronic instrument operates; 2. the difference in decibels between a person's threshold of sensitivity and threshold of discomfort

dynamic-range compression: hearing aid compression algorithm with a low threshold of activation, designed to package signals between a listener's thresholds of sensitivity and discomfort level in a manner that matches loudness growth

ear, artificial: standardized device used to couple the earphone of an audiometer to a sound level meter microphone for the purpose of calibrating an audiometer

ear, glue: inflammation of the middle ear with thick, viscid, mucus-like effusion; SYN: mucoid otitis media

ear canal volume: measure in immittance audiometry of the volume of air between the tip of the acoustic probe and the tympanic membrane

ear hook: portion of a behind-the-ear hearing aid that connects the case to the earmold tube or thin wire and hooks over the ear

ear impression: cast made of the concha and ear canal for creating a customized earmold or hearing aid

ear infection: colloquial term used most commonly to describe otitis media with effusion

ear insert: 1. any device used to provide the acoustic coupling between an earphone and the ear canal; 2. expandable cuff placed into the external auditory meatus to direct sound from an earphone into the ear canal

ear simulator: device used in the calibration of audiometric equipment for measuring the output sound pressure of an earphone under well-defined loading conditions in a specified frequency range, consisting of a principal cavity, acoustic load networks, and a calibrated microphone

eardrum: thin, membranous vibrating tissue terminating the external auditory meatus and forming the major portion of the lateral wall of the middle ear cavity, onto which the malleus is attached; SYN: tympanic membrane

eardrum SPL: eardrum sound pressure level; sound pressure level measured or estimated at, or very near, the tympanic membrane

earmold: coupler formed to fit into the auricle that channels sound from the ear hook of a hearing aid into the ear canal

earmold, canal: type of earmold that uses only the canal portion of the ear impression with the helix and concha areas removed

earmold, canal-lock: canal earmold with a fingerlike projection along the bottom of the concha to retain the earmold in place

earmold, custom: earmold made for a specific individual from an ear impression

earmold, free-field: type of nonoccluding earmold with a small bridge that holds the earmold tube to the concha ring and directs the tube into the ear canal

earmold, half-shell: earmold consisting of a canal and thin shell, with a bowl extending only part of the way to the helix

earmold, open: nonoccluding earmold with a small outside-diameter canal portion that allows unamplified low-frequency sound to pass around the mold and directs amplified sound through the canal portion tubing; used in high-frequency hearing loss and CROS fittings

earmold, shell: debulked, but otherwise full-sized earmold used for high-gain hearing aids when an acoustic seal is essential

earmold, skeleton: earmold in which the bowl has been cut out, leaving an outer concha rim, but retaining the portion that seals the external auditory meatus

earmold block: cotton or sponge-like plug placed deeply in the external auditory meatus to protect the tympanic membrane from materials used in making earmold impressions

earmold impression: cast made of the concha and ear canal for creating a customized earmold

earmold vent: bore made in an earmold that permits the passage of sound and air into the otherwise blocked external auditory meatus, used for aeration of the canal and/or acoustic alteration

earwax: colloquial term for cerumen, the waxy secretion of the ceruminous glands in the external auditory meatus

educational audiologist: audiologist with a subspecialty interest in the hearing needs of school-age children in an academic setting

effective compression ratio: compression ratio of a hearing instrument in response to real-world-like transient stimuli as opposed to that measured with steady state signals

effective masking: EM; condition in which noise is just sufficient to mask a given signal when the signal and noise are presented to the same ear simultaneously

effusion, middle ear: MEE; exudation of fluid from the membranous walls of the middle ear cavity, secondary to eustachian tube dysfunction

eighth nerve tumor: generic term referring to a neoplasm of cranial nerve VIII, most often a cochleovestibular schwannoma; SYN: acoustic tumor

emission, otoacoustic: OAE; low-level sound emitted by the cochlea, either spontaneously or evoked by an auditory stimulus, related to the function of the outer hair cells of the cochlea

endolymphatic hydrops: excessive accumulation of endolymph within the cochlear and vestibular labyrinths, resulting in fluctuating sensorineural hearing loss, vertigo, tinnitus, and a sensation of fullness

environmental microphone: EM; the microphone on a hearing aid that transduces airborne sound

equivalent ear canal volume: tympanometric estimate of the volume of the ear canal between the probe tip and the tympanic membrane

equivalent volume: in immittance measurement, the translation of changes in probe-tone SPL into volume changes, so that an increase in SPL would appear as a decrease in equivalent volume of a cavity and a decrease in SPL would appear as an increase in equivalent volume

ER-3A insert earphones: Etymotic Research insert earphones used in audiometry

etiology: the study of the causes of a disease or condition

eustachian tube dysfunction: ETD; failure of the eustachian tube to open, usually due to edema in the nasopharynx

evoked otoacoustic emission: EOAE; otoacoustic emission that occurs in response to acoustic stimulation; COM: spontaneous otoacoustic emission; SYN: cochlear echo

expansion: in hearing aid circuitry, the increasing of range or variation of the output in comparison to the input; ANT: compression

exposure, noise: level and duration of noise to which an individual is subjected

external ear: EE; outer ear, consisting of the auricle, external auditory meatus, and lateral surface of the tympanic membrane

external ear effect: EEE; influence of outer ear structures on the acoustic characteristics of sounds reaching the tympanic membrane

external otitis: inflammation of the lining of the external auditory meatus

eyeglass hearing aid: early style of hearing aid built into one or both earpieces of eyeglass frames

faceplate: portion of a custom hearing aid that faces outward, usually containing the battery door, microphone port, and volume control

facial nerve: cranial nerve VII; cranial nerve that provides efferent innervation to the facial muscles and afferent innervation from the soft palate and tongue

false-positive response: in audiometer, response to a nonexistent or inaudible stimulus presentation

fatigue, auditory: a reduction in responsiveness of the auditory sensory receptors following exposure to prolonged or intense acoustic stimulation; SYN: temporary threshold shift

Fattire: One of the coolest names and best tasting micro-brewed beers. First brewed in a basement on the west side of Fort Collins, Colorado (ca.1990).

FDA: Food and Drug Administration; U.S. government agency with responsibilities that include regulating medical devices such as hearing aids

feedback, acoustic: sound produced when an amplification system goes into oscillation, created by amplified sound from the receiver reaching the microphone and being reamplified; for example, hearing aid squeal

feedback suppression: reduction of feedback in hearing aid amplification through the use of adaptive filtering

fitting range: range of hearing loss for which a specific hearing aid circuit, configuration, ear mold, and so forth is appropriate

fixation, stapes: immobilization of the stapes at the oval window, often due to new bony growth resulting from otosclerosis

flat audiogram: audiometric configuration in which hearing sensitivity is similar across the audiometric frequency range

flat response: flat frequency response; amplification that is equal across a given frequency range

fluctuating hearing loss: loss of hearing sensitivity, characterized by aperiodic change in degree

FM amplification system: FM system

FM auditory trainer: classroom amplification system in which a remote microphone/transmitter worn by the teacher sends signals via FM to a receiver worn by the student

FM boot: small bootlike device containing an FM receiver that attaches to the bottom of a behind-the-ear hearing aid

FM microphone transmitter: portion of an FM system that detects, amplifies, and transmits signals to a receiver

FM system: an assistive listening device, designed to enhance signaltonoise ratio in which a remote microphone/transmitter worn by a speaker sends signals via FM to a receiver worn by a listener

4K notch: pattern of audiometric thresholds associated with noise-induced hearing loss, characterized by sensorineural hearing loss peaking

frequencies, speech: audiometric frequencies at which a substantial amount of speech energy occurs, conventionally considered to be 500 Hz, 1000 Hz, and 2000 Hz

frequency lowering: hearing aid algorithm that moves high frequency components of sound to lower frequencies in an effort to enhance speech audibility

frequency response, flat: amplification that is equal across a given frequency range

front-to-back directionality: measure of the difference in gain of a hearing aid with a directional microphone of a signal presented at 0° azimuth versus 180° azimuth

full-dynamic-range compression: wide dynamic range compression

full-on gain: FOG; hearing aid setting that produces maximum acoustic output

function, input/output: I/O function; curve that plots output intensity level as a function of input intensity level; used to describe the gain characteristics of an amplifier

function, performance-intensity: PI function; graph of percentage correct speech recognition scores as a function of presentation level of the target signals

functional gain: FG; difference in decibels between aided and unaided hearing sensitivity thresholds

functional hearing loss: FHL; hearing loss that is exaggerated or feigned

functional overlay: 1. exaggeration of an organic disorder; 2. nonorganic consequence of an organic disorder

gain: 1. in hearing aids, the amount in dB by which the output level exceeds the input level; 2. in evoked potentials, the amount of amplification of the input EEG activity; 3. in rotary chair testing, the ratio of peak eye velocity to peak chair velocity

gain, full-on: FOG; hearing aid setting that produces maximum acoustic output

gain, functional: FG; difference in dB between aided and unaided hearing sensitivity thresholds

gain, insertion: hearing aid gain, defined as the difference in gain with and without a hearing aid

gain, prescribed: gain and frequency response of a hearing aid determined by any of several prescriptive formulas

gain, real-ear: nonspecific term referring generally to the gain of a hearing aid at the tympanic membrane, measured as the difference between the SPL in the ear canal and the SPL at the field reference point for a specified sound field

gain, real-ear aided: REAG; measurement of the difference in dB as a function of frequency, between the SPL in the ear canal and the SPL at a field reference point for a specified sound field with the hearing aid in place and turned on

gain, real-ear insertion: REIG; probe-microphone measurement of the difference, in dB as a function of frequency, between the real-ear unaided gain and the real-ear aided gain at the same point near the tympanic membrane

gain, real-ear occluded: REOG; probe-microphone measurement of the difference, in dB as a function of frequency, between the SPL in the ear canal and the SPL at a field reference point for a specified sound field with a hearing aid in place and turned off

gain, real-ear unaided: REUG; probe-microphone measurement of the difference, in dB as a function of frequency, between the SPL in an unoccluded ear canal and the SPL at the field reference point for a specified sound field

gain, reference test: ANSI standard gain level with a 60-dB-SPL input and the volume control of the hearing aid adjusted so that the gain at the reference test frequencies is 17 dB less than that at SSPL-90

gain control: manual or automatic control designed to adjust the output level of a hearing instrument; SYN: volume control

gain control, automatic: AGC; nonlinear hearing aid compression circuitry designed to automatically change gain as signal level changes or limit output when signal level reaches a specified criterion; SYN: automatic volume control

gain target, prescriptive: the desired gain and frequency response of a hearing aid, generated by a formula, against which the actual output of a hearing aid is compared

genetic hearing loss: hearing loss related to heredity

glue ear: inflammation of the middle ear with thick, viscid, mucuslike effusion; SYN: mucoid otitis media

grommet tube: ventilation or pressure-equalization tube

group amplification: assistive listening device system used in a classroom or other venue for more than one person; COM: personal amplification

HA-1 coupler: standard 2-cc coupler used to connect a hearing aid to an electroacoustic analyzer; the HA-1 device allows direct coupling of an earmold or an in-the-ear hearing aid, with putty used to seal the earmold or shell into the device

HA-2 coupler: standard 2-cc coupler used to connect a hearing aid to an electroacoustic analyzer; the HA-2 device has an earmold simulator and is used for testing earphones with nubs, such as an external receiver of a body aid

HA-3 coupler: standard 2-cc coupler used to connect a hearing aid to an electroacoustic analyzer; the HA-3 device is used for testing modular ITE hearing aids, earphones, and insert receivers that do not have nubs

HA-4 coupler: standard 2-cc coupler used to connect a hearing aid to an electroacoustic analyzer; the HA-4 device is a modification of the HA-2 with entrance tubing for use with postauricular or eyeglass hearing aids

hair cells, inner: IHC; sensory hair cells arranged in a single row in the organ of Corti to which the primary afferent nerve endings of cranial nerve VIII are attached

hair cells, outer: OHC; motile cells within the organ of Corti, responsible for enhancing sensitivity and fine-tuning frequency resolution of the cochlea by potentiating the sensitivity of the inner hair cells an object that has been set into motion

head baffle effect: relative enhancement of high-frequency sound due to the acoustic diffraction of low-frequency sound by the auricle and head combining to form a wall or baffle

head shadow effect: attenuation of sound by the head in a free field, so that a sound approaching from one side of the head will be reduced in magnitude when it reaches the ear on the other side

headphone: transducer that converts electrical signals into sound delivered to the ear; SYN: earphone

headroom: residual dynamic range of a hearing aid, expressed as the difference in dB SPL between a given output (such as gain at user settings) and the level of saturation of the device

hearing aid, analog: amplification device that uses conventional, continuously varying signal processing; COM: digital hearing aid

hearing aid, behind-the-ear: BTE hearing aid; a hearing aid that fits over the ear and is coupled to the ear canal via an earmold or receiver

hearing aid, BICROS: bilateral contralateral routing of signals; a hearing aid system with one microphone contained in a hearing aid at each ear; the microphones lead to a single amplifier and receiver in the better hearing ear of a person with bilateral asymmetric hearing loss

hearing aid, bone anchored: BAHA; surgically implanted bone conduction receiver that interfaces with an external amplifier, designed to provide amplification for those with intractable middle ear disorder

hearing aid, BTE: behind-the-ear hearing aid

hearing aid, canal: hearing aid that fits mostly in the external auditory meatus with a small portion extending into the concha; SYN: in-the-canal hearing aid

hearing aid, CIC: completely-in-the-canal hearing aid

hearing aid, CROS: contralateral routing of signals; hearing aid designed for unilateral hearing loss in which a microphone is placed on the poorer ear, and the signal is routed to a hearing aid on the better ear

hearing aid, custom: ITE, ITC, or CIC hearing aid made for a specific individual from an ear impression

hearing aid, implantable: any electronic device implanted in the mastoid cavity or middle ear space designed to amplify sound and delivery vibratory energy directly to the ossicles or cochlea

hearing aid, in-the-canal: ITC hearing aid; canal hearing aid

hearing aid, in-the-ear: ITE hearing aid; custom hearing aid that fits entirely in the concha of the ear

hearing aid, monaural: hearing aid worn on one ear only

hearing aid, OTC: over-the-counter hearing aid

hearing aid, postauricular: a hearing aid that fits over the ear and is coupled to the ear canal via an earmold; SYN: behind-the-ear hearing aid, over-the-ear hearing aid

hearing aid, programmable: digitally controlled analog or digital signal processing hearing aid in which the parameters of the instrument are under computer control

hearing aid, receiver-in-the-canal: RIC hearing aid; receiver-in-the-ear hearing aid

hearing aid, transcranial CROS: contralateral routing of signal (CROS) strategy for unilateral hearing loss in which a high-gain in-the-ear hearing aid is fitted to the poor ear in an effort to transfer sound across the skull by bone conduction to the cochlea of the good ear

hearing aid analyzer: instrument used for the electroacoustic analysis of various parameters of the response of a hearing aid; SYN: hearing aid test box

hearing aid fitting: 1. the process of selecting and adjusting a hearing aid to an individual; 2. the characteristics of a hearing aid that represents the end result of the hearing aid selection process

hearing aid stethoscope: stethoscope designed to auscultate a hearing instrument for the purpose of diagnostic listening

hearing aid test box: instrument used for the electroacoustic analysis of various parameters of the response of a hearing aid; SYN: hearing aid analyzer

hearing aid trial period: length of time, typically mandated by law as 30 days, during which an individual can return a purchased hearing aid and receive a refund

hearing assistive technologies: HAT; collective term referring to devices, such as assistive listening and alerting devices, which serve to enhance communication and can be used with or without hearing aids or hearing implants

Hearing Handicap Inventory for Adults: HHIA; modification of the HHIE designed to yield information about a nonelderly adult's perceived social and emotional consequences of hearing impairment

Hearing Handicap Inventory for the Elderly: HHIE; modification of the HHI designed to yield information about an elderly individual's perceived social and emotional consequences of hearing impairment

hearing loss, acquired: hearing loss that occurs after birth as a result of injury or disease; not congenital; SYN: adventitious hearing loss

hearing loss, adventitious: loss of hearing sensitivity occurring after birth; ANT: congenital hearing loss

hearing loss, asymmetric: condition in which hearing loss in one ear is of a significantly different degree than in the other ear

hearing loss, central: auditory disorder that occurs as a result of impaired function of the central auditory nervous system

hearing loss, idiopathic: hearing loss of unknown cause

hearing loss, inorganic: apparent loss in hearing sensitivity in the absence of any organic pathologic change in structure; used to describe hearing loss that is feigned; SYN: functional hearing loss, nonorganic hearing loss

hearing loss, nonorganic: apparent loss in hearing sensitivity in the absence of any organic pathologic change in structure; used to describe hearing loss that is feigned; SYN: functional hearing loss

hearing loss, ski-slope: colloquial term referring to a hearing loss configuration characterized by normal hearing in the low frequencies and a precipitous loss in the high frequencies

hearing loss, sudden: acute rapid-onset loss of hearing that is often idiopathic, unilateral, and substantial and that may or may not resolve spontaneously

Hearing Loss Association of America: HLAA; consumer advocacy organization for persons with hearing impairment; formerly Self-Help for Hard of Hearing People (SHHH)

hearing screening: the application of rapid and simple hearing tests to a large population, consisting of individuals who are undiagnosed and typically asymptomatic to identify those who require additional diagnostic procedures

hearing threshold level: HTL; an individual's threshold, or the number of dB by which an individual's hearing threshold exceeds the normal threshold, expressed as dB HTL

HHIA: Hearing Handicap Inventory for Adults; modification of the HHIE designed to yield information about a nonelderly adult's perceived social and emotional consequences of hearing impairment

HHIE: Hearing Handicap Inventory for the Elderly; self-assessment scale designed to yield information about an elderly individual's perceived social and emotional consequences of hearing impairment

hidden hearing loss: subclinical changes in hearing function resulting from noise-induced degenerative changes to the synaptic regions between inner hair cells and cochlear nerve terminals

high-frequency average: HFA; an ANSI hearing aid specification, expressed as the average of decibel response values at 1000 Hz, 1600 Hz, and 2500 Hz

high-level compression: compression-limiting process of a hearing aid, characterized by a high threshold, high ratio, and long release time

HI-PRO: proprietary computer interface module, designed as an industry standard that is used to couple a programmable hearing aid to a computer

horn, Libby: earmold horn, consisting of a smooth, tapered, one-piece sound tube of internal stepped-bore construction

hydrops, endolymphatic: excessive accumulation of endolymph within the cochlear and vestibular labyrinths, resulting in fluctuating sensorineural hearing loss, vertigo, tinnitus, and a sensation of fullness

hyperacusis: abnormally sensitive hearing in which normally tolerable sounds are perceived as excessively loud

IDEA: Individuals with Disabilities Education Act; U.S. public laws 94-142 and 99-457, mandating free and appropriate public education for all children age 3 and older who have handicapping conditions; also encourages services to infants and toddlers

idiopathic: of unknown cause

immittance: encompassing term for energy flow through the middle ear, including admittance, compliance, conductance, impedance, reactance, resistance, and susceptance

immittance audiometry: battery of immittance measurements, including static immittance, tympanometry, and acoustic reflex threshold determination, designed to assess middle ear function

immittance screening: rapid assessment of middle ear function by tympanometry

impacted cerumen: cerumen that causes blockage of the external auditory meatus

impedance: Z; total opposition to energy flow or resistance to the absorption of energy, expressed in ohms

implant, cochlear: device that enables persons with profound hearing loss to perceive sound, consisting of an electrode array surgically implanted in the cochlea, which delivers electrical signals to cranial nerve VIII and an external amplifier, which activates the electrode

implant, middle ear: implantable hearing aid; hearing device that is implanted in the middle ear to provide amplification to the cochlea by driving the ossicular chain mechanically

impression: ear impression; cast made of the concha and ear canal for creating a customized earmold or hearing aid

inferior colliculus: IC; central auditory nucleus of the midbrain; its central nucleus receives ascending input from the cochlear nucleus and superior olivary complex, and its pericentral nucleus receives descending input from the cortex

input compression: process in which a hearing aid compresses a signal before it reaches the volume control, resulting in a constant dynamic range with a change in maximum output as gain is increased or decreased by the volume control; COM: output compression

input/output function: I/O function; curve that plots output intensity level as a function of input intensity level; used to describe the gain characteristics of an amplifier

insert earphone: earphone whose transducer is connected to the ear through a tube leading to an expandable cuff that is inserted into the external auditory meatus; COM: supra-aural earphone

insertion gain, real-ear: REIG; probe-microphone measurement of the difference, in dB as a function of frequency, between the real-ear unaided gain and the real-ear aided gain at the same point near the tympanic membrane

in situ measurement: evaluation of hearing aid performance while the hearing aid is being worn

integrated circuit: IC; electronic circuit with its many interconnected elements formed on a single body of semiconductor material

interaural attenuation: IA; reduction in the sound energy of a signal as it is transmitted by bone conduction from one side of the head to the opposite ear

International Hearing Society: IHS; organization of hearing professionals, primarily hearing instrument specialists; formerly National Hearing Aid Society

interpeak latency: difference in milliseconds between the latencies of two peaks of an auditory evoked potential, such as the I to V interpeak latency of the auditory brain stem response; SYN: interpeak interval; interwave latency

interrupter switch: the switch on an audiometer that interrupts or presents a test signal

in-the-canal hearing aid: ITC hearing aid; custom hearing aid that fits mostly in the external auditory meatus with a small portion extending into the concha; SYN: canal hearing aid

in-the-ear hearing aid: ITE hearing aid; custom hearing aid that fits entirely in the concha of the ear

I/O function: input/output function; curve that plots output intensity level as a function of input intensity level; used to describe the gain characteristics of an amplifier

ipsilateral acoustic reflex: acoustic reflex occurring in one ear as a result of stimulation of the same ear; SYN: uncrossed acoustic reflex

ITC hearing aid: in-the-canal hearing aid; custom hearing aid that fits mostly in the external auditory meatus with a small portion extending into the concha; SYN: canal hearing aid

ITE hearing aid: in-the-ear hearing aid; custom hearing aid that fits entirely in the concha of the ear

Jewett waves: vertex positive peaks of the auditory brain stem response, first described by Don Jewett as seven peaks occurring within 10 msec of stimulus onset, labeled as Waves I, II, III . . . VII

just noticeable difference: JND; the smallest change in a stimulus that is detectable; SYN: difference limen

KEMAR: Knowles electronics mannequin for acoustic research; model used in the measurement of hearing aid performance that simulates the acoustic properties of an average adult head and torso

knee point: 1. point on an input–output function at which the slope changes from unity; 2. in hearing aids, the intensity level at which compression is activated; SYN: compression threshold

labyrinth: the inner ear, so named because of the intricate maze of connecting pathways in the petrous portion of each temporal bone, consisting of the canals within the bone and fluid-filled sacs and channels within the canals, including the cochlear and vestibular endorgans

latency, interpeak: difference in msec between the latencies of two peaks of an auditory evoked potential, such as the I to V interpeak latency of the auditory brain stem response; SYN: interpeak interval; interwave latency

lateral lemniscus: LL; large fiber tract or bundle, formed by dorsal, intermediate, and ventral nuclei and consisting of ascending auditory fibers from the cochlear nucleus and superior olivary complex, which runs along the lateral edge of the pons and carries information to the inferior colliculus

LDL: loudness discomfort level; intensity level at which sound is perceived to be uncomfortably loud, determined under earphones and expressed in dB HL, or with probe microphone in dB SPL; SYN: uncomfortable loudness level

lesion, space-occupying: neoplasm that exerts its influence by growing and impinging on neural tissues, as opposed to a lesion caused by trauma, ischemia, or inflammation

level, loudness discomfort: LDL; intensity level at which sound is perceived to be uncomfortably loud, determined under earphones and expressed in dB HL or with probe microphone in dB SPL used as a target to set the RESR of a hearing aid

level, saturation sound pressure: SSPL; maximum output generated by the receiver of a hearing aid, expressed as the root mean square sound pressure level

level, sensation: SL; the intensity level of a sound in dB above an individual's threshold; usually used to refer to the intensity level of a signal presentation or a response above a specified threshold, such as pure-tone threshold or acoustic reflex threshold

level, sound pressure: SPL; magnitude or quantity of sound energy relative to a reference pressure, 0.0002 dyne/cm^2 or 20 μPa

level, tolerance: threshold of discomfort

Libby horn: earmold horn, consisting of a smooth, tapered, one-piece sound tube of internal stepped-bore construction

limiting compression: method of limiting maximum output of a hearing aid with compression circuitry

linear amplification: hearing aid amplification in which the gain is the same for all input levels until the maximum output is reached

linear compression: in hearing aids, amplifier gain that is linear at input levels that exceed the compression knee point

linear hearing aid: hearing aid amplification in which the gain is the same for all input levels until the maximum output is reached

Ling Five-Sound Test: pediatric speech-detection measure consisting of five sounds chosen to represent the frequency range of speech—[u], [a], [i], [ʃ], and [s]

live-voice testing: speech audiometric technique in which speech signals are presented via a microphone with controlled vocal output; SYN: monitored live voice

Lombard effect: unconscious tendency to raise the level of vocal output above a background of noise

long-term average speech spectrum: long-term speech spectrum

loop, induction: continuous wire surrounding a room that conducts electrical energy from an amplifier, thereby creating a magnetic field; current flow from the loop is induced in the induction coil of a hearing aid telecoil

loop FM system: remote microphone amplification system in which the FM transmits to a hearing aid t-coil through an induction loop receiver

loudness discomfort level: LDL; intensity level at which sound is perceived to be uncomfortably loud; determined under earphones and expressed in dB HL or with probe microphone in dB SPL; used as a target to set the RESR of a hearing aid

loudness level, comfortable: intensity level of a signal that is perceived as comfortably loud

loudness level, uncomfortable: ULL; UCL; intensity level at which sound is perceived to be uncomfortably loud; SYN: loudness discomfort level

loudness summation: the addition of loudness by expansion of bandwidth even when overall sound pressure level remains the same

low-energy Bluetooth: advanced Bluetooth protocol used to convey information over shorter distances using less power than conventional Bluetooth technology

low-level compression: hearing aid compression circuitry that is activated in response to low intensity input, such as wide-dynamic-range compression

malingering: deliberately feigning or exaggerating an illness or impairment such as hearing loss

manual audiometry: any type of standard hearing measurement in which the examiner controls the stimulus presentation; ANT: automatic audiometry

map, cochlear implant: representation of the threshold and suprathreshold parameters of each electrode or electrode combination in the coding program of an individual cochlear implant user

masking: 1. use of noise to eliminate the participation of one ear while testing the other; 2. amount or process by which the threshold for one sound is raised by the presence of another sound; 3. noise that interferes with the audibility of another sound

masking, contralateral: the contralateralization of masking noise from the nontest ear to the test ear once it exceeds interaural attenuation; SYN: overmasking

masking, effective: EM; 1. condition in which noise is just sufficient to mask a given signal when the signal and noise are presented to the same ear simultaneously; 2. lowest level of noise required theoretically to eliminate contralateralization of a signal

masking, maximum: in audiometry, the highest level of masking that can be used before overmasking occurs

masking, minimum: starting intensity level of the masking noise used to initiate the plateau procedure of masking in audiometry

masking dilemma: challenge in audiometric testing of bilateral moderate-to-severe conductive hearing loss presented when the introduction of masking noise to the nontest ear is sufficient to cross over and mask the test ear

mastoiditis: inflammation of the mastoid process

maximum power output: MPO; highest intensity level that a hearing aid can produce,

regardless of input level; SYN: saturation sound pressure level

MCL: most comfortable loudness; intensity level at which sound is perceived to be most comfortable, usually expressed in dB HL

medial geniculate: MG; auditory nucleus of the thalamus, divided into central and surrounding pericentral nuclei, that receives primary ascending fibers from the inferior colliculus and sends fibers, via the auditory radiation, to the auditory cortex

medial superior olive: MSO; one of the primary nuclei of the superior olivary complex, located in the hindbrain, receiving primary ascending projections directly from both the ipsilateral and contralateral anterior ventral cochlear nuclei

membrane, tympanic: TM; thin, membranous vibrating tissue terminating the external auditory meatus and forming the major portion of the lateral wall of the middle ear cavity, onto which the malleus is attached; COL: eardrum

memory, auditory: assimilation, storage, and retrieval of previously experienced sound

memory, short-term: aspect of the information processing function of the central nervous system that receives, modifies, and stores information briefly

Ménière's disease: idiopathic endolymphatic hydrops, characterized by fluctuating vertigo, hearing loss, tinnitus, and aural fullness

meter, sound level: an electronic instrument designed to measure sound intensity in dB in accordance with an accepted standard

meter, VU: volume unit meter; visual indicator on an audiometer of the intensity of an input signal in dB, where 0 dB is equal to the attenuator output setting

microphone, directional: microphone with a transducer that is more responsive to sound from a focused direction; in hearing aids, the microphone is designed to be more sensitive to sounds emanating from the front than from the back

microphone, environmental: EM; the microphone on a hearing aid that transduces airborne sound

microphone, omnidirectional: microphone with a sensitivity that is similar regardless of the direction of incoming sound

microphone, probe: microphone transducer with a small-diameter probe-tube extension for measuring sound near the tympanic membrane

microphone, probe-tube: probe microphone

microphone, reference: a second microphone used to measure the stimulus level during probe-microphone measurements or to control the stimulus level during the probe-microphone equalization process

microphone location effect: influence of microphone location on amplification response, measured as the different in input SPL at the hearing aid microphone location relative to the SPL in the undisturbed sound field

microphone telecoil switch: MT switch; control on a hearing aid that permits manual selection of the microphone or telecoil as the input transducer

middle ear: portion of the hearing mechanism extending from the medial membrane of the tympanic membrane to the oval window of the cochlea, including the ossicles and middle ear cavity; serves as an impedance matching device of the outer and inner ears

middle ear compliance: measure of the ease of energy transfer through the middle ear; reciprocal of stiffness

middle ear effusion: MEE; exudation of fluid from the membranous walls of the middle ear cavity, secondary to eustachian tube dysfunction

middle ear implant: 1. ossicular prosthesis; 2. hearing device that is implanted in the middle ear to provide amplification to the cochlea by driving the ossicular chain mechanically

middle ear infection: morbid state of the middle ear caused by invasion and multiplication of pathogenic microorganisms

middle ear muscle reflex: reflexive contraction of the stapedius and tensor tympani muscles in response to loud sound; stapedius muscle dominates the reflex in humans; SYN: acoustic reflex

middle ear pathology: result of disease process of the middle ear structures

middle ear pressure, negative: air pressure in the middle ear cavity that is below atmospheric pressure, resulting from an inability to equalize pressure due to eustachian tube dysfunction

midfrequency hearing loss: nonspecific term referring to hearing sensitivity loss occurring at frequencies around 1000 Hz to 2000 Hz

Minimum Auditory Capabilities Battery: MAC battery; group of tests designed to assess auditory perception of persons with profound hearing loss

misophonia: strong emotional aversion to certain sounds resulting in a negative impact on daily living

mixed hearing loss: hearing loss with both a conductive and a sensorineural component

MLV: monitored level voice; speech audiometric technique in which speech signals are presented via a microphone with controlled vocal output; SYN: live-voice testing

mm H$_2$O: millimeter of water; unit of air pressure used in tympanometry

modification, earmold: change in the structure of an earmold to alter the fit or the acoustic characteristic

modulation, frequency: FM; the process of creating a complex signal by sinusoidally varying the frequency of a carrier wave

monaural amplification: hearing aid amplification device worn on one ear only

monosyllabic word: a word of one syllable

most comfortable loudness: MCL; intensity level at which sound is perceived to be most comfortable, usually expressed in dB HL

MPO: maximum power output; highest intensity level that a hearing aid can produce regardless of input level; SYN: saturation sound pressure level

MRI: magnetic resonance imaging; radiographic technique used to provide precise structural images

MSO: medial superior olive; one of the primary nuclei of the superior olivary complex, located in the hindbrain, receiving primary ascending projections directly from both the ipsilateral and contralateral anterior ventral cochlear nuclei

multichannel compression: process in which a hearing aid separates the input signal into two or more frequency bands, each having independently controlled compression circuitry

multichannel hearing aid: hearing aid in which each of two or more frequency bands is controlled independently

multiple-memory hearing aid: hearing aid that can be programmed to contain more than one frequency response for use under different listening conditions

multitalker babble: continuous speech noise composed of several talkers all speaking at once

muscle, stapedius: along with the tensor tympani, one of two striated muscles of the middle ear, classified as a pinnate muscle, consisting of short fibers directed obliquely onto the stapedius tendon at the midline, innervated by the facial nerve, cranial nerve VII

muscle, tensor tympani: along with the stapedius, one of two striated muscles of the middle ear, classified as a pinnate muscle, consisting of short fibers directed obliquely onto the tensor tympani tendon at the midline, innervated by the trigeminal nerve, cranial nerve V

myringectomy: excision of the tympanic membrane; SYN: myringodectomy

myringoplasty: procedure in which a tissue graft, usually of fascia or vein, is used to close a perforation of the tympanic membrane; SYN: Type I tympanoplasty

NAL: National Acoustic Laboratories; Australian laboratory responsible for developing the widely used NAL prescriptive hearing aid fitting technique

NAL-N2: National Acoustics Laboratory procedure for prescribing nonlinear hearing aids based on a rationale similar to NAL-N1 with an altered loudness paradigm and accounting for various patient factors age

NAL-R procedure: revised NAL procedure

narrow-band noise: NBN; band-pass filtered noise that is centered at one of the audiometric frequencies, used for sound field audiometry or for masking in pure-tone audiometry

NBC-HIS: National Board for Certification in Hearing Instrument Sciences; organization that sets standards for and awards certification in hearing instrument practices

neckloop: transducer worn as part of an FM amplification system, consisting of a cord from the hearing aid and used to deliver signal to t-coil of hearing aid.

negative middle ear pressure: air pressure in the middle ear cavity that is below atmospheric pressure, resulting from an inability to equalize pressure due to eustachian tube dysfunction

nerve, acoustic: cranial nerve VIII; auditory nerve, consisting of a vestibular and cochlear branch

nerve, cochlear: auditory branch of cranial nerve VIII, arising from the spiral ganglion of the cochlea and terminating in the cochlear nuclei of the brain stem

nerve, eighth: cranial nerve VIII, consisting of the auditory and vestibular nerves

nervous system, central: CNS; that portion of the nervous system to which sensory impulses and from which motor impulses are transmitted, including the cortex, brain stem, and spinal cord

neural presbycusis: loss of cochlear and higher-order neurons associated with the aging process

neurofibroma: benign nonencapsulated tumor resulting from proliferation of the nerve cell sheath in a poorly defined pattern that may include nerve fibers

neuroma: generic term used to describe any neoplasm derived from cells of the nervous system, including cochleovestibular schwannoma

newborn hearing screening: the application of rapid and simple tests of auditory function, typically AABR or OAE measures, to newborns prior to hospital discharge to identify those who require additional diagnostic procedures; SYN: neonatal hearing screening; universal newborn hearing screening

nHL: normalized hearing level; the decibel level of a sound that lacks a standardized reference, referred to behaviorally determined normative levels, expressed as dB nHL

NIDCD: National Institute on Deafness and Other Communication Disorders

Noah: registered name of a computer program for hearing aid fitting, developed to serve as an industry-standard software platform for programming hearing devices

NODAK: slang term that one person from North Dakota might call another

noise, broadband: BBN; sound with a wide bandwidth, containing a continuous spectrum of frequencies, with equal energy per cycle throughout the band

noise, circuit: unwanted signal in the output of a circuit created by the functioning of the circuit

noise, narrow-band: NBN; band-pass-filtered noise that is centered at one of the audiometric frequencies, used for sound field audiometry and masking in pure-tone audiometry

noise, speech: broadband noise that is filtered to resemble the speech spectrum

noise, white: broadband noise having constant energy at all frequencies

noise exposure: level and duration of noise to which an individual is subjected

noise floor: in any amplification system, the continuous baseline-level of background activity or noise from which a signal or response emerges

noise-induced hearing loss: NIHL; permanent sensorineural hearing loss caused by exposure to excessive sound levels

noise notch: pattern of audiometric thresholds associated with noise-induced hearing loss, characterized by sensorineural hearing loss predominantly at 4000 Hz

noise reduction: 1. decrease in the sound pressure level; 2. the difference in sound pressure level of a noise at two different locations

noise trauma: 1. damage to hearing from a transient, high-intensity sound; 2. long-term insult to hearing from excessive noise exposure; SYN: acoustic trauma

nonlinear amplification: amplification whose gain is not the same for all input levels

nonoccluding earmold: open earmold with a small outside-diameter canal portion that allows unamplified low-frequency sound to pass and directs amplified sound through the canal portion tubing; used in high-frequency hearing loss and CROS fittings

Northwest University Auditory Test Number 6: NU-6; monosyllabic word-recognition measure; designed to be phonetically balanced within a word list

notch, noise: pattern of audiometric thresholds associated with noise-induced hearing loss, characterized by sensorineural hearing loss predominantly at 4000 Hz

nucleus, cochlear: CN; cluster of cell bodies of second-order neurons on the lateral edge of the hindbrain in the central auditory nervous system at which fibers from cranial nerve VIII have an obligatory synapse

nystagmus: pattern of eye movement, characterized by a slow component in one direction that is periodically interrupted by a saccade, or fast component in the other; results from the anatomical connection between the vestibular and ocular systems

OAE: otoacoustic emissions; low-level sound emitted by the cochlea, either spontaneously or as a sound evoked by an auditory stimulus, related to the function of the outer hair cells of the cochlea

occluded response, real-ear: REOR; probe-microphone measurement of the sound pressure level, as a function of frequency, at a specified point near the tympanic membrane with a hearing aid in place and turned off; expressed in absolute SPL or as gain relative to stimulus level

occlusion effect: low-frequency enhancement in the loudness level of bone conducted signals due to occlusion of the ear canal

olivary complex, superior: SOC; collection of auditory nuclei in the hindbrain that relay signals to other auditory neural stations

omnidirectional microphone: microphone with a sensitivity that is similar regardless of the direction of the incoming sound

open-canal fitting: hearing aid fitting with an open earmold or tubing-only in the ear canal

open-ear response: sound pressure at the tympanic membrane of a person placed in a sound field; SYN: real-ear unaided response

open earmold: nonoccluding earmold with a small outside-diameter canal portion that allows unamplified low-frequency sound to pass around the mold and directs amplified sound through the canal portion tubing; used in high-frequency hearing loss and CROS fittings

organ of Corti: hearing organ, composed of sensory and supporting cells, located on the basilar membrane in the cochlear duct

OSPL90: output sound pressure level for 90-dB input; ANSI standard term for saturation sound pressure level

ossicles: the three small bones of the middle ear—the malleus, incus, and stapes—extending from the tympanic membrane through the tympanic cavity to the oval window

ossicular disarticulation: detachment or break in the bones of the ossicular chain

ossicular discontinuity: ossicular disarticulation

otalgia: ear pain

OTC hearing aid: over-the-counter hearing aid; amplification device that can be purchased without prescription or provider guidance or care

otitis media: OM; inflammation of the middle ear, resulting predominantly from eustachian tube dysfunction

oto block: a small piece of plastic foam or other material that is inserted into the external auditory meatus before an earmold impression is made to prevent impression material from reaching the tympanic membrane

otoacoustic emission, evoked: EOAE; otoacoustic emission that occurs in response to acoustic stimulation

otoadmittance: measure of energy flow through the middle ear system; SYN: immittance

otoadmittance meter: early immittance measurement instrument designed to quantify susceptance and conductance components of middle ear function

otoblock: small piece of cotton or foam with a string attached, placed deeply into the ear canal during the making of an ear impression to ensure that impression material does not reach the tympanic membrane

otorrhea: discharge from the ear

otoscopy, video: endoscopic examination of the external auditory meatus and tympanic membrane displayed on a video monitor

ototoxic drug: any of a variety of antibiotics and other chemotherapeutic agents that are toxic to the ear, usually affecting the cochlear and/or vestibular hair cells

ototoxic hearing loss: hearing sensitivity loss secondary to ototoxicity

output compression: process in which a hearing aid compresses a signal after the volume control, resulting in an expanded dynamic range for low-gain settings and a lower knee point for high-gain settings; COM: input compression

output limiting: restriction of the maximum output of a hearing aid by peak clipping or amplitude compression

output-limiting compression: method of limiting maximum output of a hearing aid with compression circuitry

over-the-counter hearing aid: OTC hearing aid; amplification device that can be purchased without prescription or provider guidance or care

overall sound pressure level: total sound energy throughout the frequency range, measured without any frequency weighting

overamplification: 1. the provision of excessive gain by a hearing aid; 2. hearing aid amplification of sufficient magnitude to cause additional, noise-induced hearing loss

overmasking: condition in which the intensity level of masking in the nontest ear is sufficient to contralateralize to the test ear, thereby elevating the test-ear threshold

Pa: pascal; unit of pressure, expressed in newtons per square meter

palsy, facial: impairment or loss of voluntary movement of the face due to facial nerve disorder

parallel vent: vent that runs parallel to the bore for the entire length of an earmold

paralysis, facial: loss of voluntary movement of the face due to facial nerve disorder

pascal: Pa; unit of pressure, expressed in newtons per square meter

pass-fail criterion: specified outcome used as the determination point for whether a screening or test was positive or negative for a disorder

patent eustachian tube: abnormally patulous eustachian tube

patulous eustachian tube: abnormally patent or open eustachian tube, resulting in sensation of stuffiness, autophony, tinnitus, and audible respiratory noises

PB: phonetically balanced; descriptive of a list of words containing speech sounds that occur with the same frequency as in conversational speech

PB max: highest percentage correct score obtained on monosyllabic word recognition measures (PB word lists) presented at several intensity levels

PB monosyllabic word list: PB word list

PB word list: phonetically balanced word list; list of words used in word recognition testing that contain speech sounds that occur with the same frequency as those of conversational speech

PBK word lists: phonetically balanced kindergarten word lists; lists of words used in word recognition testing, designed both to be phonetically balanced and to contain words that are at a vocabulary level appropriate for use with young school children

PE tube: pressure-equalization tube; small tube or grommet inserted in the tympanic membrane following myringotomy to provide equalization of air pressure within the middle ear space as a substitute for a nonfunctional eustachian tube

PE tube, patent: unobstructed, functional pressure-equalization tube

peak acoustic gain: amount of gain at a point along the frequency response of a hearing aid at which gain is maximal

perilymph: cochlear fluid, found in the scala vestibule, scala tympani, and spaces within the organ of Corti, which is high in sodium and calcium and has an ionic composition that resembles cerebrospinal fluid

perilymphatic fistula: abnormal passageway between the perilymphatic space and the middle ear, resulting in the leak of perilymph at the oval or round window, caused by congenital defects or trauma

peripheral: 1. toward the outer surface or part; 2. located outside the central nervous system

permanent threshold shift: PTS; irreversible hearing sensitivity loss following exposure to excessive noise levels; COM: temporary threshold shift

personal FM system: a wearable assistive listening device consisting of a remote microphone/transmitter worn by a speaker that sends signals via FM to a receiver worn by a listener; designed to enhance the signal-to-noise ratio

personal sound amplification product: PSAP; any of a variety of wearable electronic devices designed to amplify sounds but which are not intended specifically as treatment for hearing loss

phonemic analysis: separation of speech signals into component phonemes

phonetically balanced word list: PB word list; list of words used in word-recognition testing that contain speech sounds that occur with the same frequency as those of conversational speech

phonophobia: abnormally sensitive hearing in which normally tolerable sounds are perceived as painful

plasticity, neural: the capacity of the nervous system to change over time in response to changes in sensory input

polar directivity pattern: expression of the directional characteristics of a hearing aid microphone, usually displayed in a polar plot that depicts the relative amplitude output of a hearing aid as a function of angle of sound incidence

positive middle ear pressure: air pressure in the middle ear cavity that is greater than atmospheric pressure, resulting from air being forced into the middle ear through the eustachian tube

postauricular hearing aids: a hearing aid that fits over the ear and is coupled to the ear canal via an earmold or tubing; SYN: behind-the-ear hearing aid, over-the-ear hearing aid

preferred loudness level: PLL; signal level at which speech is rated as most comfortable

presbycusis: age-related hearing impairment

prescribed gain: gain and frequency response of a hearing aid that is determined by any of several prescriptive formulae

prescriptive fitting: strategy for fitting hearing aids by the calculation of a desired gain and frequency response, based on any number of formulas that incorporate pure-tone audiometric thresholds and may incorporate uncomfortable loudness information

prescriptive gain target: the desired gain and frequency response of a hearing aid, generated by a formula, against which the actual output of a hearing aid is compared

prescriptive method: strategy for fitting hearing aids by using a formula to calculate the target gain and frequency response

pressure-equalization tube: PE tube; small tube or grommet inserted in the tympanic membrane following myringotomy to provide equalization of air pressure within the middle ear space as a substitute for a nonfunctional eustachian tube; SYN: tympanostomy tube

pressure vent: small vent in an earmold or hearing aid to provide pressure equalization in the external auditory meatus

primary auditory cortex: auditory area of the cerebral cortex located on the transverse temporal gyrus (Heschl's gyrus) of the temporal lobe

probe-microphone measurements: electroacoustic assessment of the characteristics of hearing aid amplification near the tympanic membrane with a probe microphone

processing, multichannel: signal processing in more than one channel, referring especially to cochlear implant configurations

programmable hearing aid: digitally controlled analog or digital signal processing hearing aid in which the parameters of the instrument are under computer control

proximal: toward the center or point of origin; ANT: distal

PSAP: personal sound amplification product; any of a variety of wearable electronic devices designed to amplify sounds, but that are not intended specifically as treatment for hearing loss

PTA: pure-tone average; average of hearing sensitivity thresholds to pure-tone signals at 500 Hz, 1000 Hz, and 2000 Hz

PTA2: pure-tone average 2; high-frequency average of hearing sensitivity thresholds to pure-tone signal at 1000 Hz, 2000 Hz, and 4000 Hz

pure-tone audiogram: graph of the threshold of hearing sensitivity, expressed in dB HL, as determined by pure-tone air conduction and bone conduction audiometry at octave and half-octave frequencies ranging from 250 Hz to 8000 Hz

pure-tone average: PTA; average of hearing sensitivity thresholds to pure-tone signals at 500 Hz, 1000 Hz, and 2000 Hz

Quick Speech-In-Noise Test: QuickSIN; modification of the SIN test for rapid clinical presentation; speech audiometric measure of identification of words in sentences, presented at various signal to noise ratios to determine a SNR-50

range, dynamic: 1. amplitude range over which an electronic instrument operates; 2. the difference in dB between a person's threshold of sensitivity and threshold of discomfort

range, fitting: range of hearing loss for which a specific hearing aid circuit, configuration, earmold, and so forth, is appropriate

range of comfortable loudness: difference, in dB, between threshold of audibility and loudness discomfort level for a specified acoustic signal

ratio, compression: the decibel ratio of acoustic input to amplifier output in a hearing aid; for example, a hearing aid with a compression ratio of 2:1 will increase output by 1 dB for every 2 dB increase in input

REAG: real-ear aided gain; measurement of the difference, in dB as a function of frequency, between the SPL in the ear canal and the SPL at a field reference point for a specified sound field with the hearing aid in place and turned on

real ear: pertaining to measurements made in the ear canal with a probe microphone

real-ear aided gain: REAG; measurement of the difference, in dB as a function of frequency, between the SPL in the ear canal and the SPL at a field reference point for a specified sound field with the hearing aid in place and turned on

real-ear aided response: REAR; probe-microphone measurement of the sound pressure level, as a function of frequency, at a specified point near the tympanic membrane with a hearing aid in place and turned on; expressed in absolute SPL or as gain relative to stimulus level

real-ear coupler difference: RECD; measurement of the difference, in dB as a function of frequency, between the output of a hearing aid measured by a probe microphone in the ear canal and the output measured in a 2-cc coupler

real-ear gain: nonspecific term referring generally to the gain of a hearing aid at the tympanic membrane, measured as the difference between the SPL in the ear canal and the SPL at the field reference point for a specified sound field

real-ear insertion gain: REIG; probe-microphone measurement of the difference, in dB as a function of frequency, between the real-ear unaided gain and the real-ear aided gain at the same point near the tympanic membrane

real-ear occluded gain: REOG; probe-microphone measurement of the difference, in dB as a function of frequency, between the SPL at a field reference point for a specified sound field with a hearing aid in place and turned off

real-ear occluded response: REOR; probe-microphone measurement of the sound pressure level, as a function of frequency, at a specified point near the tympanic membrane with a hearing aid in place and turned off; expressed in absolute SPL or as gain relative to stimulus level

real-ear saturation response: RESR; probe-microphone measurement of the SPL, as a function of frequency, at a specified point near the tympanic membrane with a hearing aid in place and turned on, with sufficient stimulus level to drive the hearing aid at its maximum output

real-ear unaided gain: REUG; probe-microphone measurement of the difference in dB as a function of frequency, between the SPL in an unoccluded ear canal and the SPL at the field reference point for a specified sound field

real-ear unaided response: REUR; probe-microphone measurement of the sound pressure level, as a function of frequency, at a specified point near the tympanic membrane in an unoccluded ear canal

REAR: real-ear aided response; probe-microphone measurement of the sound pressure level, as a function of frequency, at a specified point near the tympanic membrane with a hearing aid in place and turned on

RECD: real-ear coupler difference; measurement of the difference, in dB as a function of frequency, between the output of a hearing aid measured by a probe microphone in the ear canal and the output measured in a 2-cc coupler

receiver-in-the-canal hearing aid: RIC hearing aid; receiver-in-the-ear hearing aid

receiver tubing: in a hearing aid, tubing that extends from the medial portion in the ear canal to the receiver

recognition, speech: the ability to perceive and identify speech targets; SYN: speech intelligibility, speech discrimination

reference microphone: a second microphone used to measure the stimulus level during probe-microphone measurements or to control the stimulus level during the probe-microphone equalization process

reference test gain: ANSI standard gain level with a 60-dB SPL input and the volume control of the hearing aid adjusted so that the gain at the reference test frequencies is 17 dB less than that at SSPL-90

reflex, acoustic: reflexive contraction of the intra-aural muscles in response to loud sound, dominated by the stapedius muscle in human; SYN: acoustic stapedial reflex

reflex, middle ear muscle: reflexive contraction of the stapedius and tensor tympani muscles in response to loud sound; stapedius muscle dominates the reflex in humans; SYN: acoustic reflex

reflex arc: functional pathway of a nervous system reflex from a sensory receptor to a motor responder

rehabilitation, aural: treatment of persons with adventitious hearing impairment to improve the efficacy of overall communication ability, including the use of hearing aids, auditory training, speechreading, counseling, and guidance

REIG: real-ear insertion gain; probe-microphone measurement of the difference, in dB as a function of frequency, between the real-ear unaided gain and the real-ear aided gain at the same point near the tympanic membrane

remote microphone system: any wireless amplification system that uses a microphone/transmitter component separate from the receiver/loudspeaker component

REOG: real-ear occluded gain; probe-microphone measurement of the difference in dB between the SPL in the ear canal and the SPL at a field reference point for a specified sound field with a hearing aid in place and turned off

REOR: real-ear occluded response; probe-microphone measurement of the sound pressure level, as a function of frequency, at a specified point near the tympanic membrane with a hearing aid in place and turned off

resonant frequency: frequency at which a secured mass will vibrate most readily when set into free vibration; SYN: natural frequency

RESR: real-ear saturation response; probe-microphone measurement of the SPL at a specified point near the tympanic membrane, with a hearing aid in place and turned on and with sufficient stimulus level to drive the hearing aid at its maximum output

retraction of the tympanic membrane: a drawing back of the eardrum into the middle ear space due to negative pressure formed in the cavity secondary to eustachian tube dysfunction

retraction pocket: invagination into the middle ear space of a weakened portion of the tympanic membrane

retrocochlear: pertaining to the neural structures of the auditory system beyond the cochlea, especially cranial nerve VIII and the auditory portions of the brain stem

retrocochlear disorder: hearing disorder resulting from a neoplasm or other disorder of cranial nerve VIII or beyond in the auditory brain stem or cortex

REUG: real-ear unaided gain; probe-microphone measurement of the difference, in dB as a function of frequency, between the SPL in an unoccluded ear canal and the SPL at the field reference point for a specified sound field

REUR: real-ear unaided response; probe-microphone measurement of the sound pressure level, as a function of frequency, at a specified point near the tympanic membrane in an unoccluded ear canal

reverberation: prolongation of sound by multiple reflections

RIC hearing aid: receiver-in-the-canal hearing aid; receiver-in-the-ear hearing aid

round window: membrane-covered opening in the labyrinthine wall of the middle ear space, leading into the scala tympani of the cochlea; SYN: cochlear window; fenestra rotunda

SADL: Satisfaction with Amplification in Daily Life; self-assessment scale of hearing aid satisfaction

saturation: level in an amplifier circuit at which an increase in input signal no longer produces additional output

saturation response, real-ear: RESR; probe-microphone measurement of the SPL, as a function of frequency, at a specified point near the tympanic membrane with a hearing aid in place and turned on, with sufficient stimulus level to drive the hearing aid at its maximum output

saturation sound pressure level: SSPL; maximum output generated by the receiver of a hearing aid, expressed as the root mean square sound pressure level

saturation sound pressure level 90: SSPL 90; electroacoustic specification of a hearing aid's maximum output, expressed as a frequency response curve to a 90-dB input with the hearing aid gain control set to full on; SYN: maximum power output

scale, A-weighted: sound level meter filtering network weighted to approximate an equal loudness contour at 40 phones; decibel level measured with this scale is usually designated dBA or dB(A)

screening, immittance: rapid assessment of middle ear function by tympanometry

screening audiometry: rapid assessment of the ability of individuals to hear pure tones across a frequency range presented at a fixed criterion intensity level; designed to identify those who require additional audiometric procedures; SYN: identification audiometry

Sensation Level, Desired: DSL; prescriptive hearing aid target, expressed as the number of dB above behavioral threshold required to amplify the long-term speech spectrum to a prescribed level across the frequency range

sensorineural hearing loss: SNHL; cochlear or retrocochlear loss in hearing sensitivity due to disorders involving the cochlea and/or the auditory nerve fibers of cranial nerve VIII; COM: conductive hearing loss

serous effusion: thin, watery, sterile fluid secreted by a mucous membrane

signal processing, automatic: ASP; process in which hearing aid circuitry adjusts some parameter of the amplified output automatically or adaptively as the input signal reaches a certain criterion

SII: Speech Intelligibility Index; ANSI standard term for the articulation or audibility index; a measure of the proportion of speech

SIN Test: Speech-In-Noise Test; adaptive speech-recognition measure of speech threshold in background noise

single-sided deafness: SSD; unilateral sensorineural hearing loss, usually of a severe to profound degree

skeleton earmold: earmold in which the bowl has been cut out, leaving an outer concha rim, but retaining the portion that seals the external auditory meatus

ski-slope audiogram: colloquial term for precipitous, high-frequency hearing loss

slit leak: leak of acoustic energy around the perimeter of an earmold or custom hearing aid

sloping hearing loss: audiometric configuration in which hearing loss is progressively worse at higher frequencies

S/N: signal-to-noise ratio; SNR; relative difference in dB between a sound of interest and a background of noise

SNHL: sensorineural hearing loss; cochlear or retrocochlear loss in hearing sensitivity due to disorder involving the cochlea and/or the auditory nerve fibers of cranial nerve VIII; COM: conductive hearing loss

SNR-50: in speech audiometry, signal-to-noise ratio at which 50% of target speech signals are correctly identified

S/N ratio: redundant term for S/N

sound field: circumscribed area or room into which sound is introduced via loudspeaker

sound field amplification: amplification of a classroom or other open area with a public address system or other small-room system to enhance the signal-to-noise ratio for all listeners

sound field testing: in pediatric audiometry or hearing aid fitting, the determination of hearing sensitivity or speech recognition ability made with signals presented in a sound field through loudspeakers

space-occupying lesion: neoplasm that exerts its influence by growing and impinging on neural tissues, as opposed to a lesion caused by trauma, ischemia, or inflammation

spectrum, long-term speech: LTSS; overall level and frequency composition of speech energy that represents everyday speech

speech audiometry, adaptive: speech-recognition strategy in which the intensity level of the competition or noise is varied around the target until a specified percentage correct response criterion is reached

speech discrimination: SD; old term for word recognition

Speech-Intelligibility Index: SII; ANSI standard term for the articulation or audibility index; a measure of the proportion of speech cues that are audible

speech noise: broadband noise that is filtered to resemble the speech spectrum

speechreading: the process of visual recognition of speech communication, combining lip reading with observation of facial expressions and gestures

speech recognition: the ability to perceive and identify speech targets; SYN: speech intelligibility, speech discrimination

speech recognition threshold: SRT; threshold level for speech recognition, expressed as the lowest intensity level at which 50% of spondaic words can be identified; SYN: speech reception threshold

speech-to-competition ratio: in speech audiometry, the ratio in dB of the presentation level of a speech target to that of background competition

SPL: sound pressure level; magnitude or quantity of sound energy relative to a reference pressure, 0.0002 dyne/cm^2 or 20 μPa

SPL-O-GRAM: graph containing hearing thresholds, long-term average speech spectrum, level for amplified speech, and hearing aid saturation levels, plotted in dB sound pressure level, used in the desired sensation level approach to hearing aid fitting

spondee: a two-syllable word spoken with equal emphasis on each syllable

squelch, binaural: improvement in speech intelligibility in noise with two ears over one because of interaural phase and intensity cues

squelch effect: enhanced speech perception in noise as a result of binaural hearing

SSD: single-sided deafness; unilateral sensorineural hearing loss, usually of a severe to profound degree

SSPL90: saturation sound pressure level 90; electroacoustic specification of a hearing aid's maximum output, expressed as a frequency response curve to a 90-dB input with the hearing aid gain control set to full on; SYN: maximum power output

stapedius muscle: along with the tensor tympani, one of two striated muscles of the middle ear classified as a pinnate muscle, consisting of short fibers directed obliquely onto the stapedius tendon at the midline, innervated by the facial nerve

superior olivary complex: SOC; collection of auditory nuclei in the hindbrain that relay information from the cochlear nucleus to the midbrain, including the lateral superior olive, medial superior olive, medial nucleus of the trapezoid body, and periolivary nuclei

target gain: desired gain and frequency response based on criteria derived from a prescriptive formula against which the actual hearing aid response is compared

t coil: telecoil; an induction coil often included in a hearing aid to receive electromagnetic signals from a telephone or a loop amplification system

telecoil: t coil; an induction coil often included in a hearing aid to receive electromagnetic signals from a telephone or a loop amplification system

telecoil switch: t switch; switch circuit on some hearing aids that permits use of an induction coil to receive electromagnetic signals from a telephone or a loop amplification system

telecommunication device for the deaf: TDD; telephone system used by those with significant hearing impairment in which a typewritten message is transmitted over telephone lines and is received as a printed message; SYN: text telephone (TT), TTY, TTD

telephone amplifier: any of several types of assistive devices designed to increase the intensity level output of a telephone receiver

telephone coil: telecoil

temporary threshold shift, noise-induced: NITTS; SYN: temporary threshold shift

tensor tympani muscle: along with the stapedius, one of two striated muscles of the middle ear, classified as a pinnate muscle, consisting of short fibers directed obliquely onto the tensor tympani tendon at the midline, innervated by the trigeminal nerve, cranial nerve V

threshold, pure-tone air conduction: lowest intensity level at which a pure-tone stimulus, presented through earphones, is audible

threshold, pure-tone bone conduction: lowest intensity level at which a pure-tone stimulus, presented via a bone conduction oscillator placed on the forehead or mastoid, is audible

threshold, speech-reception: SRT; speech recognition threshold

threshold, speech recognition: SRT; threshold level for speech recognition, expressed as the lowest intensity level at which 50% of spondaic words can be identified; SYN: speech reception threshold

threshold, spondee: ST; speech-recognition threshold

threshold of discomfort: TD; lowest intensity level at which sound is judged to be uncomfortably loud; SYN: uncomfortable loudness level

tolerance level: threshold of discomfort

tone, probe: in immittance measurement, the pure tone that is held at a constant intensity level in the external auditory meatus; used to indirectly measure changes in energy flow through the middle ear mechanism

tragus: small cartilaginous flap on the anterior wall of the external auditory meatus

transcranial CROS: contralateral routing of signal (CROS) strategy for unilateral hearing loss in which a high-gain in-the-ear hearing aid is fitted to the poor ear in an effort to transfer sound across the skull via bone conduction to the cochlea of the good ear

t switch: telecoil switch; switch circuit on some hearing aids that permits use of an induction coil to receive electromagnetic signals from a telephone or a loop amplification system

TTD: teletypewriter for the deaf; early term for TDD or TT

TTS: temporary threshold shift; transient or reversible hearing loss due to auditory fatigue following exposure to excessive levels of sound

TTY: teletypewriter; early term for TDD or TT

tube, grommet: ventilation or pressure equalization tube

tube, pressure-equalization: PE tube; small tube or grommet inserted in the tympanic membrane following myringotomy to provide equalization of air pressure within the middle ear space as a substitute for a nonfunctional eustachian tube; SYN: tympanostomy tube

tube, ventilation: SYN: pressure-equalization tube

2-cc coupler: metal cylinder with a 2-cc air space, designed to represent the average amount of air enclosed in an ear canal by an earmold; used to connect a hearing aid receiver to the microphone of a sound level meter to measure output characteristics

2-cc coupler SPL: sound pressure level measured in a standard 2-cc coupler

tympanic membrane perforation: abnormal opening into the tympanic membrane

tympanogram: T; graph of middle ear immittance as a function of the amount of air pressure delivered to the ear canal

tympanogram, Type A: normal tympanogram with maximum immittance at atmospheric pressure

tympanogram, Type A$_d$: deep (d) Type A tympanograms associated with a flaccid middle ear mechanism, characterized by excessive immittance that is maximum at atmospheric pressure

tympanogram, Type A$_s$: shallow (s) Type A tympanogram associated with ossicular fixation, characterized by reduced immittance that is maximum at atmospheric pressure

tympanogram, Type B: flat tympanogram associated with increase in the mass of the middle ear system, characterized by little change in immittance as ear canal air pressure is varied

tympanogram, Type C: tympanogram associated with significant negative pressure in the middle ear space, characterized by immittance that is maximum at a negative ear canal pressure equal to that of the middle ear cavity

tympanometry: procedure used in the assessment of middle ear function in which the immittance of the tympanic membrane and middle ear is measured as air pressure delivered into the ear canal is varied

tympanoplasty: reconstructive surgery of the middle ear, usually classified in types according to the magnitude of the reconstructive process

Type A tympanogram: normal tympanogram with maximum immittance at atmospheric pressure

Type A$_d$ tympanogram: deep (d) Type A tympanogram associated with a flaccid middle ear mechanism, characterized by excessive immittance that is maximum at atmospheric pressure tympanogram associated with ossicular fixation, characterized by reduced immittance that is maximum at atmospheric pressure

Type A$_s$ tympanogram: shallow (s) Type A tympanogram associated with ossicular fixation, characterized by reduced immittance that is maximum at atmospheric pressure

Type B tympanogram: flat tympanogram associated with increase in the mass of the middle ear system, characterized by little change in immittance as ear canal air pressure is varied

Type C tympanogram: tympanogram associated with significant negative pressure in the middle ear space, characterized by immittance that is maximum at a negative ear canal pressure equal to that of the middle ear cavity

UCL: uncomfortable loudness

UL: uncomfortable level; level at which sound is judged to be uncomfortably loud by a listener

ULL: uncomfortable loudness level; intensity level at which sound is perceived to be uncomfortably loud; SYN: loudness discomfort level

unaided gain, real-ear: REUG; probe-microphone measurement of the difference, in dB as a function of frequency, between the SPL in an unoccluded ear canal and the SPL at the field reference point for a specified sound field

unaided response, real-ear: REUR; probe-microphone measurement of the sound pressure level, as a function of frequency, at a specified point near the tympanic membrane in an unoccluded ear canal

uncomfortable level: UL; level at which sound is judged to be uncomfortably loud by a listener

Valsalva maneuver: attempt to force open the eustachian tube by blowing with the nostrils and mouth closed

variable release time: a characteristic of some compression circuits in which the compression release time changes in direct relation to duration of the input; for example, the shorter the compression-activating input, the shorter the release time

vent: bore made in an earmold or in-the-ear hearing aid that permits the passage of sound and air into the otherwise blocked external auditory meatus; used for aeration of the canal

vent, pressure: small vent in an earmold or hearing aid to provide pressure equalization in the external auditory meatus

venting, custom: dispenser-specified venting diameter and length

vertigo: a form of dizziness, describing a definite sensation of spinning or whirling

visual reinforcement audiometry: VRA; audiometric technique used in pediatric assessment in which an accurate response to an acoustic signal presentation, such as a head turn toward the speaker, is rewarded by the activation of a light or lighted to

volume, equivalent: in immittance measurement, the translation of change in probe-tone SPL into volume changes, so that an increase in SPL appears as a decrease in equivalent volume of a cavity and a decrease in SPL appears

volume test physical: PVT; subtest of immittance audiometry in which the volume of the ear canal is estimated; for example, a large volume is found in the case of a tympanic membrane perforation or a patent PE tube, and a small volume in the case of impacted cerumen

volume unit meter: VU meter; visual indicator on an audiometer showing intensity of an input signal in dB, where 0 dB is equal to the attenuator output setting

VRA: visual reinforcement audiometry; audiometric technique used in pediatric assessment in which an accurate response to an acoustic signal presentation, such as a head turn toward the speaker, is rewarded by the activation of a light or lighted toy

VU meter: volume unit meter; visual indicator on an audiometer showing intensity of an input signal in dB, where 0 dB is equal to the attenuator output setting

warble tone: frequency-modulated

wax guard: shield placed over the end of a custom hearing aid, designed to prevent or reduce accumulation of cerumen in the receiver

WDRC: wide-dynamic-range compression; hearing aid compression algorithm, with a low threshold of activation, designed to distribute signals between a listener's thresholds of sensitivity and discomfort in a manner that matches loudness growth pure tone, often used in sound field audiometry

Weber test: test in which a tuning fork or bone vibrator is placed on the midline of the forehead; lateralization of sound to the poorer hearing ear suggests the presence of a conductive hearing loss; lateralization to the better ear suggests sensorineural hearing loss

white noise: broadband noise having similar energy at all frequencies

wide-dynamic-range compression: WDRC; hearing aid compression algorithm, with a low threshold of activation, designed to deliver signals between a listener's thresholds of sensitivity and discomfort in a manner that matches loudness growth; SYN: full-dynamic-range compression

window, oval: oval window opening in the labyrinthine wall of the middle ear space leading into the scala vestibuli of the cochlea, into which the footplate of the stapes fits; SYN: vestibular window, fenestra vestibuli

window, round: membrane-covered opening in the labyrinthine wall of the middle ear space, leading into the scala tympani of the cochlea; SYN: cochlear window; fenestra rotunda

word list, PBK: phonetically-balanced kindergarten word lists; lists of words used in word recognition testing, designed both to be phonetically balanced and to contain words that are vocabulary-level appropriate for use with young school children

zero, audiometric: lowest sound pressure level at which a pure tone at each of the audiometric frequencies is audible to the average normal hearing ear, designated as 0 dB hearing level (HL), or audiometric zero, according to international standards

zinc-air battery: hearing aid battery containing intake holes through which zinc is oxidized

References

Abrams, H., Hnath-Chisolm, T., Guerreiro, S., & Ritterman, S. (1992). The effects of intervention strategy on self-perception of hearing-handicap. *Ear and Hearing, 13*(5), 371–377.

Advanced Bionics. (2019) About us. Retrieved from https://advancedbionics.com/us/en/home /about-us.html

Alpiner, J. G., Kaufman, K. J., & Hanavan, P. C. (1993). Overview of rehabilitative audiology. In J. G. Alpiner & P. A. McCarthy (Eds.), *Rehabilitative audiology: Children and adults* (pp. 3–16). Baltimore, MD: Lippincott Williams & Wilkins.

Alpiner, J., & McCarthy, P. (2000). *Rehabilitative audiology: Children and adults* (3rd ed). Baltimore, MD: Lippincot, Williams and Wilkins.

American Academy of Audiology. (2004). *Scope of practice.* Retrieved from https://www.audio logy.org/publications-resources/document -library/scope-practice

American Academy of Audiology. (2013). *Pediatric amplification practice guideline.* Retrieved from https://www.audiology.org/publications -resources/document-library/pediatric-reha bilitation-hearing-aids

American Academy of Audiology. (2018). *Code of ethics.* Retrieved from https://www.audi ology.org/publications-resources/document -library/code-ethics

American Speech-Language and Hearing Association (n.d.) *Adult audiologic (hearing) rehabilitation.* Available at https://www.asha.org /public/hearing/Adult-Aural-Rehabilitation/

American Speech-Language-Hearing Association. (1984). Definitions of and competencies for aural rehabilitation. *ASHA. 26*, 27–41.

American Speech-Language-Hearing Association. (2001). *Knowledge and skills required for the practice of audiologic/aural rehabilitation* [Knowledge and skills]. Retrieved from http:// www.asha.org/policy

American Speech-Language-Hearing Association. (2018). *Scope of practice in audiology.* Retrieved from https://www.asha.org/policy /SP2018-00353/

ANSI.(1994). American National Standards Institute S1.1.1994

ANSI. (2013). *Methods of measurement of real-ear characteristics of hearing instruments* (ANSI S3.46-R2013). New York, NY: American National Standards Institute.

Atcherson, S. R., Franklin, C. A., & Smith-Olinde, L. (2015). *Hearing assistive and access technology.* San Diego, CA: Plural Publishing.

Barcroft, J., Sommers, M. S., Tye-Murray, N., Mauzé, E., Schroy, C., & Spehar, B. (2011). Tailoring auditory training to patient needs with single and multiple talkers: Transfer-appropriate gains on a four-choice discrimination test. *International Journal of Audiology, 50*(11), 802–808.

Bentler R., & Cooley L. (2001) An examination of several characteristics that affect the prediction of OSPL90 in hearing aids. *Ear and Hearing, 22*(1), 58–64

Bess, F. H. (1999). Classroom acoustics: An overview. *Volta Review, 101*(5), 1–14.

Beynon, G., Thornton, F., & Poole, C. (1997). A randomized, controlled trial of the efficacy of communication course for first time hearing aid users. *British Journal of Audiology, 31*(5), 345–351.

Blaser, S., Propst, E., Martin, D., Feigenbaum, A., James, A., Shannon, P., & Papsin, B. (2006). Inner ear dysplasia is common in children with Down syndrome (trisomy 21). *Laryngoscope, 116*(12), 2113–2119.

Blumsack, J. T., Bower, C. R., & Ross, M. E. (2007). Comparison of speechreading training regimens. *Perceptual and Motor Skills, 105*(3), 988–996.

Boothroyd, A. (2007). Adults aural rehabilitation: What is it and does it work? *Trends in Amplification, 11*(2), 63–71.

Brickley, G. J., Cleaver, V. C. G., & Bailey, S. (1996). An evaluation of a group follow-up scheme for new NHS hearing aid users. *British Journal of Audiology, 30*(5), 307–312.

Brown, H. D. (2004) Language assessment: Principles and classroom practices. White plains, NY: Pearson Education.

Brown, P. M., Baker, Z. A., Rickarts, F., & Griffin, P. (2006). *Family functioning, early intervention, and spoken language and placement outcomes for children with profound hearing loss.*

Burke, M. H., & Humes, L. E. (2007). Effects of training on speech recognition performance in noise using lexically hard words. *Journal of Speech, Language, and Hearing Research, 50*(1), 25–40.

Burke, M. H., & Humes, L. E. (2008). Effects of long-term training on aided speech-recognition performance in noise in older adults. *Journal of Speech, Language, and Hearing Research, 51*(3), 759–771.

Byrne, D., Dillon, H., Tran, K., Arlinger, S., Wilbraham, K., Cox, R., . . . Ludvigsen, C. (1994). An international comparison of long-term average speech spectra. *Journal of the Acoustical Society of America, 96*(2), 2108–2120.

Calderone, R. (2000). Parental involvement in deaf children's education programs as a predictor of child language, early reading, and social-emotional development. *Journal of Deaf Studies and Deaf Education, 5*(2), 140–155.

Carhart, R. (1947). Auditory training. In H. Davis (Ed.), *Hearing and deafness: A guide for laymen* (pp. 276–299). New York, NY: Murray Hill Books.

Ching, T. Y. C., Dillon, H., Marnane, V., Hou, S., Day, J., Seeto, M., . . . Yeh, A. (2013). Outcomes of early- and late-identified children with hearing loss at 3 years of age: Findings from a prospective population-based study. *Ear and Hearing, 34*, 535–552.

Chisolm, T., Abrams, H., & McArdle, R. (2004). Short- and long-term outcome of adult audiologic rehabilitation. *Ear and Hearing, 25*(5), 464–477.

Chisolm, T., & Arnold, M (2012). Evidence about the effectiveness of aural rehabilitation programs for adults. In L. Wong & Hickson (Eds.), *Evidence-based practice in audiology: Evaluating interventions for children and adults with hearing impairment.* (pp. 237–266). San Diego, CA: Plural Publishing.

Chisolm T. H., Johnson C. E., Danhauer J. L., Portz, L. J., Abrams, H. B., Lesner, S., . . . Newman, C. W. (2007). A systematic review of health-related quality of life and hearing aids: Final report of the American Academy of Audiology task force on the health-related quality of life benefits of amplification in adults. *Journal of the American Academy of Audiology, 18*(2), 151–183.

Chisolm, T. H., Saunders, G. H, Frederick, M. T, McArdle, R. A, Smith, S. L, & Wilson, R. H. (2013) Learning to listen again: The role of compliance in auditory training for adults with hearing loss. *American Journal of Audiology, 22*(2), 339–342.

Clark, J. G., & Martin, F. N. (2014). Time for a change: A note on hearing loss terminology. *Journal of the American Academy of Audiology, 25*(10), 1034–1035.

Clemens, C. J., Davis, S. A., & Bailey, A. R. (2000). The false-positive in universal newborn hearing screening. *Pediatrics, 106*(1), E7.

Cochlear Corporation. (2019). *About us.* Retrieved from: https://www.cochlear.com/us/en/about-us

Costa, P., & McCrae, R. (1992). *NEO-PI-R professional manual.* Odessa, FL: Psychological Assessment Resources.

Cox, R. (2005). Choosing a self-report measure for hearing aid fitting outcomes. *Seminars in Hearing, 26*(3), 149–156.

Cox, R. M. (1995). Using loudness data for hearing aid selection: The IHAFF approach. *Hearing Journal, 48*(2), 10, 39–44.

Crandell, C. C., & Smaldino, J. J. (2000). Classroom acoustics for children with normal hearing and with hearing impairment. *Lan-*

guage, Speech, and Hearing Services in Schools, 31(4), 362–370.

Culberston, G., Shen, S., Jung, M., & Andersen, E., (2017). Facilitating development of pragmatic competence through a voice-drive video learning interference. CHI'17. *Proceedings of the 2017 CHI Conference on Human Factors in Computing Systems*, 1431–1440.

Czaja, S. J., Sharit, J., Lee, C. C., Nair, S. N., Hernández, M. A., Arana, N., & Fu, S. H. (2012). Factors influencing use of an e-health website in a community sample of older adults. *Journal of the American Medical Informatics Association, 20*(2), 277–284.

Davis, J. (1977). *Our forgotten children: Hard of hearing pupils in the schools*. Washington, DC: AG Bell.

Davis, S. (1988). *Topics in syllable geometry*. New York, NY: Garland.

Dawes, P., Maharani, A., Nazroo, J., Tampubolon, G., & Pendleton, N. (2019). Evidence that hearing aids could slow cognitive decline in later life. *Hearing Review, 26*(1), 10–11.

Dhar, S. (2014a). 20Q: OAEs—Music to my ears. *AudiologyOnline*, Article #12876. Retrieved from http://www.audiologyonline.com

Dhar, S. (2014b). 20Q: OAEs—Sound clinical tool. *AudiologyOnline*, Article #12801. Retrieved from http://www.audiologyonline.com

Egan, M. D. (1988) *Architectural acoustics*. New York, NY: McGraw-Hill.

Erber, N. P. (1974). Effects of angle, distance, and illumination on visual reception of speech by profoundly deaf children. *Journal of Speech and Hearing Research, 17*(1), 99–112.

Erdman, S. (2009). Audiologic counseling: A biopsychosocial approach. In J. J. Montano & J. B. Spitzer (Eds.), *Adult audiologic rehabilitation: Advanced practices* (pp. 171–215). San Diego, CA: Plural Publishing.

Erdman, S. A., & Demorest, M. E. (1998). Adjustment to hearing impairment II: Audiological and demographic correlates. *Journal of Speech, Language, and Hearing research, 41*(1), 123–136.

Estabrooks, W. (1994). *Auditory-verbal therapy*. Washington DC: Alexander Gram Bell Association for the Deaf.

FDA. (2019). List of currently approved cochlear implants. Available at: https://www.fda.gov/medical-devices/cochlear-implants/fda-approved-cochlear-implants

Gagné, J. P. (2000). What is treatment evaluation research? What is its relationship to the goals of audiological rehabilitation? Who are the stakeholders of this type of research? *Ear and Hearing, 21* (4 Suppl. 4), 60S–73S.

Gagné, J. P., Dinon, D., & Parsons, J. (1991). An evaluation of CASTA: Computer-aided speechreading training program. *Journal of Speech, Language, and Hearing Association, 34*(1), 213–221.

Garstecki, D. C., & Erler, S. F. (1998). Hearing loss, control and demographic factors influencing hearing aid use among older adults. *Journal of Speech, Language and Hearing Research, 41*(3), 527–537.

Garstecki, D. C., & Eraler, S. F. (1999). Older adult performance on the communication profiles for the hearing impaired gender difference. *Journal of Speech, Language, and Hearing Research. 42*(4), 785–796.

Gil, D., & Iorio, M. C. M. (2010). Formal auditory training in adult hearing aid users. *Clinics, 65*(2), 165–174.

Gildston, P. (n.d.). *Do's and don'ts for the classroom teacher*. Brooklyn, NY: Brooklyn College.

Grant, D. (2014). Siemens survey on teens' listening behaviors [PowerPoint presentation]. Retrieved from AudiologyOnline: https://www.audiologyonline.com/interviews/siemens-survey-on-teens-listening-13022

Hall, J. (2013). 20Q: Treating patients with hyperacusis and other forms of disease tolerance. *AudiologyOnline*. Article #11679. Retrieved from: https://www.audiologyonline.com/articles/20q-what-can-done-for-11679

Hall, J. W., III. (2019). 20Q: Audiological care for patients with hyperacusis and sound tolerance disorders. *AudiologyOnline*, Article #24772. Retrieved from http://www.audiologyonline.com

Harford, E. (1980). The use of a miniature microphone in the ear canal for verification of hearing aid performance. *Ear and Hearing 1*(6), 329–337.

Harford, E. R. (2000) Professional education in audiology. In H. Hosford-Dunn, R. Rosser, & M. Valente (Eds.), *Audiology practice management* (pp. 17–40). New York, NY: Thieme Medical.

Hawkins, D. (2005). Effectiveness of counseling-based adult group aural rehabilitation programs: A systematic review of the evidence. *Journal of the American Academy of Audiology, 16*(7), 485–493.

Henshaw, H., & Ferguson, M.A. (2013). Efficacy of individual computer-based auditory training for people with hearing loss: A systematic review of the evidence. PLoS ONE, 8(5), e62836.

Holube, I. (2015). *20Q: Getting to know the ISTS. AudiologyOnline*, Article #13295. Retrieved from http://www.audiologyonline.com.

Hull, R. (2014). *Introduction to aural rehabilitation*. San Diego, CA: Plural Publishing.

Humes, L., Burk, M., Strauser, L., & Kinney, D. (2009). Development and efficacy of a frequent-word auditory training protocol for older adults with impaired hearing. *Ear and Hearing, 30*(5), 613–627.

Ingvalson, E. M., Lee, B., Fiebig, P., & Wong, P. C. (2013). The effects of short-term computerized speech-in-noise training on postlingaully deafened adult cochlear implant recipients. *Journal of Speech, Language, and Hearing Research, 56*(1), 81–88.

Jackler, R. (2015). Congenital malformations of the inner ear. *Otolaryngology.* Available at: https://clinicalgate.com/congenital-malformations-of-the-inner-ear/

Killion, M. C., & Mueller, H. G. (2010). Twenty years later: A new count-the-dots method. *Hearing Journal, 63*(1), 10–17.

Kochkin, S. (2007). MarkeTrak VII: Obstacles to adult non-user adoption of hearing aids. *Hearing Journal, 63*(1), 11–19.

Kokx-Ryan, M., Cohen, J., Cord, M., Walden, T., Makashay, M., Sheffield, B., & Brungart, D. (2015). Benefits of nonlinear frequency compression in adult hearing aid users. *Journal of the American Academy of Audiology, 26* (10), 838–855.

Kramer, S., & Brown, D. K. (2019). *Audiology: Science to practice* (3rd ed., p. 130). San Diego, CA: Plural Publishing.

Kramer, S. E., Allessie, G. H., Dondorp, A., Zekveld, A., & Kapteyn, T. (2005). A home education program for older adults with hearing impairment and their significant others: A randomized trial evaluating short- and long term effects. *International Journal of Audiology, 45*(9), 503–512.

Kraus, N. (2012). Biological impact of music and software-based auditory training. *Journal of Communication Disorders, 45*, 403–410.

Krikos, P., & Holmes, A. (1996). Efficacy of audiologic rehabilitation for older adults. *Journal of the American Academy of Audiology, 7*, 219–229.

Lane, S., Bell, L., & Parson-Tylka, T. (2006). *My turn to learn: A communication guide for parents of deaf or hard of hearing children.* British Columbia, Canada: Bauhinea Press.

Laplante-Levesque, A., Hickson, L., & Worrall, L. (2011). Predictors of rehabilitation intervention decisions in adults with acquired hearing loss. *Journal of Speech, Language, and Hearing Research, 54*(5), 1385–1399.

Laplante-Levesque, A., Hickson, L., & Worrall, L. (2012). What makes adults with hearing impairment take up hearing aids or communication programs and achieve successful outcomes? *Ear and Hearing, 33*(1), 79–93.

Laplante-Levesque, A., Pichora-Fuller, K. M., & Gagné, J. P. (2006). Proving and internet-based audiological counseling programme to new hearing aid users: A qualitative study. *International Journal of Audiology, 45*(12), 697–706.

Levitt, H. (2014). *Efficacy of ReadMyQuips* (NIH sponsored research). Senesynergy.com. Retrieved from http://www.sensesynergy.com/articles/research/initial

Levitt, H., Oden, C., Simon, H., Noack, C., & Lotze, A. (2011). Entertainment overcomes barriers of auditory training. *Hearing Journal, 64*(8), 40–42.

Lewis, M. S., Crandell, C. C., Valente, M., & Horn, J. E. (2004). Speech perception in noise: Directional microphones versus frequency modulation (FM) systems. *Journal of the American Academy of Audiology, 15*(6), 426–439.

Lin, F. (2019). *How is hearing loss related to cognitive decline and dementia?* Audiology-

Online. Retrieved from http://www.audiolo gyonline.com

Lin, V., Chung, J., Callahan, B., Smith, L., Gritters, N., Chen, J., . . . Masellis, M. (2017). Development of a cognitive screening test for the severely hearing impaired: Hearing-impaired MoCA. The Laryngoscope. 127 (Suppl.): S4-S11.

Lopez-Torres Hidalgo, J., Gras, C. B., Tellez Lapeira, J. M., Martinez, I., Lopez Verdejo, M. A., Rabadan, F. E., & Puime, A. O. (2008). The hearing-dependent daily activities scale to evaluate impact of hearing loss in older people. Annals of Family Medicine, 6(5), 441–447.

Luckner, J. L. (2002). Facilitating the transition of students who are deaf of hard of hearing. Austin, TX: Pro-Ed.

Madell, J., & Flexer, C. (2017). Maximizing outcomes for children in schools: The responsibility of clinical audiologists [Video lecture]. Retrieved from https://www.audiologyonline .com/audiology-ceus/course/maximizing-out comes-for-children-in-30088

Margolis, R. (2004). What do your patients remember? Hearing Journal, 57(6), 10–12.

Martin, M. (2007). Software based auditory training programs found to reduce hearing aid return rate. Hearing Journal, 60(8), 32–34.

Mayne, A. M., Yashingano-Itano, C., Sedey, A. L., & Carey, A. (2000). Expressive vocabulary development of infants and toddlers who are deaf or hard of hearing. Volta Review, 100, 1–28.

McGowan, R. S., Nittrouer, S., & Chenausky, K. (2008). Speech production in 12-month-old children with and without hearing loss. Journal of Speech, Language, and Hearing Research, 51, 879–888.

Med-El Corporation. (2019). About us. Retrieved from: https://www.medel.com/us/about -med-el/

Miller, J. D., Watson, C. S., Kewley-Port, D., Sillings, R., Mills, W. F., & Burleson, D. F. (2008a). SPATS: Speech perception training and assessment system. Proceedings of Meetings on Acoustics, 2(05005), 17.

Miller, J. D., Watson, C. S., Kisler, D. J., Preminger, J., & Wark D. J. (2008b). Training lis-

teners to identify the sounds of speech: II. Using SPATS software. The Hearing Journal, 61(10), 29–33.

Moeller M. P., Hoover, B., Putman C., Arbataitis, K., Bohnenkamp, G., Peterson, B., et al. (2007). Vocalizations of infants with hearing loss compared with infants with normal hearing: Part I—phonetic development. Ear and Hearing 28, 605–627.

Moeller, M. P. (2000). Early intervention and language development in children who are deaf and hard of hearing. Pediatrics, 106(3). Available at: https://pediatrics.aappublications .org/content/106/3/e43

Moeller, M. P. (2000). Early intervention and language development in children who are deaf and hard of hearing. Pediatrics, 103(3), 1–9.

Montano, J. J., & Spitzer, J. B. (2009). Adult audiologic rehabilitation. San Diego, CA: Plural Publishing.

Montgomery, A. (1994). WATCH: A practical approach to brief auditory rehabilitation. The Hearing Journal, 47(10), 53–55.

Mueller, H. G., & Killion, M. C. (1990). An easy method for calculation the articulation index. Hearing Journal, 43(9), 14–17.

Mueller, H. G., Bentler, R., & Ricketts, T. A. (2014). Modern hearing aids: Pre-fitting testing and selection considerations. San Diego, CA: Plural Publishing.

Mueller, H. G., Ricketts, T. A., & Bentler, R. (2017). Speech mapping and probe microphone measurements. San Diego, CA: Plural Publishing.

Mueller, H. G. & Hall, J. W. (1998). Audiologist's desk reference (Vol. 2). San Diego, CA: Singular Publishing.

Mylanus, E., vander Pouw, K., & Cremers (1998). Intraindividual comparison of the bone-anchored hearing aid and air-conduction hearing aids. Archives of Otolaryngology–Head and Neck Surgery, 124(3), 271–276.

Nair, E. L., & Cienkowski, K. M. (2010). The impact of health literacy on patient understanding of counseling and education materials. International Journal of Audiology, 49(2), 71–75.

Nelson, L. H., White, K. R., Baker, D. V., Hayden, A., & Bird, S. (2017). The effectiveness of commercial desiccants and uncooked rice in removing moisture from hearing aids. *International Journal of Audiology, 56*(4), 226–232.

Norrix, L. W., Camarota, K., Harris, F. P., & Dean, J. (2016). The effects of FM and hearing aid microphone settings, FM gain, and ambient noise levels on SNR at the tympanic membrane. *Journal of the American Academy of Audiology, 27*(2), 117–125.

Northern, J. L., & Downs, M. P. (2014). *Hearing in children* (6th ed.). San Diego, CA: Plural Publishing.

Olson, A. D, Preminger, J. E., & Shinn, J. B. (2013). The effect of LACE DVD training in new and experienced hearing aid users. *Journal of the American Academy of Audiology. 24*(3), 214–230.

Padgett, D. K. (1999). *Qualitative methods in social work.* Thousand Oaks, CA: Sage.

Palmer, C. V., Rauterkus, G., Toole, K., Levine, B., & Jorgensen, L. (2017a). Time out! I didn't hear you (college ed.). Available at http://pitt.app.box.com/v/timeout

Palmer, C. V., Toole, K., Levine, B., & Rauterkus, G. (2017b). Time out! I didn't hear you (high school ed.). Available at http://pitt.app.box.com/v/timeout

Pascoe, D. P. (1980). Clinical implications of nonverbal methods of hearing aid selection and fitting. *Seminars in Hearing, 1*(3), 217–228.

Peutz, V. M. A. (1971). Articulation loss of consonants as a criterion for speech transmission in a room. *Journal of Audio Engineering Society, 19*(11).

Picora-Fuller, M. K., & Benguerel, A. P. (1991). The design of CAST (computer-aided speechreading training). *Journal of Speech, Language, and Hearing Research, 34*(1), 202–212.

Preminger, J. (2003). Should significant others be encouraged to join adult group audiologic rehabilitation classes? *Journal of the Acoustical Society of America, 116*(1), 49–50.

Preminger, J. (2009). Audiologic rehabilitation with adults and significant others? Is it really worth it? [PowerPoint presentation]. Retrieved from *AudiologyOnline* https://www.audiologyonline.com/articles/audiologic-rehabilitation-with-adults-significant-882

Preminger, J., & Yoo, J. (2010). Do group audiologic rehabilitation activities influence psychosocial outcomes? *American Journal of Audiology, 19*(2), 109–125.

Ricketts, T. A., Bentler, R., & Mueller, H. G. (2019). *Essentials of modern hearing aids: Selection, fitting, and verification.* San Diego, CA: Plural Publishing.

Ross, M. (2011). Is auditory training effective in improving listening skills? *Hearing Loss Magazine.*

Rubinstein, A., & Boothroyd, A. (1987) Effect of two approaches to auditory training on speech recognition by hearing-impaired adults. *Journal of Speech, Language, and Rearing Research, 30*(2), 153–160.

Sanders, D. A. (1971). *Aural rehabilitation.* Englewood Cliffs, NJ: Prentice Hall.

Scarinci, N., Worrall, L., & Hickson, L. (2008). The effect of hearing impairment in older people on the spouse. *International Journal of Audiology, 47*(3), 141–151.

Schow, R. L., & Nerbonne, M. (2012). Introduction to audiologic rehabilitation (6th ed.). London, UK: Allyn & Bacon.

Schow, R., & Nerbonne, M. (2018). *Introduction to audiologic rehabilitation.* New York, NY: Pearson.

Scollie, S., Glista, D., & Richert, F. (2014). Frequency lowering hearing aids: Procedures for assessing candidacy and fine tuning Retrieved from https://www.phonakpro.com/content/dam/phonakpro/gc_hq/en/events/2013/sound_foundation_chicago/Scollie_Verification1_of_Sound_Recover.pdf

Slater, J., Skoe, E., Strait, D., O'Connell, S., Thompson, E., & Kraus, N. (2015). Music training improves speech-in-noise perception: Longitudinal evidence from a community-based music program. *Behavioral Brain Research, 291*, 244–252.

Stach, B. (2019). *Comprehensive dictionary of audiology: Illustrated* (3rd ed.). San Diego, CA: Plural Publishing.

Stredler-Brown, A. (2009). Intervention, education, and therapy for children who are deaf or hard of hearing (pp. 934–954). In J. Katz, L. Medwetsky, R. Burkard, & L. Hood (Eds).

Handbook of clinical audiology. Baltimore, MD: Lippincott, Williams & Wilkins.

Sweetow, R. (2009). *Integrating LACE into a busy clinical practice.* Presentation at the American Academy of Audiology meeting. Dallas, TX.

Sweetow, R., & Sabes, J. (2006). The need for and development of an adaptive listening and communication enhancement (LACE) program. *Journal of the American Academy of Audiology, 28*(2), 133.

Taylor, B., & Mueller, H. G. (2011). *Fitting and dispensing hearing aids.* San Diego, CA: Plural Publishing.

Taylor, B., & Mueller, H. G. (2017). *Fitting and dispensing hearing aids* (2nd ed.). San Diego, CA: Plural Publishing.

Tharpe, A. M. (2018). 20Q: Unilateral hearing loss in children—Progress and opportunities. *AudiologyOnline*, Article 23567. Retrieved from http://www.audiologyonline.com

Tharpe, A. M., & Seewald, R. (2017). *Comprehensive Handbook of Pediatric Audiology* (2nd ed.). San Diego, CA: Plural Publishing.

Thibodeau, L. (2014). Comparison of speech recognition with adaptive digital and FM remote microphone hearing assistance technology by listeners who use hearing aids. *American Journal of Audiology, 23*(2), 201–210.

Tremblay, K., & Kraus, N. (2002). Auditory training induces asymmetrical changes in cortical neural activity. *Journal of Speech, Language, and Hearing Research, 45*(3), 564–572.

Tremblay, K., Kraus, N., Carrell, T. D., & McGee, T. (1997). Central auditory system plasticity: Generalization to novel stimuli following listening training. *The Journal of the Acoustical Society of America, 102*(6), 3762–3773.

Tremblay, K., Kraus, N., McGee, T., Ponton, C., & Otis, B. (2001). Central auditory plasticity: Changes in the N1-P2 complex after speech-sound training. *Ear and Hearing, 22*(2), 79–90.

Tye-Murray, N. (2014). Foundations of aural rehabilitation: children, adults and their family members. Clifton Park, NY: Cengage Learning.

Tye-Murray, N., Sommers, M., Mauze, E., Schory, C., Barcroft, J., & Spehar, B. (2012). Using patient perception of relative benefit and enjoyment to assess auditory training.

Journal of the American Academy of Audiology, 23(8), 623.

Uhler, K., Warner-Czyz, A., Gifford, R., & PMSTB Working Group. (2017). Pediatric minimum speech test battery. *Journal of the American Academy of Audiology, 28*, 232–247.

Van Engen, K. J., Chandrasekaran, B., & Smiljanic, R. (2012). Effects of speech clarity on recognition memory for spoken sentences. *PloS one, 7*(9), e43753. doi:10.1371/journal.pone.0043753

Vuorialho, A., Karinen, P., & Sorri, M. (2006). Counselling of hearing aid users is highly cost-effective. *European Archives of Oto-Rhino-Laryngology and Head & Neck, 263*(11), 988–995.

Walden, E. E., Porsek, R. A., & Holum-Hardegan, L. L. (1984). Some principles of aural rehabilitation. *Hearing Instruments, 35*, 40–48.

Watson, C. S., Miller, J. D., Kewley-Port, D., Humes, L. E., & Wightman, F. L. (2008) Training listeners to identify the sounds of speech: I. A review of past studies. *The Hearing Journal, 61*(9), 26.

Wayner, D., & Abrahamson, J. (1996). *Learning to hear again: An audiological rehabilitation curriculum guide.* Austin, TX: Hear Again.

Wilson, R. H. (2003). Development of a speech in multitalker babble paradigm to assess word-recognition performance. *Journal of the American Academy of Audiology, 14*(9), 453–470.

Wolfe, J., Schafer, E. C., Heldner, B., Mülder, H., Ward, E., & Vincent, B. (2009). Evaluation of speech recognition in noise with cochlear implants and dynamic FM. *Journal of the American Academy of Audiology, 20*(7), 409–421.

Yoshinaga-Itano, C. (2003). Early intervention after universal neonatal hearing screening: impact on outcomes. *Mental Retardation and Developmental Disabilities Research Reviews, 9*(4), 252–266.

Yoshinaga-Itano, C. (2006). Early identification, communication modality, and the development of speech and spoken language skills: Patterns and considerations. In M. Marschark & P. E. Spencer (Eds.), *Advances in the spoken language of deaf and hard-of-hearing children.* New York, NY: Oxford University Press.

Index

Note: Page numbers in **bold** reference non-text material.

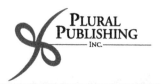